BY THE EDITORS OF
CONSUMER GUIDE™

Complete Book of
VITAMINS
&
MINERALS

SUSAN MALE SMITH, M.A., R.D.
ARLINE McDONALD, PH.D.
DENSIE WEBB, PH.D., R.D.

PUBLICATIONS INTERNATIONAL, LTD.

Contributing Writers:
Susan Male Smith, M.A., R.D., is a freelance writer and consultant who specializes in nutrition and health. She has written for *American Health, Family Circle, McCall's,* and *Redbook* and has co-authored the books *Foods for Better Health* and *All-New Family Medical Guide to Health & Prevention.* **Arline McDonald, Ph.D.,** is a nutritionist with Scientific Nutrition Consulting in Chicago. She serves as adjunct assistant professor with the Department of Preventive Medicine at Northwestern University Medical School in Chicago and the Department of Human Nutrition and Dietetics at the University of Illinois, Chicago. **Densie Webb, Ph.D., R.D.,** serves on the editorial advisory board for *Eating Well* magazine and is the editor of *Environmental Nutrition* newsletter. She has authored or co-authored several books, including *Foods for Better Health: Prevention & Healing of Diseases,* and contributes to numerous consumer magazines, including *American Health, Woman's Day, Longevity, Family Circle,* and *Weight Watchers.* **Annette Natow, Ph.D., R.D.,** is professor emeritus at the Adelphi University School of Nursing and is the editor of *The Journal of Nutrition for the Elderly.* **Jo-Ann Heslin, M.A., R.D.,** is the associate editor of *The Journal of Nutrition for the Elderly* and has written extensively on nutrition for numerous health publications.

Illustrations: Leonid Mysakov

Cover photo: Sacco Photography

Acknowledgments:
Vitamin and Mineral Counter (version 22) information provided by the Nutrition Coordinating Center at the University of Minnesota.

Nutritional analysis of recipes provided by Linda Yoakam, M.S., R.D., Naperville Nutrition Network.

The publishers would like to thank the following organizations for the use of their recipes in this publication: Almond Board of California; American Celery Council; American Lamb Council; California Apricot Advisory Board; California Cling Peach Advisory Board; California Tree Fruit Agreement; Canned Food Information Council; Florida Department of Citrus; Minnesota Cultivated Wild Rice Council; National Broiler Council; National Live Stock & Meat Board; National Pasta Association; National Turkey Federation; The Sugar Association, Inc.; Walnut Marketing Board; Washington Apple Commission; Western New York Apple Growers; and Wisconsin Milk Marketing Board.

Contents

Introduction

The year is 1700. It's almost dawn. At last count, 25 more sailors aboard His Majesty's ship have taken ill. The journey has been long and treacherous. Many months have passed since the crew of hale and hearty men set sail across the high seas. Now, as the captain looks around him, his men are slowly dying, one by one. Mysterious, irregular patches of red and purple skin cover their weakened bodies. Their gums are swollen and bleeding, and their teeth are falling out.

This scene was all too common on sailing ships of the time. In fact, the mysterious condition had plagued many since the time of Hippocrates, in 400 B.C. Yet it wasn't until 1747 that a British doctor, James Lind, began to solve the puzzle of this elusive killer by recognizing that men who were at sea for extended periods of time were deprived of certain foods, particularly fresh fruits. And not until 1795 did the British remedy the situation by issuing lime juice to the sailors aboard their naval vessels, earning them the nickname "limeys." Miraculously, it seemed, the elusive killer disappeared.

Why? What had this doctor discovered? What possible role could lime juice play in warding off a centuries-old killer? We know now that the men on those long ocean voyages were suffering from a deficiency of vitamin C—the dreaded killer was scurvy.

Throughout most of history, no one knew vitamins or minerals existed—at least, not by name. People knew only the results of not having certain foods in their diets.

Deciding what to eat back then was relatively simple. You ate whatever food was around. If you were lucky, nutrients balanced themselves in the available food, keeping you and your neighbors healthy. But at times, inevitably, the diet lacked various essential nutrients, and the entire population suffered the consequences. By trial and error, people improved their diets, recognizing in some elementary way the connection between good food and good health.

Today, of course, we have a wealth of knowledge about essential nutrients. We know what each nutrient does for us when taken in normal amounts, as well as effects they may have when taken in large doses. Now we have a new problem—too much information. There are so many reports about vitamins—which should we believe? Should we follow the one that says megadoses of vitamin A can cure cancer, or the other that says the same nutrient can be toxic and is dangerous for pregnant women?

Some of the claims you see in vitamin and mineral advertisements, books, newspaper articles, and magazine stories may tempt you. Take a little of this mineral or a large dose of that vitamin, they say, and you'll be able to grow hair, smooth wrinkles, avoid cancer, and stop the aging process. Being seduced by such promises is easy.

But if it were really that easy—if all these claims were true—no one would ever go bald, develop wrinkles, get cancer, or look a day over 25. This is hardly the case. Such fantastic claims are often anecdotal—the "it worked for me, so you try it" type of advice. The testing of such claims is rare, so there's no way to know if coincidence was responsible for the outcome. If it was just a fluke, you could actually endanger your health, and you'll most certainly waste your money.

Scientific evidence, not hearsay, is the type of advice you can use and trust—evidence that's supported by repeated studies, tests, and long, hard hours of research. The confusing part is that more and more of this kind of hard evidence supports what we used to think was simply hearsay. So, where do you turn to separate the good advice from the bad?

Right here. CONSUMER GUIDE™ and a team of recognized experts in the field of nutrition provide you with a thorough, medically sound, up-to-date source book. We've cut through the confusion and have come up with a clear explanation of the function, value, and possible dangers of deficiency and overdose for each nutrient.

In the *Complete Book of Vitamins & Minerals* you can find answers to such questions as:

- Which nutrients do I need?
- How much of each should I take?
- What foods are rich sources?
- What about supplements?
- Will large doses help prevent or cure diseases?
- Are there any dangers?
- What's the latest research?

We'll first explain how the challenge of eating right is up to you. Then, we'll tell you everything you need to know about vitamins and minerals. Finally, we'll tackle everything you should know about over-the-counter supplements, in case your doctor determines you need them. We emphasize throughout that you should meet recommended nutrient intakes by eating a balanced diet. It's our hope that the information in this book will compel you to select foods that will contribute to a healthier life.

CHAPTER 1

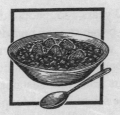

Eating Right Is Up to You

Studying only vitamins and minerals in the school of nutrition is like studying only verbs and nouns in an English class—they're only part of the overall picture. We must also understand what other elements food contains, why we need them, and how they're used in our bodies. Once we understand the intricate workings of essential nutrients, we'll have the knowledge we need to eat better and live a healthier life.

HISTORY

Human beings have walked the face of the earth for at least 250,000 years. For the vast majority of that time, our ancestors were hunters and gatherers, scrounging for food among the plants and animals available in the immediate area. When the local food sources became scarce, tribes and individuals either moved on to greener pastures or perished.

About 10,000 years ago, people developed agriculture. They began to farm and domesticate animals, thereby working with the environment to take care of themselves. From ignorance evolved curiosity about how food sustains life. With the dawning of the scientific age, people began to ask even more questions: What happens to food when it's eaten? How does food generate energy? What foods are important for growth and the maintenance of health? These and other questions remained unanswered until chemistry, biochemistry, physiology, and other related sciences advanced.

In the late 1700s, Antoine Lavoisier, a Frenchman often considered to be the "Father of Nutrition," investigated the relationship between respiration and energy production. His studies showed that our bodies use the oxygen we inhale to produce body heat and energy. He also observed that carbon dioxide is created and exhaled in the process. Lavoisier concluded that food acts as fuel, which the body oxidizes, or burns up, to release energy.

In a coal furnace, for example, coal burns in the presence of oxygen, releasing carbon dioxide and energy as heat. The oxidation of food is similar: In the presence of oxygen, the food we eat is burned to release carbon dioxide and energy. Lavoisier's work was the first step toward uncovering how food sustains life. But the oxidation of food is only a part of a complex series of reactions that occur in the body—reactions we refer to as metabolism.

METABOLISM AND ENERGY

Metabolism encompasses all the chemical reactions that take place in the body's trillions of cells. Our cells break down the molecules of some substances and build up the molecules of others. These chemical reactions are necessary to produce proteins, hormones, enzymes, fats, and stored forms of sugar that are vital to life. The reactions produce chemical waste products that the body must eliminate. And, of course, all-important energy is either stored or released.

What is energy? Energy is simply the ability to do work. We get energy from burning food as fuel, and we can determine how much energy a certain food supplies. We talk about the energy value of foods by comparing the number of calories foods provide. A calorie is the unit of heat energy. The energy value of individual foods depends on the amount of carbohydrates, fats, and proteins present. Carbohydrates and proteins supply four calories per gram, while fats yield nine calories per gram. (One gram is about equal to the mass of a paper clip. For comparison to more meaningful measures: There are 28.3 grams in an ounce and 453 grams in a pound. A milligram (mg) is 1/1,000 of a gram; a microgram (μg) is

1/1,000,000 of a gram, or 1/1,000 of a milligram.)

Different types of energy are interchangeable. For example, the chemical energy of carbohydrates, which are important body fuels, can be converted into heat energy to help maintain a constant body temperature. It can also change to kinetic energy necessary for muscle action, or it can be trapped as chemical energy and stored in other body compounds.

THE ESSENTIAL NUTRIENTS

As the science of chemistry developed in the 18th and 19th centuries, so did procedures to analyze what we eat. Scientists soon discovered the great variety of chemically distinct compounds in foods. Their experiments determined which parts of foods are best suited for growth and health.

The English physician William Prout was probably among the first to define an "adequate diet." In 1827, he described the three "staminal principles" of foods necessary to support life:

- the oily
- the saccharin
- the albuminous

Today, we recognize these three basic components as fats, carbohydrates, and proteins.

The study of food chemistry became increasingly sophisticated. By the latter part of the 19th century, the definition of Prout's "adequate diet" was expanded to include inorganic elements, known as minerals. Today, we recognize about 17 minerals as essential nutrients for humans, and the list continues to grow. In fact, some 20 or 30 other minerals found in foods that are now thought to be contaminants may, in the future, prove to be essential.

But something was still missing. By the dawn of the 20th century, scientists found that experimental animals perished when fed diets containing only highly purified preparations of fats, carbohydrates, proteins, and the known minerals. The missing vital nutrients turned out to be vitamins, the fifth class of nutrients discovered. (Previous researchers had failed to recognize the existence of vitamins because the diets prepared for experimental animals were not sufficiently "pure"—they were "contaminated" with vitamins.) Thirteen necessary vitamins are now known. The last, vitamin B_{12}, was discovered in the 1940s. The phrase "adequate diet" has been updated to refer to one that supplies all of the essential nutrients in appropriate amounts.

CLASSES OF ESSENTIAL NUTRIENTS

Carbohydrates (Starches; sugars): Used primarily to supply energy; carbohydrates furnish four calories per gram.

Fats and Oils (Fatty acids): Also called lipids; used to supply energy; fats furnish nine calories per gram. Dietary fat supplies the two "essential fatty acids," important components of cells that the body cannot synthesize. A layer of fat under the skin insulates the body. Fat around internal organs cushions and protects them. Accumulation of too much fat leads to being overweight or obese.

Proteins (Amino acids): Used primarily in the growth and maintenance of lean body tissues— muscle. If necessary, our bodies use proteins for energy, furnishing four calories per gram. Proteins are made up of smaller units called amino acids— nine of which are essential and must come from food.

Vitamins: Regulators of metabolism necessary for normal formation and breakdown of body carbohydrates, fats, and proteins. Many vitamins play roles as coenzymes, helping to trigger important reactions.

Inorganic Elements (Minerals; water): Used for various functions. Elements like calcium and phosphorus contribute to body structure as an important part of bones. Iron is a part of hemoglobin, the red pigment in blood that transports oxygen from the lungs to body tissues. Some inorganic elements are essential for optimum nerve and muscle response to stimuli. Others are essential for normal enzyme action. The elements in body fluids help maintain the acid-base balance and water balance. Water is a component of every cell in the body, accounting for 60 percent of body weight. Blood, a water solution, carries nutrients to cells and waste products away from them.

RECOMMENDED DIETARY ALLOWANCES

The Food and Nutrition Board of the National Research Council—an arm of the National Academy of Sciences—establishes and periodically updates the Recommended Dietary Allowances (RDAs). The first RDA table was an outgrowth of the need to determine the U.S. population's food and nutrition status as it related to national defense during World War II. The productivity of the American people depended on good health, and good health depended on good nutrition.

The RDAs are estimates, based on available scientific knowledge, of the amount of nutrients that people need to maintain good health over a period of time. The RDAs are useful when planning menus for groups of people, such as those in schools, hospitals, or nursing homes. The government also uses them to evaluate food programs at the federal, state, and local levels.

Evaluating an individual's food intake was never the intention of the RDAs, though it is not uncommon for them to be used that way. RDAs

Table 1
FOOD AND NUTRITION BOARD, NATIONAL ACADEMY OF SCIENCES—NATIONAL RESEARCH COUNCIL RECOMMENDED DIETARY ALLOWANCES,[a] Revised 1989

Designed for the maintenance of good nutrition of practically all healthy people in the United States.

Category	Age (years) or Condition	Weight[b] (kg)	Weight[b] (lb)	Height[b] (cm)	Height[b] (in)	Protein (g)	Minerals Calcium* (mg)	Phosphorus* (mg)	Magnesium* (mg)	Iron (mg)	Zinc (mg)	Iodine (µg)	Selenium (µg)
Infants	0.0–0.5	6	13	60	24	13	—	—	—	6	5	40	10
	0.5–1.0	9	20	71	28	14	—	—	—	10	5	50	15
Children	1–3	13	29	90	35	16	—	—	—	10	10	70	20
	4–6	20	44	112	44	24	—	—	—	10	10	90	20
	7–10	28	62	132	52	28	—	—	—	10	10	120	30
Males	11–14	45	99	157	62	45	—	—	—	12	15	150	40
	15–18	66	145	176	69	59	—	—	—	12	15	150	50
	19–24	72	160	177	70	58	—	—	—	10	150	150	70
	25–50	79	174	176	70	63	—	—	—	10	15	150	70
	51–	77	170	173	68	63	—	—	—	10	15	150	70
Females	11–14	46	101	157	62	46	—	—	—	15	12	150	45
	15–18	55	120	163	64	44	—	—	—	15	12	150	50
	19–24	58	128	164	65	46	—	—	—	15	12	150	55
	25–50	63	138	163	64	50	—	—	—	15	12	150	55
	51–	65	143	160	63	50	—	—	—	10	12	150	55
Pregnant						60	—	—	—	30	15	175	86
Lactating	1st 6 months					65	—	—	—	15	19	200	75
	2nd 6 months					62	—	—	—	15	16	200	75

[a] The allowances, expressed as daily intakes over time, are intended to provide for individual variations among most normal persons as they live in the United States under usual environmental stresses. Diets should be based on a variety of common foods in order to provide other nutrients for which human requirements have been less well defined.

[b] Weights and heights of reference adults are actual medians for the U.S. population of the designated age, as reported by NHANES II. The median weights and heights of those under 19 years of age were taken from Hamill et al (1979). The use of these figures does not imply that the height-to-weight ratios are ideal.

Tables 1–4 reprinted with permission from Recommended Dietary Allowances, 10th Edition, ©1989, by the National Academy of Sciences, National Academy Press, Washington, D.C.

*See page 23–26 for new dietary reference intake in this category.

FOOD AND NUTRITION BOARD, NATIONAL ACADEMY OF SCIENCES—NATIONAL RESEARCH COUNCIL RECOMMENDED
DIETARY ALLOWANCES,ª Revised 1989

Table 1 (cont.)

Designed for the maintenance of good nutrition of practically all healthy people in the United States.

Category	Age (years) or Condition	Fat-Soluble Vitamins				Water-Soluble Vitamins						
		Vitamin A (µg RE)ᶜ	Vitamin D* (µg)ᵈ	Vitamin E (mg α-TE)ᵉ	Vitamin K (µg)	Vitamin C (mg)	Thiamin (mg)	Riboflavin (mg)	Niacin (mg NE)ᶠ	Vitamin B6 (mg)	Folate (µg)	Vitamin B12 (µg)
Infants	0.0-0.5	375	—	3	5	30	0.3	0.4	5	0.3	25	0.3
	0.5-1.0	375	—	4	10	35	0.4	0.5	6	0.6	35	0.5
Children	1-3	400	—	6	15	40	0.7	0.8	9	1.0	50	0.7
	4-6	500	—	7	20	45	0.9	1.1	12	1.1	75	1.0
	7-10	700	—	7	30	45	1.0	1.2	13	1.4	100	1.4
Males	11-14	1,000	—	10	45	50	1.3	1.5	17	1.7	150	2.0
	15-18	1,000	—	10	65	60	1.5	1.8	20	2.0	200	2.0
	19-24	1,000	—	10	70	60	1.5	1.7	19	2.0	200	2.0
	25-50	1,000	—	10	80	60	1.5	1.7	19	2.0	200	2.0
	51-	1,000	—	10	80	60	1.2	1.4	15	2.0	200	2.0
Females	11-14	800	—	8	45	50	1.1	1.3	15	1.4	150	2.0
	15-18	800	—	8	55	60	1.1	1.3	15	1.5	180	2.0
	19-24	800	—	8	60	60	1.1	1.3	15	1.6	180	2.0
	25-50	800	—	8	65	60	1.1	1.3	15	1.6	180	2.0
	51-	800	—	8	65	60	1.0	1.2	13	1.6	180	2.0
Pregnant		800	—	10	65	70	1.5	1.6	17	2.2	400	2.2
Lactating	1st 6 months	1,300	—	12	65	95	1.6	1.8	20	2.1	280	2.6
	2nd 6 months	1,200	—	11	65	90	1.6	1.7	20	2.1	260	2.6

ᶜRetinol equivalents. 1 retinol equivalent = 1 µg retinol or 6 µg beta-carotene. To calculate IU: for fruits and vegetables, multiply the RE value by 10; for foods from animal sources, multiply the RE value by 3.3.

ᵈAs cholecalciferol. 10 µg cholecalciferol = 400 IU of vitamin D.

ᵉα-Tocopherol equivalents. 1 mg d-α tocopherol = 1 α-T.E.

ᶠNE (niacin equivalent) is equal to 1 mg of niacin or 60 mg of dietary tryptophan.

Tables 1-4 reprinted with permission from Recommended Dietary Allowances, 10th Edition, ©1989, by the National Academy of Sciences, National Academy Press, Washington, D.C.

*See page 23-26 for new dietary reference intake in this category.

are also not minimum dietary requirements. They were set as representative amounts of nutrients that meet the needs of most healthy people. Except for calories, the RDAs contain a sizable margin of safety. Officials deliberately set them at levels higher than what's needed for the average person. This allows room for the occasional anomalous individual requirement and for those infrequent but inevitable stress situations in life that boost our nutrient needs. The RDAs also take into account differences in the absorption level of nutrients from various sources. They are not, however, intended to meet the needs of seriously ill people or of those with genetic or metabolic disorders that cause profound changes in nutrient needs.

The very first RDAs, established in 1943, recommended intakes for 6 vitamins, 2 minerals, calories, and protein. The 10th edition, issued in 1989, gave an RDA for 11 vitamins, 7 minerals, and protein, divided into 15 different age and gender categories (see Table 1, pages 16–17).

In addition, it gave "Estimated Safe and Adequate Daily Dietary Intakes of Additional Selected Vitamins and Minerals" for seven more vitamins and minerals (see Table 2, page 20). Less information was available about the nutrients in this table; therefore, no definite allowances were made. The 1989 RDAs gave estimations, as ranges, instead. The same was true for the three minerals listed in "Estimated Sodium, Chloride, and Potassium

Minimum Requirements of Healthy Persons" (see Table 3, page 20).

The 10th edition of the RDA, published in 1989, differed from previous editions in several ways. It used actual height and weight measures of American adults of different ages, taken from the most recent National Health and Nutrition Examination Survey (NHANES II). Previous editions of the RDAs used arbitrary weight-for-height standards.

For the first time, the 1989 edition featured RDAs for vitamin K and selenium, reflecting the availability of better research. Another first: Smokers were given an additional allowance for vitamin C to reflect their higher needs (see Chapter 5 on antioxidants). And breast-feeding mothers now had two sets of requirements to differentiate needs specific to the first six months after delivery versus the second six-month period.

The 1989 RDAs also signaled changes for seven nutrients—one value was raised; six were lowered. The RDA for calcium increased from 800 mg to 1,200 mg for women aged 22 to 24 years— expanding the years for peak bone growth. The RDAs decreased for vitamin B_6, folate, vitamin B_{12}, magnesium, iron, and zinc. In addition, the low ends of the ranges for the Estimated Safe and Adequate Daily Dietary Intake fell even lower for four additional nutrients—biotin, manganese, copper, and molybdenum.

Table 2
SUMMARY TABLE
Estimated Safe and Adequate Daily Dietary Intakes of Additional Selected Vitamins and Minerals[a]

Category	Age (years)	Vitamins	
		Biotin µg	Pantothenic Acid
Infants	0-0.5	10	2
	0.5-1	15	3
Children and adolescents	1-3	20	3
	4-6	25	3-4
	7-10	30	4-5
	11+	30-100	4-7
Adults		30-100	4-7

Category	Age (years)	Trace Elements[b]				
		Copper (mg)	Manganese (mg)	Fluoride (mg)	Chromium (µg)	Molybdenum (µg)
Infants	0-0.5	0.4-0.6	0.3-0.6	0.1-0.5	10-40	15-30
	0.5-1	0.6-0.7	0.6-1.0	0.2-1.0	20-60	20-40
Children and adolescents	1-3	0.7-1.0	1.0-1.5	0.5-1.5	20-80	25-50
	4-6	1.0-1.5	1.5-2.0	1.0-2.5	30-120	50-150
	7-10	1.0-2.0	2.0-3.0	1.5-2.5	50-200	75-250
	11+	1.5-2.5	2.0-5.0	1.5-2.5	50-200	75-250
Adults		1.5-3.0	2.0-5.0	1.5-4.0	50-200	75-250

[a] Because there is less information on which to base allowances, these figures are not given in the main table of RDA and are provided here in the form of ranges of recommended intakes.

[b] Since the toxic levels for many trace elements may be only several times usual intakes, the upper levels for the trace elements given in this table should not be habitually exceeded.

Table 3
Estimated Sodium, Chloride, and Potassium Minimum Requirements of Healthy Persons[a]

Age	Weight		Sodium (mg)[a,b]	Chloride (mg)[a,b]	Potassium (mg)[c]
	(lb)[d]	(kg)[d]			
Months					
0-5	9.9	4.5	120	180	500
6-11	19.6	8.9	200	300	700
Years					
1	24.2	11.0	225	350	1,000
2-5	35.2	16.0	300	500	1,400
6-9	55.0	25.0	400	600	1,600
10-18	110.0	50.0	500	750	2,000
>18[d]	154.0	70.0	500	750	2,000

[a] No allowance has been included for large, prolonged losses from the skin through sweat.

[b] There is no evidence that higher intakes confer any health benefit.

[c] Desirable intakes of potassium may considerably exceed these values (~3,500 mg for adults).

[d] No allowance included for growth. Values for those below 18 years assume a growth rate at the 50th percentile reported by the National Center for Health Statistics (Hamill et al., 1979) and averaged for males and females.

Some experts in nutrition expressed concern that the 1989 edition lowered so many RDAs. Clearly, the RDAs' focus has been on preventing deficiency diseases more than protecting against chronic diseases of current importance to public health. Our need for some vitamins and minerals certainly would be greater than these recommendations if the stated goal was to prevent chronic disease. This growing belief led to some outspoken criticism about the usefulness of the 1989 RDAs and, just recently, the release of new RDAs for five nutrients. These new RDAs at last go beyond minimum standards by setting recommended nutrient intakes that aim to prevent chronic disease and optimize health. Unlike previous editions, these newly revamped RDAs will be released in stages, with nutrients having similar functions grouped together. The first group, released in the summer of 1997, included calcium, phosphorous, magnesium, vitamin D, and fluoride, all of which are related to bone health. The new recommended allowances for these nutrients are listed in tables 4–7 on pages 23–26. There are several changes in age groupings and in the grouping-together of some recommendations for men and women. Note that there has also been a change in terminology. Here's a glossary of the new nutrition buzz words:

Dietary Reference Intakes (DRVs)—an umbrella term that includes RDAs, AIs, and UIs, which are defined below.

Recommended Dietary Allowance (RDA)—though the term is the same, the meaning has changed. It now indicates the amount of a nutrient that should reduce the risk of developing certain chronic diseases for most healthy people of a certain age and gender.

Adequate Intake (AI)—has the same meaning as RDA, but at this time there is not enough evidence to officially set an RDA.

Tolerable Upper Intake Level—the upper safe intake level for a nutrient. It is not intended as a recommended level of intake.

In particular, the requirements for folate in women of child-bearing age, and for vitamin B_{12} and zinc in the elderly, are under discussion. The National Academy of Sciences convened a special session of the Food and Nutrition Board to consider the merit of these criticisms.

The 10th edition of the RDA is on pages 16–17 of this chapter. Individual vitamin and mineral profiles appear in Chapters 7 and 11, with discussions of allowances for adults. For information about allowances for infants, children, teenagers, young adults, and women who are pregnant or breast-feeding, refer to the complete tables earlier in this chapter.

THE FOOD GUIDE PYRAMID

After World War II, officials developed the Basic Four Food Groups because of a concern that peo-

Table 4
Dietary Reference Intakes for Calcium and Vitamin D

Life Stage Group*	Calcium	Vitamin D
	AI (mg/day)	AI (mg/day)
0 to 6 months	210	5
6 to 12 months	270	5
1 through 3 years	500	5
4 through 8 years	800	5
9 through 13 years	1,300	5
14 through 18 years	1,300	5
19 through 30 years	1,000	5
31 through 50 years	1,000	5
51 through 70 years	1,200	10
>70 years	1,200	10
Pregnancy		
<18 years	1,300	5
19 through 50 years	1,000	5
Lactation		
<18 years	1,300	5
19 through 50 years	1,000	5

*All groups except Pregnancy and Lactation include both males and females.

ple were not getting enough protein, vitamins, and minerals in their diets. (Meat, milk, and eggs anchored diets of that time.) Little attention was paid to the fat, sugar, and calories we worry about today.

To help people plan and evaluate their diets for adequate nutrition, the United States Department of Agriculture (USDA) developed the "Food

Table 5
Dietary Reference Intakes for Magnesium

Life Stage Group*	Magnesium	
	Male AI (mg/day)	Female AI (mg/day)
0 to 6 months (AI)	30	30
6 to 12 months	75	75
	RDA	RDA
1 through 3 years	80	5
4 through 8 years	130	130
9 through 13 years	240	240
14 through 18 years	410	360
19 through 30 years	400	310
31 through 50	420	320
51 through 70	420	320
>70 years	420	320
Pregnancy		
<18 years	335	400
19 through 30 years	290	350
31 through 50 years	300	360
Lactation		
<18 years	300	360
19 through 30 years	255	310
31 through 50 years	265	320

Guide Pyramid" (see page 29) in 1992. This food guide is an updated version of the familiar Basic Four Food Groups, or Daily Food Guide of the 1950s, except that the number of food groups is now five instead of four. The new Pyramid also reflects a concern for moderation in intakes of fats, oils, and sweets.

Table 6
Dietary Reference Intakes for Phosphorus

Life Stage Group*	Phosphorus
	AI
	(mg/day)
0 to 6 months	100
6 to 12 months	275
	RDA
1 through 3 years	460
4 through 8 years	500
9 through 13 years	1,300
14 through 18 years	1,300
19 through 30 years	1,000
31 through 50 years	1,000
51 through 70 years	1,200
>70 years	1,200
Pregnancy	
<18 years	1,300
19 through 50 years	1,000
Lactation	
<18 years	1,300
19 through 50 years	1,000

*All groups except Pregnancy and Lactation include both males and females.

GROUPING BY NUTRIENT

The Basic Four Food Groups lumped fruits and vegetables into one group. The Pyramid created two distinct groups, emphasizing the specific contributions each brings to the table. Fruit provides some vitamins and minerals in amounts not necessarily found in vegetables, and vice versa. For

Table 7
Dietary Reference Intakes for Fluoride

Life Stage Group*	Fluoride
	AI (mg/day)
0 to 6 months	0.01
6 to 12 months	0.5
1 through 3 years	0.7
4 through 8 years	1.1
9 through 13 years	2.0
14 through 18 years	2.9
19 through 30 years	3.1
31 through 50 years	3.1
51 through 70 years	3.1
>70 years	3.1
Pregnancy	
<18 years	2.9
19 through 50 years	3.1
Lactation	
<18 years	2.9
19 through 50 years	3.1

*All groups except Pregnancy and Lactation include both males and females.

example, without citrus fruit it would be difficult to get enough vitamin C. Likewise, without a serving of a yellow-orange or dark-green, leafy vegetable, it might be difficult to get enough beta-carotene in the diet.

Moreover, citrus fruits are richer than vegetables in the water-soluble fiber that may help to lower blood cholesterol. But vegetables have more of the insoluble fiber—the kind that may protect the colon from cancer.

Other than separating fruits from vegetables, the food groups in the Pyramid are identical to those in the Basic Four. The particular groupings of foods are determined by the nutrients they share. The vegetable group provides potassium, magnesium, folate, vitamin E, vitamin K, and sometimes calcium, in addition to vitamin A and fiber, depending on your choice of vegetable. Fruits offer potassium as well as vitamin C and fiber.

The milk group includes yogurt and cheese—good sources of calcium, phosphorus, vitamin D, and riboflavin (vitamin B_2), as well as protein. Grains include breads, cereals, rice, and pasta—important sources of B vitamins and fiber, along with such minerals as iron, potassium, zinc, copper, and selenium.

Most eclectic is the meat group, which includes poultry, fish, eggs, dried beans, and nuts as concentrated sources of protein. Dried beans and nuts are good alternative protein sources—for anyone, not just vegetarians. Dried beans, like meat, are also a source of iron and zinc. In addition, they provide folate, calcium, and fiber. Nuts also furnish magnesium and vitamin E.

Grouping foods according to the nutrients they provide allows you to choose from a variety of different foods. Just remember to include items from each of the food groups. The Pyramid offers an easy way to plan a healthful diet with a balanced intake of nutrients, while avoiding the rigid approach and monotony of fixed menus.

By balancing foods from each of the food groups, the Pyramid eating plan also ensures adequate amounts of vitamins and minerals in the diet, with a few exceptions. Women in their child-bearing years and teenage girls may have difficulty getting enough iron unless they make an effort to include extra servings of such iron-rich foods as whole-grain or enriched breads and cereals in their diets.

These women, as well as postmenopausal women, also have special requirements for calcium. The recommended number of servings from the milk group may not completely meet their needs, nor will extra servings of other calcium sources such as dried beans and broccoli. Such instances might call for the use of dietary supplements.

EATING FROM THE BOTTOM UP

The Pyramid's triangular shape better represents the relative proportion of foods in your diet than the old square Basic Four, which implied equality among the groups. However, you should not interpret the position of the food groups on the Pyramid to mean that one group is paramount over another. The groups on top are not more important than the lower ones. Each food group's placement on the Pyramid visually portrays its ideal proportion in the diet. You should eat more from the bottom of the Pyramid and less from the top. Yet selecting foods from each group is necessary to obtain a balanced diet with all the vitamins, minerals, and other nutrients you need.

The number of recommended servings from each group reflects the difference nutritionists place on the proportional value of the different groups.

The low end of the range given for number of servings is sufficient for older adults and inactive

Food Guide Pyramid
A Guide to Daily Food Choices

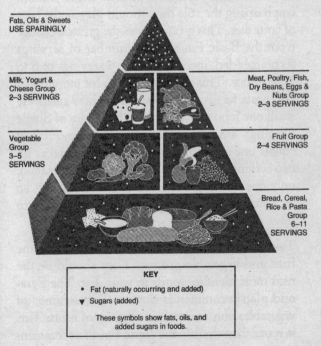

Fats, Oils & Sweets
USE SPARINGLY

Milk, Yogurt & Cheese Group
2–3 SERVINGS

Meat, Poultry, Fish, Dry Beans, Eggs & Nuts Group
2–3 SERVINGS

Vegetable Group
3–5 SERVINGS

Fruit Group
2–4 SERVINGS

Bread, Cereal, Rice & Pasta Group
6–11 SERVINGS

KEY

• Fat (naturally occurring and added)

▼ Sugars (added)

These symbols show fats, oils, and added sugars in foods.

29

women who eat about 1,600 calories per day. The middle number meets the needs for most children, teenage girls, active adult women, and inactive adult men; it provides about 2,200 calories per day. Teenage boys, active adult men, and women who are very active need about 2,800 calories daily and should aim for the highest number of servings listed. No one should eat fewer than the lowest number of servings listed for each food group. Small children who may need less than 1,600 calories should simply eat smaller portions.

Grains form the foundation of the Pyramid, emphasizing the role they should play as the base of your diet. This group shows the greatest change from the Basic Four in the number of servings recommended, increasing from 4 servings to 6 to 11 servings. This may seem like a lot more bread and pasta to eat, until you realize how relatively small one food serving is (see "Examples of Single Servings" on page 34). Since one slice of bread equals one serving, a sandwich already makes up two servings of grains. According to the Pyramid, only one-half cup of pasta equals one serving, so an average plate of spaghetti easily translates into three or four Pyramid servings.

Take a step up from grains and you'll find the fruit and vegetable groups. They should be the next most plentiful foods in your diet. The Pyramid plan recommends three to five servings of vegetables plus two to four servings of fruits. This is more than double the Basic Four's recommendation, which called for only four servings from a combined group of fruits and vegetables. This change is based on new research that shows fruits and vegetables can prevent chronic diseases, whether through their rich nutrient content or their contribution of phytochemicals—the natural disease-fighting chemicals found in plants (see Chapter 5).

Near the top of the Pyramid are the milk and meat groups, signaling their smaller roles relative to grains, fruits, and vegetables. They share a step because the proportions they contribute to the total diet should be about the same. The Pyramid plan recommends two to three servings from each group. This recommendation is unchanged from the Basic Four plan.

At the very top of the Pyramid are fats, oils, and sweets. These items are not considered a food group. Their position on the Pyramid conveys the message that they should be used sparingly because fat and sugar are already present in the other groups.

The guidelines for fat are based on limiting your fat intake to 30 percent of your total calories. If you choose to eat foods with the lowest fat contents from each food group, the Pyramid eating plan will provide approximately half of the fat you need in your diet. You can then use the remainder of your fat allowance for cooking oils, spreads, or salad dressings.

The guidelines for sugar suggest limiting intake to 6 teaspoons for a 1,600-calorie diet, 12 teaspoons for a 2,200-calorie diet, and 18 teaspoons for a 2,800-calorie diet. This allowance includes any amount you might be getting from sweetened fruit juices, presweetened breakfast cereals, candy, and baked goods. Reading labels becomes essential (remember, four grams of sugar equal one teaspoon).

There are fat traps in almost all the groups. The meat group contains the most, because meats are more likely to be high in fat. But grain-based foods such as cookies, cakes, and pastries are also high in fat, and you shouldn't meet the recommendations for grains by eating a lot of these foods. Fat in the milk group comes from whole-milk products, ice cream, and most cheeses. Vegetables can also be sources of fat if fried or eaten with cream sauces. (Fruits eaten in the form of sweetened fruit sauce, canned fruit, juice drinks, jellies, jams, or preserves can also add sugar to the diet.)

These Pyramid recommendations mirror those promoted in the Dietary Guidelines for Americans, published jointly by the USDA and the Department of Health and Human Services, as well as in the U.S. Surgeon General's 1988 Report on Nutrition and Health. These dietary guidelines stress the need to lower your fat intake to protect against heart disease, cancer, and overweight.

Keep in mind that foods rich in fat and sugar are often devoid of vitamins and minerals. You should direct yourself toward foods rich in the nutrients you need. These are the food choices most likely to supply the vitamins and minerals necessary for good health.

FOOD LABELING

The "Nutrition Facts" food label includes a measurement called Percent Daily Value, or %DV, which provides information about a food's nutrient content. The %DV reflects the RDA values for the age and gender that has the greatest needs.

In 1990, Congress passed the Nutrition Labeling and Education Act to clear up confusion over food labels. All packaged foods and meat and poultry products must have nutrition information on their labels (see sample label, page 37). For unpackaged raw foods, such as fruits, vegetables, and raw fish, look for voluntary information provided by posters or pamphlets in the produce sections and at seafood counters.

There are strict definitions now about what claims manufacturers can make. A food has to meet strict guidelines to use words such as lite or light, low, high, less, more, reduced, good source, or free. Even casual use of the word "fresh" is taboo. A food claiming to be a good source of vitamin E, for example, must provide ten percent of the recommended amount of vitamin E per serving. If a food claims to be cholesterol free, it cannot con-

EXAMPLES OF SINGLE SERVINGS

Food Group	
Milk, Yogurt, and Cheese	1 cup of milk or yogurt 1½ ounces of natural cheese 2 ounces of processed cheese
Meat, Poultry, Fish, Dry Beans, Eggs, and Nuts	2–3 ounces of cooked lean meat, poultry, or fish ½ cup of cooked beans, 1 egg, or 2 tablespoons of peanut butter count as 1 ounce of lean meat
Vegetables	1 cup of raw leafy vegetables ½ cup of other vegetables, cooked or chopped raw ¾ cup of vegetable juice
Fruit	1 medium apple, banana, or orange ½ cup of chopped, cooked, or canned fruit ¾ cup of fruit juice
Bread, Cereal, Rice, and Pasta	1 slice of bread 1 ounce of ready-to-eat cereal ½ cup of cooked cereal, rice, or pasta

tain more than 2 mg of cholesterol per serving. But even a truly cholesterol-free food cannot make this claim if it is high in fat, because the message would be too confusing for consumers. The labeling on a food that naturally contains zero cholesterol, such as pinto beans, can make only general statements about being cholesterol-free.

To make comparisons easier, nutrition information is expressed in exactly the same way from package to package, with only a few exceptions. Foods that contain insignificant amounts of many nutrients are allowed to use an abbreviated version of the label. Foods that come in very small packages only are required to provide a toll-free number where consumers can call for nutrition information.

Serving sizes are now standardized for similar types of foods. The size of a serving is based on details from food consumption surveys and thus is more realistic than the old serving sizes made up by the manufacturers. The label states the total number of calories per serving, along with the number of calories from fat in a serving.

Amounts of total fat, saturated fat, cholesterol, sodium, carbohydrate, dietary fiber, sugars, and protein are expressed in grams or milligrams per serving of the food. The relative amounts or percentages of vitamin A, vitamin C, calcium, and iron provided by one serving are also on the label. Other nutrients can also appear on the label as long as the Food and Drug Administration (FDA) has included them on its authorized list.

Preventing heart disease and cancer is a current health concern responsible for the shift in emphasis on the food label. The label relegates nutrients we might be underconsuming to a lesser status, not mentioning some of them at all. At this time, evidence is not sufficient that vitamin and mineral deficiencies—except for deficiencies of vitamin A, vitamin C, calcium, and iron—cause significant health problems. But as researchers complete more comprehensive studies on the health benefits of vitamins such as folate and vitamin E, or minerals such as selenium or chromium, this position could change. (See Chapters 6 and 10 for more information on the roles of vitamins and minerals in fighting diseases.)

Although the food label is now more informative about fat, sugar, and calories, it is less informative about vitamins and minerals. Now the nutrient information just lists the 2 vitamins and 2 minerals a food is highest in, instead of the 11 vitamins and 3 or 4 minerals it did before. However, if a food claims to be high in a particular vitamin or mineral, then that nutrient must also appear on the label in addition to the required vitamins and minerals.

Despite these limitations, the label information is still useful in selecting foods to make up a healthful diet. The new term Daily Value (DV) now

Nutrition Facts

Serving Size ½ cup (114g)
Servings per Container 4

Amount Per Serving

Calories 90   **Calories from Fat** 30

                                         % Daily Value*

Total Fat 3g	5%
Saturated Fat 0g	0%
Cholesterol 0mg	0%
Sodium 300mg	13%
Total Carbohydrate 13g	4%
Dietary Fiber 3g	12%
Sugars 3g	
Protein 3g	

Vitamin A 80%	•		Vitamin C 60%
Calcium 4%	•		Iron 4%

---

*Percent Daily Values are based on a 2,000 calorie diet.
Your daily values may be higher or lower depending on your
calorie needs.

	Calories:	2,000	2,500
Total Fat	Less than	65g	80g
Sat Fat	Less than	20g	25g
Cholesterol	Less than	300mg	300mg
Sodium	Less than	2,400mg	2,400mg
Total Carbohydrate		300g	375g
Fiber		25g	30g

Calories per gram:
Fat 9   •   Carbohydrate 4   •   Protein 4

appears on the label. The DV replaces the U.S.
RDA. All nutrients on the label are expressed as
a percentage of the DV (%DV) that one serving
of the food contributes to a 2,000-calorie diet. If
your daily caloric intake is more or less than 2,000

calories, the percentages applying to your diet will vary from the percentage listed. For diets of 2,000 and 2,500 calories, the actual %DV for some nutrients appears on the label.

Some foods claim specific health benefits on their labels. If a food meets certain requirements, its label is allowed to state a relationship between particular foods and certain diseases, as long as it stresses the importance of the food as part of an overall healthful diet.

For example, labels can identify foods low in sodium (less than 140 mg per serving) as an important part of a diet aimed at lowering the risk of high blood pressure. Foods that are good sources of calcium or provide ten percent of the DV for this mineral (120 mg per serving) may carry a message about calcium's importance in the diets of young adult women to help prevent osteoporosis.

Fruits and vegetables can carry a statement saying they offer protection against cancer as part of a balanced diet that is low in fat. Before their labeling can make this statement, these foods must meet the definition of a good source of vitamin A, vitamin C, or dietary fiber—that is, they must provide ten percent of the DV for these nutrients.

Fruit, vegetable, and whole-grain products that are good sources of fiber and are also low in fat can make claims about lowering the risk of cancer. Foods low in total fat, saturated fat, and cholesterol can make claims about preventing heart disease. Foods that supply a critical amount of soluble fiber, such as oats, oranges, and peaches, can also claim to benefit the heart. And foods rich in the B vitamin folate can now make claims about protecting against neural tube defects in pregnant women.

These health claims have been approved by the FDA for current use on food labels. As more clinical research accumulates, you may see additional claims on food labels to alert you to foods that may protect against disease. Although not yet approved, possible health claims on the horizon could include:

- zinc to benefit immune system function in the elderly
- vitamin E to lower risk of heart disease
- calcium to combat high blood pressure

(For more information on the links between these vitamins and disease prevention, see Chapters 6 and 10.)

CHAPTER 2

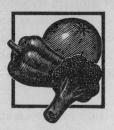

The Story of Vitamins

With all this talk about the importance of vitamins to good nutrition and healthy living, it's time to ask, "What are vitamins anyway?" Vitamins are organic substances that are necessary in very small amounts to maintain normal metabolism in the body.

In 1912, Dr. Casimir Funk, a Polish chemist working at the Lister Institute in London, coined the word *vitamine*. He derived it from *vita*, meaning "life," and *amine*, referring to a class of nitrogen-containing organic compounds. At the time, Dr. Funk was investigating thiamin—vitamin B_1—which is an amine. Later, scientists realized that not all vitamins are amines, so the final *e* in *vitamine* was dropped. The word vitamin reflects the vital life-giving importance of these substances.

Vitamins and Their Chemical Names

Vitamin	Chemical Name
A	carotenoids; beta-carotene; retinol; vitamin A acetate; vitamin A palmitate
B_1	thiamin; thiamin hydrochloride; thiamin mononitrate
B_2	riboflavin; riboflavin 58-phosphate; sodium riboflavin phosphate; disodium riboflavin phosphate
B_3	niacin; nicotinic acid; nicotinamide; niacinamide
B_6	pyridoxine hydrochloride
B_{12}	cobalamin; cyanocobalamin; cyanocobalamin concentrate
C	ascorbic acid; sodium ascorbate; erythorbic acid (isoascorbic acid)
D	cholecalciferol; calciferol; ergocalciferol
E	tocopherol; alpha-tocopherol; alphatocopheryl acetate; alphatocopheryl acid succinate
K	naphthoquinone; menadione (K_3); phylloquinone (K_1, phytonadione); menaquinone (K_2)
Biotin	biotin
Folate	folic acid; folacin
Pantothenic acid	panthenol; calcium pantothenate

The phrase "in very small amounts" included in the definition of vitamins sets them apart from the other classes of essential organic compounds. For example, proteins, fats, and carbohydrates are also organic substances, but we require them in considerably greater quantities. We measure vitamins in milligrams (mg) and micrograms (μg); in contrast, we measure proteins, fats, and carbohydrates in grams (g).

We've only known about the existence of vitamins since Dr. Funk's research in 1912. Since that time, scientists have identified 13 vitamins. The last to be isolated was vitamin B_{12} in the late 1940s. Upon its discovery, researchers assigned a letter designation to each vitamin in alphabetical order. It turned out, however, that some of the vitamins were actually several substances. The compound vitamin B, for example, turned out to be a group of compounds. So we now have vitamin B_1, vitamin B_2, vitamin B_6, and so forth. Although vitamins' alphabetical designations are still in common use, they also have chemical names. (The table on page 41 identifies the 13 vitamins and their chemical names.)

All vitamins are essential to life and must be supplied in the diet. As with any rule, though, there are exceptions. The body does produce small amounts of biotin, vitamin B_{12}, and vitamin K from intestinal bacteria, but in such negligible quantities that we still need more from the foods we eat.

Furthermore, if the body is supplied with the proper raw materials, it is capable of manufacturing certain other vitamins. For example, plant foods such as fruits and vegetables don't actually contain vitamin A but instead have vitamin A "activity." In other words, they are "precursors" to vitamin A because they contain substances called carotenes that our bodies can convert to vitamin A. Carotenes, or carotenoids, are the yellow-orange pigments that give the characteristic color to vegetables and fruits such as carrots, squash, and cantaloupe. These precursors are sometimes called provitamin A. Carotenes may also function as antioxidants, giving them importance beyond their conversion to vitamin A (see Chapter 5).

We have a provitamin D in our skin. Sunlight triggers a chemical reaction in skin that begins the provitamin's complex conversion to vitamin D—a process that is later completed in the kidneys. This explains vitamin D's nickname, the "sunshine vitamin." Often, though, the amount produced this way isn't enough to meet our bodies' needs, and we still need a dietary source. The body also meets some of its niacin needs by conversion from the amino acid tryptophan. Because we must rely on diet to fulfill our requirements for these vitamins, they are all essential.

Another way to classify vitamins is by solubility. Fat-soluble vitamins—A, D, E, and K—require fat for absorption. Water-soluble vitamins include biotin, folate, niacin, pantothenic acid, and vitamins B_1, B_2, B_6, B_{12}, and C. (Information about each of the 13 vitamins is provided in Chapter 7.)

So Much from So Little

Many vitamins, especially those of the B complex, act as coenzymes, or small molecules attached to enzymes that help the enzymes do their job. An enzyme is a catalyst—a substance that regulates the speed of a chemical reaction without being used up or changed in that reaction. So our bodies can use enzymes over and over again to control specific reactions. The body can also repeatedly use vitamins that act as coenzymes.

However, the body still needs a regular supply of these and the other vitamins to replace those excreted in the urine or destroyed or changed by the body during certain metabolic processes.

Subclinical Deficiency

Concern about vitamin deficiencies is rapidly being replaced with concern about the effects of marginally adequate vitamin intakes—amounts that may not cause a vitamin-deficiency disease but might interfere with normal body functions.

A subclinical deficiency can sneak up on you when the amount of a nutrient in your diet or your total "body pool" of a nutrient is only marginally adequate. Biochemical and metabolic changes can begin to take place, and then you become at risk for a vitamin deficiency.

Subclinical deficiencies can be deceptive. Outward signs are not apparent, but symptoms can develop rapidly if intake of the nutrient suddenly drops or if your nutrient requirement suddenly increases because of an illness or surgery. You could appear to be the picture of health, even though the process leading to disease may already be set in motion. And once a disease is present, it isn't always possible to reverse the effects of a longtime inadequate vitamin intake.

Sometimes symptoms never develop or aren't recognized when they do. For example, a vitamin E deficiency does not have any clear symptoms to identify it. If you are subclinically deficient in vitamin E, your immune system suffers the effects of operating at less-than-optimal capacity and may be unable to protect you fully against infections or cancer.

Only laboratory tests can confirm subclinical vitamin deficiencies. Depending on the vitamin, these laboratory tests may measure the amount of the vitamin circulating in the blood or the amount of the vitamin's breakdown products excreted in the urine.

In some instances, tests measure metabolic by-products of a vitamin. The amount of these compounds in the blood or urine often indicates the vitamin status of the individual. That's because certain compounds accumulate if the vitamin they need to function is in low supply.

It is also possible to measure the activity of certain enzymes that require vitamins as coenzymes. For example, the enzyme transketolase (present in red blood cells) exhibits below-normal activity when not enough thiamin, its coenzyme, is available.

Waiting to act on your nutrient needs until you have a clear deficiency or a disease is not a prudent approach. Fortunately, severe vitamin deficiencies are rare in the United States today, but they do still exist in developing areas of the world, where food shortages and malnutrition are more prevalent.

One way to protect yourself from the dangers of undetectable subclinical deficiencies is to eat a wide variety of foods. If you do not eat enough calories, or if your eating habits are not as good as you would like, you may want to consider taking a multivitamin/mineral supplement. The supplement should balance what you are already getting from your diet.

TOXICITY

We know that large doses of vitamins can have harmful effects on the body. In fact, an overdose of a vitamin can be as serious as a vitamin deficiency. Overdoses are more likely to occur with fat-soluble vitamins, which are stored in body fat and the liver and used as needed. The more fat-soluble vitamins you take, the more of them your body stores. If too much is stored, serious consequences result. Cases of toxicity from excesses of vitamins A and D are occasionally reported (see the profiles in Chapter 7).

Our bodies cannot store large amounts of water-soluble vitamins, so we need a more constant supply of them. Overdoses are unlikely, because we excrete any excess of these vitamins in urine if too much is consumed. Because of this, nutritionists used to believe you couldn't take in a dangerous amount of water-soluble vitamins. We now know, however, that large quantities of vitamin C and some of the B vitamins—particularly B6—can trigger toxic effects.

Moreover, high doses of vitamins can create vitamin imbalances. That is, large amounts of one vitamin can cause a deficiency of another. For example, animal studies have shown that high doses of vitamin E may adversely affect a person's vitamin K status.

Hypervitaminosis is the clinical term for a vitamin overdose. The danger of this condition exists whenever you take large doses—called megadoses—of vitamins. (For more information about megadoses, see Chapter 4.)

THERAPEUTIC USES: VITAMINS AS DRUGS

Many situations increase vitamin needs. For example, from infancy to the end of puberty—a period of growth and development—children often need extra vitamins. Since pregnant women are eating for two (or more), they also usually require extra nutrients. When people cannot consume a regular diet because of severe illness, surgery, or allergies, they may need vitamin supplements. Vitamin requirements are higher for those taking birth control pills, those who are on very restrictive diets, and those taking drugs that may interfere with vitamin function or absorption. In rare instances, a person may be born with an inherited disorder requiring higher vitamin intakes. A qualified physician would need to carefully evaluate and treat all these situations.

Currently popular is "megavitamin therapy" or "orthomolecular therapy," based on the premise that large doses of vitamins are useful for the treatment or cure of many diseases. It's true that large doses of certain vitamins can be medically useful. For example, nicotinic acid—a form of niacin—is often prescribed to reduce blood cholesterol levels. Unfortunately, most claims haven't been substantiated by carefully controlled studies.

Any druglike action of a vitamin is unrelated to its nutritional function. When taken in megadoses, a vitamin is no longer acting as a nutrient because the amount far exceeds what's necessary to meet the body's nutritional requirements. Rather, the vitamin is acting as a drug. It is not yet clear whether moderately high doses of vitamins are active as nutrients or as drugs.

Caution: Self-treatment of real or suspected diseases with massive doses of vitamins is potentially hazardous. Not only does the danger of overdose exist, but self-diagnosis and self-treatment can only delay appropriate medical attention. Supplements that contain doses 500 to 1,000 times more than the amounts recommended by the RDA require proper medical supervision.

VITAMINS IN A
PREVENTIVE ROLE

Any benefits of vitamin megadoses in the treatment of medical conditions remain largely unproved and cannot take the place of standard medical treatment. Nevertheless, interest has grown in the possibility that certain vitamins can prevent some diseases from developing in the first place. (For more about prevention, see Chapters 5 and 6.)

Prevention does not need to be as aggressive as treatment. Prevention is similar to buying an insurance policy to protect yourself from something that might happen. But because you are not sure it actually will happen, you do not want to risk any unwanted side effects. So before you consider consuming higher-than-recommended amounts of particular vitamins, you need to be sure that scientific evidence supports it.

Much of what we know about the role of vitamins in protecting against diseases comes from studying people who exhibit fewer diseases than other people and comparing the foods they eat. One of the most striking differences in dietary habits is the abundance of fruits and vegetables eaten by groups with low rates of cancer and heart disease. Fruits and vegetables are the major sources of many vitamins and minerals—particularly antioxidants. This suggests a tentative link between these nutrients and protection from various diseases. But fruits and vegetables are also full of fiber and phytochemicals (see page 85), so no one knows for sure if one component—or all of them together—is what's responsible.

The possibility that some vitamins may help prevent disease is reflected in the current updating of the RDAs (see Chapter 1). Some evidence points to the potential for disease prevention from levels much higher than what you could get from foods, especially for vitamin E. Whether this will be reflected in the updated RDAs to come remains to be seen.

Much of the debate revolves around the new roles recently identified for vitamins in the body. The RDAs have always been based on traditional vitamin-dependent functions, but recent discoveries are forcing us to reevaluate our vitamin needs in light of newly defined functions for vitamins. Most of these functions protect us against disease processes.

No matter which way the debate is resolved, or whether the new information is reflected in the new RDAs, we may need more of certain vitamins than previously thought if we want to protect ourselves against disease.

VITAMINLIKE SUBSTANCES

Certain substances, though not true vitamins, closely resemble vitamins in their activity. When these vitaminlike substances appear in vitamin preparations, a footnote on the label usually reads: "Need in human nutrition has not been established."

The nutritional status and biological role of vitaminlike substances are murky even today. At one time, for example, choline, inositol, and para-aminobenzoic acid (PABA) were thought to be vitamins. It was later discovered that each of these substances could be synthesized in the body, and a lack of them did not cause symptoms of any type of deficiency in the body. Therefore, they do not meet the scientific definition of a vitamin.

Claims made about these substances can sometimes be misleading. Para-aminobenzoic acid (PABA) is an ingredient in some sunscreens, but taking PABA internally will not prevent sunburn. PABA also appears to affect the hair, because when it is lacking in some animals, their dark fur loses its pigment. However, PABA cannot reverse or prevent the graying of hair in human beings. Once a person's hair has turned gray, nothing short of a bottle of dye will restore his or her natural color.

Other vitaminlike substances include: bioflavonoids (often sold in combination with vitamin C), carnitine (sometimes called vitamin B-T), coenzyme Q, and lipoic acid.

Current widespread promotion of vitaminlike supplements for the treatment or cure of serious diseases lacks sufficient scientific basis. Bioflavonoids have shown promise as phytochemicals, but research is only preliminary. Based on current scientific knowledge, itaminlike substances certainly are not essential for good health. Only the 13 vitamins discussed in the following chapters are essential in the human diet.

CHAPTER 3

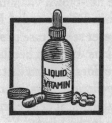

Vitamin
Supplements

Confusion and misinformation surround the use of vitamin supplements. People hear stories about our food supply being robbed of its nutritional value and about it being impossible to get the required vitamins through food alone. Vitamin supplement manufacturers encourage these fears by using such expressions as "just to be sure you get all the vitamins you need" in their promotions. In addition, supplements—especially in massive doses—are promoted to prevent and cure diseases unrelated to known deficiencies.

The notion that vitamins are endowed with miraculous powers is a popular one. This idea, combined with a misunderstanding about how vitamins work, leads many to believe that daily supplements are essential for good health.

VITAMIN STATUS—USA

We seldom see full-blown vitamin deficiency diseases in the United States today. Most practicing doctors have never seen a case of scurvy, beriberi, pellagra, or rickets. But just because vitamin deficiencies are rare doesn't mean that the vitamin status of the population is satisfactory. There is evidence that subclinical deficiencies are probably not uncommon in the United States.

From 1971 to 1974, the National Center for Health Statistics conducted its first Health and Nutrition Examination Survey (HANES I) to evaluate the nutritional status of Americans. The more than 20,000 people surveyed represented a broad cross-section of the population, unlike previous surveys that concentrated on low-income populations. The HANES I survey uncovered nutrient deficiencies for vitamin A and iron in addition to protein and calcium. But, unlike previous surveys, a simple lack of calories could not explain the deficiencies.

In 1977, HANES II was conducted to see if the physical condition and laboratory test results of HANES II subjects correlated with the low nutrient intakes found in HANES I. Some of the participants did exhibit low laboratory values for such nutrients as protein, vitamin A, thiamin, riboflavin, and iron. Yet not everyone with a low intake of a nutrient had low laboratory values. Investigators determined that some of those with low intakes were probably at the very beginning stages of subclinical deficiency.

In 1977 and 1978, the U.S. Department of Agriculture (USDA) conducted a Nationwide Food Consumption Survey. Like earlier surveys, it found that dietary adequacy was related to income. But, although Americans' weight had increased significantly (probably as a result of inactivity), calories had not. This meant that to keep weight from increasing, a person would have to reduce calories, thus reducing nutrient intake. Yet the survey indicated that for vitamins A, C, and B6 and the minerals calcium, iron, and magnesium, about one third of the participants were already getting only 70 percent or less of the Recommended Dietary Allowance (RDA). Moreover, most of those surveyed were eating foods high in fat, sugar, and cholesterol.

A second Nationwide Food Consumption Survey was conducted in 1987 and 1988. It confirmed that most adults were not meeting the dietary guidelines. Those who ate foods rich in fat were most likely to have a low intake of vitamins and minerals. One third of the women were getting less than 67 percent of the RDA for vitamin A, vitamin E, vitamin B6, folate, calcium, magnesium, iron, and zinc. Men were lacking in vitamin B6, calcium, zinc, and magnesium.

Unfortunately, promotions for vitamin supplements often misuse findings from such nutrition surveys. Advertisements for vitamins may include statements like, "Surveys show that a large number of people in our country don't get all the vitamins they need." The implication is that these people need vitamin supplements. Statements of this sort ignore the fact that most people do not need 100 percent of the RDA for vitamins and minerals. And it presumes that supplements are the only answer. Yet most nutrition problems in the United States can be corrected by providing more food to those in need and by improving the food selections or eating habits of those who already take in sufficient calories.

WHO NEEDS VITAMIN SUPPLEMENTS?

"Do I need vitamin supplements?" you may ask. No firm answer is possible without a thorough analysis of your lifestyle and eating habits.

You need to treat true vitamin deficiencies with vitamin supplements, whether the deficiency results from a faulty diet or a health condition. In either case, a qualified physician can diagnose the deficiency. If precipitated by disease, the doctor also will treat the disease to correct the underlying problem. If the problem is poor eating habits, you may be able to discontinue the supplements once they restore you to a healthy nutritional state and your dietary habits improve. If you are taking supplements to treat a disease, continue them until your physician advises otherwise.

Whether using vitamin supplements can successfully prevent conditions other than deficiency diseases is difficult to prove or disprove. Much of what we know about the effects of vitamins on disease is from studies of food, not supplements. A person who takes vitamins and does not develop a certain disease may attribute the good fortune to the supplement, but the mere absence of disease is not sufficient evidence to prove anything. It could have been coincidence.

Many people end up taking vitamin supplements as a kind of "nutrition insurance." They don't know what their actual vitamin status is, and they don't know the amount of vitamins in the foods they eat, so they take vitamin supplements "just to be sure."

Most nutritionists agree that people can get all the vitamins they need from foods—if they make the right food choices. However, nutritionists often do not argue with the use of supplements for extra insurance, as long as the supplements do not exceed 100 percent of the RDAs. Some nutrition experts, such as those representing The American Dietetic Association, do not support the use of supplements, especially if they contain megadoses of vitamins.

If you want to know if you really need to take vitamin supplements, CONSUMER GUIDE™ recommends that you consult a registered dietitian or your doctor. With help from qualified professionals, you can determine your nutrient needs based on your health, diet, activity, and lifestyle.

FOODS VERSUS SUPPLEMENTS

Wouldn't it be nice to meet all your nutritional needs by swallowing a single pill? If you think so, you probably care about your health but do not want to worry about what you eat. Unfortunately, it doesn't work that way. Food is essential to good health. Although we know something about food and the components that are vital to good health, we will never know everything. For example, scientists have already identified more than 10,000 nonnutrient compounds in plant foods. These compounds may not be essential, but each has shown some positive effects on health.

Food is also preferable to supplements as a primary source of vitamins because it's much more difficult to get too much of a vitamin from food, making overdosing unlikely. At the very high doses typical of megadose supplements, the druglike effects of vitamins can be harmful. Although vitamin toxicity rarely causes death, it can cause considerable discomfort and interfere with the healthy functioning of the body.

Some people think that as long as they take vitamin supplements, they don't need to worry about how or what they eat. This is unfortunate. To ensure good nutrition and good health, all essential nutrients, not just vitamins, must be supplied in adequate amounts.

Nutrients are all part of a team, and vitamins are some of the players. Vitamin supplements are not substitutes for good food. Do not use them as an excuse for making poor food choices or developing bad eating habits.

VITAMINS AND DIETERS

Diets that include a variety of foods usually supply an adequate amount of vitamins. In attempting to lose weight, however, many people follow weight-reduction diets that do not include the variety of foods outlined in the Pyramid eating plan. (If you need a quick review of the Pyramid plan, see Chapter 1.) Even without restricting the types of foods you eat, when you cut down on calories, you inevitably find yourself eating less food. And less food means missed chances to meet nutrient needs.

For this reason, vitamin intakes may be less than desirable among calorie-conscious people. Vitamin supplements may provide a bit of insurance against possible deficiency in this situation. However, your doctor should evaluate your general health before you begin any

- weight-reduction diet
- exercise program accompanying a diet plan
- vitamin supplementation

VITAMINS AND THE ELDERLY

Concern is growing among nutrition experts about the threat of inadequate or inappropriate diets and their effects on the vitamin status of elderly people. Data from several surveys suggest that many older people's diets contain less than two thirds of the RDAs for many vitamins and minerals. And in a continuing study of more than 700 senior citizens in the Boston area, researchers are finding that the seniors' diets provide less than two thirds of the RDAs for vitamins B_6, B_{12}, and D, as well as folate and the minerals zinc, calcium, and magnesium.

Elderly people often do not eat well for a variety of reasons, including economic problems, loneliness, physical handicaps, and reduced mobility. Many also cut down on the amount of food they eat to avoid becoming overweight. Even when elderly people do eat well, changes that occur with age can make it difficult for their bodies to absorb or use vitamins properly. Moreover, some medications, including those commonly prescribed for controlling blood pressure, can interfere with vitamin use.

For the elderly, daily multivitamin/mineral supplements that supply 100 percent of the RDAs may be the answer. A doctor's supervision in both the choice and the dosage of these supplements is necessary to ensure their proper use and effectiveness. Even so, supplements can never substitute for food. Supplements obviously lack carbohydrate, fat, protein, fiber, and many other substances that the elderly may also have trouble obtaining. Older individuals should make every attempt to eat a balanced diet, whether they regularly take supplements or not.

VITAMINS FOR PREGNANT WOMEN, INFANTS, AND CHILDREN

Vitamin supplements are almost routinely prescribed for pregnant women, since pregnancy increases the need for vitamins. The use of supplements provides a certain degree of assurance that vitamin requirements will be met.

Vitamin supplements are often prescribed for infants as well. At birth, newborns receive a vitamin K injection to hold them over until they develop the intestinal bacteria that will make their own vitamin K. Also, an infant who is breast-fed may not get enough vitamin D because breast milk does not contain vitamin D. Unless the baby is exposed to sufficient amounts of sunshine, which causes a natural production of vitamin D in the skin, pediatricians frequently prescribe a supplement that contains vitamin D. Often, this supplement also includes vitamins C and A.

Chewable vitamin supplements are popular for young children. They're available in a variety of flavors, sizes, and shapes to entice children into taking them. However, this very appeal—their candylike appearance and taste—has caused concern about possible accidental ingestion. Even though they're sold with childproof caps, chewable children's vitamins can cause accidental poisoning from overconsumption. They have also been known to cause a number of choking deaths. Small children—younger than three years old—should be given only liquid supplements or chewable tablets that have been crushed. These, as well as any other vitamin/mineral supplements or drugs—particularly iron-containing supplements, which can be deadly—must be kept capped and out of the reach of children.

Like adults, children can ordinarily acquire most of the vitamins they need from food. Nutritionists emphasize the importance of introducing children to the Food Guide Pyramid to foster good eating habits early in life. Still, children can and do go on eating jags, when variety is hardly the name of the game, providing reason for a daily supplement. Indeed, pediatricians frequently recommend the use of vitamin and mineral supplements during a child's formative years. Still, don't use supplements as an excuse to allow a child to develop bad eating habits. There is no subsititute for good nutrition.

SUPPLEMENTS AND ATHLETIC PERFORMANCE

With fitness and training programs at a peak, it is no wonder that many athletic hopefuls are searching for additional ways to get an edge over their rivals. Dietary supplements have always held an allure for athletes, beginning with the myth that salt tablets would help improve performance.

Many athletes believe that vitamin supplements can boost their energy. The truth is, only carbohydrates, fat, and protein can provide energy. The only way energy can be derived from supplements is if the supplement corrects a deficiency of a vitamin involved in the metabolism of carbohydrates, fat, or protein.

Athletes do have greater needs for some nutrients than less-active individuals. For one, their needs for energy can be considerable, ranging up to 6,000 calories a day for marathon runners. As a result, thiamin, riboflavin, niacin, iron, and copper requirements are higher to support the increase in energy metabolism. But these athletes also consume greater quantities of foods than nonathletes, which should be enough to provide them with the additional amounts of the vitamins and minerals they need.

Athletes who do not require such large amounts of calories do need to watch their intake of the vitamins and minerals that support energy metabolism. Concentrating on nutrient-rich, low-calorie foods—such as skim milk, broccoli, tomatoes, strawberries, whole-grain breads and cereals, kidney beans, turkey, chicken, and fish—is a good idea.

Female athletes may also have special needs for iron and calcium. The requirement for iron is greater for female athletes than it is for male athletes. They need more iron to make the greater number of red blood cells needed to transport the larger amount of oxygen that they require during strenuous exercise. Furthermore, in the blood vessels of the feet, the force of activity can destroy red blood cells, which then need to be replaced. These things happen to male athletes, too, but men do not lose blood through menstrual flow and, therefore, rarely have to concern themselves with iron loss.

Athletes may also benefit from higher intakes of antioxidant nutrients because they are exposed to large volumes of oxygen during exercise. (For more about antioxidants, see Chapter 5.)

SYNTHETIC VERSUS NATURAL

If you're going to take supplements, here's something to think about. Vitamins derived from foods are obviously natural. Those created in a laboratory are synthetic. Both are sold in supplement form. Which is better?

Synthetic vitamins are copies of the natural vitamins isolated from food. They're usually cheaper in price than natural vitamin supplements, and their potency can be controlled. Yet a vitamin is a vitamin regardless of its source. A vitamin made by a plant is essentially identical to one made by a drug company. As far as we know, our bodies cannot tell the difference once absorbed into the blood. Foods do, however, have additional ingredients that can either enhance or depress the amount of vitamin absorbed. For example, to absorb beta-carotene efficiently, some fat must be present.

Synthetic supplements sometimes have the advantage of being able to offer a vitamin in a more chemically stable form or in a form more readily usable by the body, but these advantages should be balanced by other considerations. For example, alpha-tocopherol acetate, a form of vitamin E found in supplements, is more stable than forms of vitamin E found in foods. However, the body retains the natural form of vitamin E longer than the synthetic form.

Folate in its supplement form, pteroylmonoglutamic acid, does not require modification first by an intestinal enzyme before being absorbed into the body, but the forms more commonly found in foods do. However, the supplement form of the vitamin is also found in fortified foods. Orange juice is rich in this form of folate.

CHECKING THE LABEL

Just as the labels on food have been changed to a uniform style, labels on supplements will soon have to conform to a particular style as well. The FDA published final dietary supplement labeling regulations in September 1997. They become effective 18 months from that date. The new supplement labels will look much like food labels and will bear the title: Supplement Facts (see sample label, page 67).

The serving size will be clearly listed in common units, such as one tablet, one teaspoonful, or one capsule.

As proposed, the "Amount Per Serving" section will contain the actual nutrient information. In this section, the ingredient, the amount per serving, and the percent of the Daily Value will be listed. The amounts of the nutrients in a supplement will be listed in a separate column, making them easier to read. They will be given in milligrams (mg), micrograms (µg or mcg), or international units (IU).

Another column will provide the percentage of the Daily Value (%DV) for each nutrient. The %DV reveals how the amount of a nutrient in one serving of the supplement relates to the amount you should get in an entire day. For most nutrients, the Daily Values are the highest RDA for all age and sex categories, excluding pregnant and lactating women. Unfortunately, this won't be as useful as it could be since supplement labels will still express vitamin and mineral doses in terms of the outdated 1968 RDAs, as do food labels (except for the six nutrients for which standards were added). This will not change until the Daily Values for nutrients are updated to reflect the most recent RDAs.

Until then—which is probably not in the near future—iron, for example, will be labeled 100%DV only when a serving of food or supple-

DIRECTIONS: One (1) tablet daily as a dietary supplement.

Supplement Facts
Serving Size 1 tablet

Amount Per Tablet		% Daily Value
Vitamin A (100% as beta-carotene)	5000 I.U.	100%
Vitamin C	250 mg	417%
Vitamin E	200 I.U.	667%
Selenium	35 mcg	50%
Lutein	6 mg	*
Fresh Bilberry Fruit Extract 4:1 extract in 70% ethanol	100 mg	*

*Daily Value not established

INGREDIENTS: ascorbic acid, dl-alpha tocopheryl acetate, bilberry fruit extract, lutein, beta-carotene, microcrystalline cellulose, sodium selenate

STORAGE: Keep tightly closed in dry place; do not expose to excessive heat.

KEEP OUT OF REACH OF CHILDREN
EXPIRATION DATE: Nov. 1999
Manufacturer or distributor's name, address, and zip code

ment contains 18 milligrams, even though the currently used 1989 RDA for iron lowered the maximum RDA to 15 milligrams. Such confusion will continue for all nutrients that have had their RDAs changed drastically. The new proposals do establish standards for six nutrients that were included in the 1989 RDAs but were not included in the 1968 RDAs at all: vitamin K, selenium, manganese, chromium, molybdenum, and chloride.

As before, when the supplement is for a specific group—such as infants, children less than four years of age, or pregnant or lactating women—the %DV column will have to state specifically the intended group and provide percentages based on that particular group's needs.

The new labels may also provide certain extra information. The vitamin A listing, for example, will be allowed to reveal what percentage of the vitamin A is provided as beta-carotene.

Labels may also include

- ingredients that supply each vitamin or mineral (listed in descending order by weight of the nutrient)
- ingredients used to form the tablet or capsule—for example, cornstarch may be used as a filler, binder, or disintegrating agent; propylparaben may be used as a coating; and vanillin may be used as a flavoring agent

- a warning—for example, "Keep out of the reach of children"
- the Latin name for botanicals
- a statement of nutritional support that describes the effect of the product on structure or function of the body or on well-being
- an expiration date. Taking a vitamin past its expiration date is not dangerous, but the supplement's potency may be reduced. If you notice any change in the color, smell, or taste of a vitamin supplement, discard it. Minerals, on the other hand, are very stable and may be used for an indefinite period
- storage instructions. Store vitamins in their original container in a cool, dry place. The kitchen and bathroom are not the best places to store vitamins because heat and humidity may hasten deterioration

Read all supplement labels carefully. It is best to choose a supplement that provides about 100 percent of the U.S. RDA (100%DV on new labels) for vitamins. Avoid those supplements that supply excessive or unbalanced quantities of vitamins.

CHAPTER 4

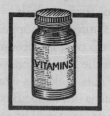

Megavitamin Therapy

We've all heard claims for megavitamin therapy: "You should take extra B vitamins when your body is under stress," they say, or "Schizophrenia can be controlled with large amounts of niacin," or even "You can eliminate the symptoms of menopause by taking lots of vitamin E."

Today, claims for miracle cures bombard us from all directions. Some megavitamin therapy promoters say that vitamin supplements—some of them containing as much as several thousand percent of the recommended amount—are effective in treating many physical and mental disorders. Although some of these claims may have merit, many are not supported by controlled clinical research.

70

Just what is megavitamin therapy? A megavitamin is a vitamin in a dose ten or more times its Recommended Dietary Allowance (RDA). For example, the RDA for vitamin C for adults is 60 mg, so 600 mg or more of vitamin C is a megavitamin dose. And by definition, therapy refers to a treatment. So megavitamin therapy does not usually mean the use of vitamins for protection from disease.

The popular but misguided idea that "if a little is good, a lot must be better" needs a particular caveat when applied to vitamins. As discussed in Chapter 2, when you take in much larger amounts of a vitamin than you need, the excess acts more like a drug in the body and less like a nutrient. This is why you run the risk of experiencing side effects, just as you would if you overdosed on a drug. And some of these side effects may be toxic.

Vitamin and mineral supplements are not labeled as drugs. They are considered "food supplements"—subject to no more scrutiny than any other health food store cure-all. There are a few exceptions. The Food and Drug Administration (FDA) does have the authority to limit the potency or composition of folate, as well as vitamin and mineral supplements used by children and pregnant or nursing women. But all other vitamins in supplements are essentially unregulated. Vitamin and mineral supplements that are considered to be drugs, such as prenatal vitamins, are controlled by other divisions of the FDA.

The FDA and the Federal Trade Commission jointly police the advertising of vitamin and mineral supplements. However, only minimal regulation polices supplement advertising. When the Food Supplement Act of 1994 categorized most supplements as food supplements and not as drugs, the development of needed regulations suffered a setback.

Some people may be able to take megadoses of some vitamins without serious side effects. But there are definite potential hazards associated with the intake of large doses of some vitamins. We'll talk about some of these hazards in the individual vitamin profiles that appear later in this book (see Chapter 7).

When promoters of megavitamin therapy raise false hopes, they are little better than hawkers at a frontier medicine show. *Life Extension*, the book by Durk Pearson and Sandy Shaw, suggests that taking megadoses of about 25 different supplements daily can prevent or significantly delay heart disease and cancer. Jack Z. Yetiv, M.D., Ph.D., in his book *Popular Nutritional Practices: A Scientific Appraisal*, evaluates the Pearson-Shaw book and finds it ". . . extremely inaccurate; some of the recommendations in the book are potentially life threatening."

The references given in the Pearson-Shaw book do not support the claims they make—and at times they even contradict them. The book is typical of many of those that promote megavitamin therapy. They tempt the public with false claims and false hopes, while in reality, they offer little more than unproven, expensive regimens that might even be harmful.

Perhaps the most serious danger in using unsubstantiated megavitamin therapies to treat disease is the possible delay of necessary medical treatment. If you have a medical problem, do not use vitamin and mineral supplements in place of legitimate medical treatment.

Large amounts of vitamins are not cure-alls. And large amounts of vitamins can be very dangerous. Indeed, almost anything can be poisonous if you take enough, even water. And vitamins are no exception.

Because vitamins in large doses might have drug-like effects, they may actually compromise the effectiveness of standard medical treatment in the same way that taking two different drugs might. It is safest to seek medical care first if you have a disease or other condition. And be sure to let your doctor know that you are interested in taking vitamins to augment your treatment. Forms of vitamins that are effective in treating diseases, such as the vitamin A–like retinoids, often are not available without a prescription from your doctor.

The bottom line is that a vitamin supplement can cure a deficiency of a vitamin, and it may even offer some protection against certain diseases.

However, excessive amounts of vitamins—especially the thousand-percent megadoses some supplements contain—can do the following:

- interfere with medications
- interfere with the absorption of other vitamins
- disrupt body functions
- be toxic to your body

So, the simple rule to remember about the use of vitamins is—DON'T OVERDOSE.

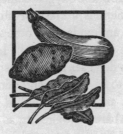

Antioxidants

Oxygen is essential for sustaining life. Without it, we could not support the basic functions of our bodies. But every breath of oxygen-laden air we take in exposes us to one of the most toxic of all biological compounds.

How can oxygen be so lethal? Oxygen itself is not the problem, but once it transforms into a free radical, it assumes destructive powers. Free radicals are unstable forms of oxygen—they have lost an electron from their molecular structures. Normally these electrons exist in pairs. To replace the lost electron, free radicals actively seek out electrons from other substances in the body. When these materials give up an electron to the free radical, their structures, in turn, become damaged. Sometimes these damaged materials themselves steal electrons from other nearby substances, creating a dominolike path of destruction.

Fortunately, our bodies are armed with the means to protect us from the oxygen damage. A key part of our armament is a class of molecular compounds called antioxidants. These substances can neutralize free radicals. Our cells have a number of antioxidant defenses at their disposal, some of which happen to be vitamins and minerals. Vitamin C, vitamin E, and the carotenoid beta-carotene (provitamin A) are antioxidants, as are three minerals: selenium, manganese, and zinc.

Among the favorite targets of free radicals are cell proteins, enzymes, the fatty acids in cell membranes, and the genetic material DNA. Damage to these structures can trigger the development of conditions as diverse as cataracts, arthritis, diabetes, heart disease, and cancer. Much of the illness and loss of vitality we experience with age may result from the unchecked accumulation of free-radical damage to cells.

The forces that act on oxygen to create free radicals are called oxidative stresses. Some of these stresses arise as a normal part of cell reactions. Everyday reactions that remove drugs or other chemicals from the body and help fight infection are also capable of causing oxidative stress.

Although we can't eliminate all oxidative stresses, the good news is we can take steps to avoid some of them. Habits like smoking cigarettes, drinking excessive amounts of alcohol, and eating excessive amounts of unsaturated fat impose unnecessary free-radical burdens on us. Air pollution and ultraviolet radiation from sunlight add even more. We can't avoid them entirely. However, we can try to minimize our exposure to them by using sunscreens and not exercising on heavily polluted days. Lead coverings also protect us from oxidative stress produced by X rays.

Luckily, antioxidants can protect us from unavoidable oxidative stresses. Our exposure to these stresses is probably much higher today than even a few years ago because of the pollution produced by our crowded, high-technology world. Thinning of the ozone layer has left us more vulnerable to ultraviolet radiation than before. So our need for antioxidant nutrients is greater than ever. Yet our intake of these nutrients is at an all-time low.

How Do Antioxidants Work?

Antioxidants tackle free radicals by using a variety of tactics. One strategy is to run interference between the free radical and the cell material it has targeted to attack for an electron. By giving the free radical one of its own electrons, the antioxidant spares the cell material from damage. Antioxidants that work this way are called free-radical scavengers. Vitamin C, beta-carotene, and vitamin E all work as scavengers.

Mineral antioxidants use another tactic. These minerals are attached to cell proteins called enzymes.

The enzymes take out the free radicals through chemical reactions. Selenium works with an enzyme called glutathione peroxidase, while zinc works with superoxide dismutase, or SOD. A protein in the blood called ceruloplasmin, which contains copper, may also act as an antioxidant. Each of these enzymes has a particular free radical it keeps under surveillance.

The various antioxidants cooperate with one another to achieve their goal of protection against free-radical damage. They require this team effort because antioxidants exist in different places in the cell and attack different free radicals. Vitamin E usually protects the fat in the cell membranes, while vitamin C protects mostly proteins. Beta-carotene is the most powerful defense we have against free radicals formed by ultraviolet light. Selenium enzymes protect the cell machinery that generates energy. Zinc enzymes take up stations at other points to halt free radicals that might have slipped by other antioxidants.

Vitamin C also helps put vitamin E back in action by giving it another electron once vitamin E loses its electron to a free radical. Likewise, vitamin E steps in to help out if selenium supplies are insufficient. So taking in enough selenium frees vitamin E to be more effective in its other duties.

FREE-RADICAL DISEASES

The vast array of diseases and conditions believed to have a free-radical connection is daunting.

From heart disease and cancer to arthritis and cataracts, a role for free radicals or material damaged by a free radical has been found. In fact, you can trace the aging process itself to lifelong free-radical damage. By squelching free radicals, antioxidants come as close as anything ever has to the fountain of youth.

HEART DISEASE

Several clinical trials have recently reported evidence that vitamin E can protect against heart disease. We already know about the link between blood levels of cholesterol—in particular low-density lipoprotein (LDL) cholesterol—and coronary heart disease. But now scientists know that only oxidized LDL cholesterol damages the walls of arteries. And it's thought that vitamin E may be able to prevent that oxidation.

Other clinical studies are now testing whether beta-carotene and vitamin C can also reduce heart disease. We know fruits and vegetables provide such protection, but until a few years ago we thought the reason was that these foods are low in fat. Low-fat diets work by keeping LDL cholesterol levels low. Now it appears these foods may be just as important for the antioxidant protection they provide.

CANCER

All cancers begin with an injury to a cell's genetic material, DNA. As these injured cells reproduce with the wrong genetic blueprint, a tumor forms. Our immune systems fight cancer by destroying tumor cells while tumors are still very small, but free radicals deal a double blow in promoting the growth of cancer. Not only can they cause the initial damage to DNA, but they can also sabotage the immune system, making it a less effective defense against tumors. Every one of the chemicals we know to cause cancer is either a free radical itself or triggers the formation of one.

CATARACTS

The eye is particularly vulnerable to free radicals that form as a result of exposure to sunlight. Unless we wear eye protection that screens out ultraviolet radiation, we are constantly exposing our eyes to these penetrating rays from the sun. The free radicals formed from ultraviolet radiation most likely damage the protein-rich lens of the eye. Ordinarily, protective enzymes remove these damaged proteins from the eye. But as we age, these enzymes become less efficient. If the amount of damaged protein is large, it begins to build up in the lens. As it accumulates, it forms an opaque, solid mass—a cataract—that does not allow light to pass through. The diminished vision can lead to blindness. About 45 percent of adults over age 75 develop cataracts.

ARTHRITIS

Not as much is known about free-radical links to other diseases, but researchers suspect a link between free radicals and arthritis. Free-radical damage to important organs and tissues may contribute to loss of function, with subtle consequences such as energy loss or lack of mobility.

ANTIOXIDANTS AND ATHLETES

An athlete's level of activity creates a greater need for energy and, thus, a much greater demand for oxygen than that of less-active people. Heavy exercise generates an additional free-radical burden because of the extra energy produced. Indeed, free-radical damage may trigger some of the muscle soreness that develops after strenuous exercise.

But do athletes have special needs for antioxidants to give them protection? This question is unanswered as yet, though many researchers think they do. The United States Olympic Committee offers the following antioxidant recommendations for athletes: 3–20 milligrams of beta-carotene, 250–100 milligrams of vitamin C, and 100–400 IU of vitamin E each day. And one study from Tufts University Human Nutrition Research Center on Aging found that taking an antioxidant supplement appeared to benefit active people over the age of 50 after they exercised more than it benefited younger active people.

MEASURING UP TO THE DIETARY REQUIREMENTS

The richest dietary sources of vitamin C and beta-carotene are fruits and vegetables. A recent study on the dietary habits of Americans revealed that most of us aren't eating enough fruits and vegetables to get the levels of antioxidants needed to protect us against free-radical–related diseases. According to the Second National Health and Nutrition Examination Survey, on a given day only 21 percent of Americans ate any fruits or vegetables rich in carotenoids and only 28 percent consumed a good source of vitamin C.

Breads and cereals made from whole grains also provide antioxidants, but most people eat bread made from refined or white flours. Some nutritionists conclude that most Americans do not consume in adequate amounts of these key nutrients for them to serve as antioxidants.

ARE WE GETTING ENOUGH?

Even if you eat food sources of antioxidants, it does not always guarantee that your body will get sufficient amounts. Citrus fruits, strawberries, potatoes, green peppers, and tomatoes contain substantial amounts of vitamin C, but high temperatures destroy the vitamin when these foods are heated.

Yellow-orange fruits and vegetables, such as carrots, squash, apricots, and mangoes, are concentrated sources of beta-carotene. Dark-green, leafy vegetables such as spinach, broccoli, asparagus, and mustard or beet greens are also rich in beta-carotene. High temperatures do not destroy this compound, and cooking may, in fact, make beta-carotene in plant foods more available. Extended storage in sunlight or exposure to the air, however, can destroy beta-carotene.

Whole grains provide vitamin E, selenium, and zinc. (The body does not absorb zinc well from whole grains, however, because zinc is tightly bound to a substance in the grains.) Vegetable oils made from corn, safflower, sunflower, and soybean are rich sources of vitamin E, but they also deliver a potential oxidative stress because they are polyunsaturated fats.

At a time when so many Americans are not choosing the right foods to provide the antioxidants they need, scientists are beginning to believe our requirements for these compounds may be higher than previously thought.

SUPPLEMENT PITFALLS

Although taking an antioxidant supplement can help meet your needs for these nutrients, take care not to rely on supplements alone. That's because most studies that have uncovered health benefits for antioxidants actually measured intake of foods, not antioxidants. Many researchers have just assumed that because these foods—mostly fruits and vegetables—are rich in antioxidants, then antioxidants must be the protective factor. But then again, maybe not.

Fruits and vegetables are also rich in fiber and low in fat. They also sport phytochemicals (see page

85). It could be any one of these, or all of them together, that helps prevent disease.

If you take an antioxidant supplement on the assumption that it holds the key, you eliminate the possible benefits these other substances might contribute. Besides, antioxidants work as a team to protect the body from free-radical damage. Taking extra amounts of one will not substitute for the lack of another. Take care to ensure that you consume sufficient quantities of all the antioxidants—vitamins and minerals—to receive their full benefits.

A word of caution: If you take extra antioxidants, don't get a false sense of security. For optimal health, you need a total commitment to eliminating unhealthy behaviors such as smoking, eating a high-fat diet, and not exercising. Taking an antioxidant without tackling these other problems will not get you far.

Indeed, some research has cast doubt on the benefits of antioxidant supplements. A 1994 Finnish study showed that supplementation with beta-carotene had no protective effect against lung cancer. This study was far from conclusive, however. Other researchers severely criticized it because the volunteers were all heavy smokers and the supplementation may have been a case of too little, too late. Those who did the best were those who had the highest level from dietary sources before the study began. Score another one for real food.

Because all these questions are still up in the air, for now it seems best to stick with food sources of antioxidants. Just be sure to eat lots of fruits and vegetables—you can't overdose on them. And one thing you'll be sure of getting is plenty of phytochemicals.

PHYTOCHEMICALS TO
THE RESCUE

Just what are phytochemicals? Phyto means plant. So phytochemicals are natural substances—chemicals—found in plants. Researchers believe that many of them have disease-fighting properties. If that sounds preposterous, just think of all the medicines we have isolated from plants.

Sure enough, foods long rumored to protect from disease—like garlic—have turned out to contain chemicals that appear to fight disease in lab conditions. In garlic's case, there are allylic sulfides, plus dozens more. In tea, that miracle beverage your grandma foisted on you to make you well, there are polyphenols. While soy has genistein and apples and strawberries contain ellagic acid, broccoli includes sulforaphane and celery contains psoralens. And there are hundreds, probably even thousands, more that are undiscovered. Scientists estimate that a single orange may contain about 150 different phytochemicals.

Take beta-carotene, for instance. It's actually a phytochemical, as are all the carotenoids, also known as carotenes. Study after study has linked foods high in beta-carotene to a lower risk of cancer, particularly lung cancer, while suggesting protection against heart disease as well.

Now, researchers admit the foods high in beta-carotene that are associated with better health may be high in other carotenoids, too. Unfortunately, even though other carotenoids might be more powerful than beta-carotene, we know relatively little about their content in foods. This illustrates the potential pitfall of relying on beta-carotene supplements, because by doing so, you're missing out on almost 500 other members of the carotenoid family. Such tunnel vision may come back to haunt you, in the names of other carotenoids like alpha-carotene, beta-cryptoxanthin, canthaxanthin, and lutein.

Lycopene is another example. This carotenoid, found particularly in tomatoes, has twice the antioxidant power of beta-carotene. A study of 47,000 men recently found tomatoes and tomato products to be protective against prostate cancer. Men who ate ten or more servings a week of tomato products—tomatoes, tomato sauce, pizza—were 45 percent less likely to develop prostate cancer than those who rarely ate them. Cooked tomatoes were particularly protective because heat can release carotenoids.

Previously, raw tomatoes were cited as lowering the risk of cancers of the mouth, esophagus, stomach, colon, and rectum. In a study of 3,000 people, those who ate seven or more servings of tomatoes per week had only half the cancer risk of those eating two servings or less. Researchers assume the protective substance in this case is lycopene, though they cannot be sure. Still, scientists have gone to the trouble to develop a tomato with extraordinarily high levels of loose lycopene.

How can phytochemicals quell cancer? Scientists have suggested that these natural substances exert double-barreled action by blocking pro-cancer enzymes in the body and stimulating anti-cancer enzymes at the same time.

Some researchers hope that by isolating phytochemicals, they can then create phyto-fortified foods, or so-called "designer" foods, "functional" foods, or "nutraceuticals." But this poses the same potential trap that taking supplements of vitamins and minerals does. How do we know we've isolated the important ones? And what if certain phytochemicals need to work together to be effective? Or maybe they work best with vitamins and minerals? Isolating them may be the worst thing we could do. Better to take them in their natural form—as fruits and vegetables.

Indeed, there is no lack of studies linking fruit and vegetable consumption to lower risk of cancer. And phytochemicals may even help prevent heart disease, high blood pressure, cataracts, and infection. One class of phytochemicals called flavonoids—present in high amounts in tea, wine, apples, and some vegetables—may protect against heart disease. In a study of more than 800 men, those who consumed the most flavonoids suffered half the heart attacks of those who consumed the least. Researchers speculate that flavonoids, which are antioxidants, prevent LDL cholesterol from becoming oxidized LDL cholesterol—the form that clogs arteries.

In light of all the evidence pointing more to fruits and vegetables than to single nutrients or phytochemicals, the National Institutes of Health instituted a program called Five A Day. It encourages the public to eat five to nine servings of fruits and vegetables each day for better health. Surprisingly, most people eat only a total of two or three servings a day, even though juice and potatoes count toward that total. A banana alone counts as two servings; for other fruits, one piece or a half cup is a serving. Why not see how close you can come to the five to nine optimal range? It's almost guaranteed to reduce your risk of disease.

CHAPTER 6

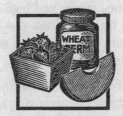

Vitamins and Disease

After years in the background, diet has finally entered the ring as a serious contender in the fight against disease. First, the focus was on the leading roles of fat, cholesterol, sodium, and calories, while the supporting roles of vitamins and minerals went largely unnoticed. Because such small amounts of these nutrients are found in the body, our understanding of their functions had to await improvement in research technology. Now that we can detect and observe these substances, we can explore the activities of vitamins and minerals that we never knew existed.

These explorations have led to a startling revelation: Vitamins (and minerals, too) may be more important than we ever dreamed in protecting us against some of the most common and deadly diseases. We have known for a while that the healthiest populations in the world eat diets that are low in fat and refined sugars and high in fiber. Now we realize it is no coincidence that these diets are also rich in fruit, vegetables, and whole grains as well as vitamins and minerals.

This chapter reviews the latest findings on vitamins and their roles in protecting against disease. Chapter 10 reviews the findings for minerals. As you read through these fascinating discoveries, keep in mind that research is ongoing. New discoveries may change current thinking.

Before you run out to stock up on supplements, remember that foods should always be your primary source of nutrition. Supplements cannot provide you with the spectrum of benefits you receive from foods because they contain only a fraction of the natural compounds foods possess—that is, the ones we know about. We are still learning about the promising potential of the other natural substances in foods called phytochemicals.

HEART DISEASE

As the leading cause of death in the United States, heart disease is the perfect target for prevention efforts. The dietary approach has traditionally centered around lowering dietary fat, saturated fat, and cholesterol; increasing fiber intake; and maintaining a lean body weight.

Now it appears that increasing your intake of vitamins—particularly antioxidants and certain B vitamins—may be just as important. Antioxidant vitamins play a key role in protecting the heart and blood vessels because low-density lipoprotein (LDL) cholesterol must be oxidized before it can do damage. And antioxidants prevent that oxidation.

The blood carries vitamin E, an antioxidant, along with LDL cholesterol—perhaps nature's way of protecting us. But when LDL cholesterol levels get too high or when vitamin E levels are too low, the protection may not be sufficient. Two recent studies, one in men and one in women, found that those who consumed the most vitamin E had the lowest risk of heart disease. In the studies, vitamin E came from both food and supplements, though protection didn't require megadoses. The average intake among those with the lowest risk of heart disease was 60 to 100 IU, or six to ten times the Recommended Dietary Allowance (RDA) for an adult man.

Vitamin C is another antioxidant vitamin that appears to protect against heart disease. People at higher risk for heart disease have lower vitamin C levels. For instance, men have lower levels than women, smokers have lower levels than non-smokers, and older adults have lower levels than younger adults. It also happens that heart disease peaks during the winter and spring months, just when the availability of fruits and vegetables that are rich in vitamin C is lowest. A coincidence? Maybe. Maybe not.

One way vitamin C apparently works is by diminishing the tendency for blood clots to form. These clots can block blood flow in the heart or brain, causing a heart attack or stroke. Reactions that rid the body of cholesterol may also involve vitamin C. Even in animals with satisfactory but marginal intakes of vitamin C, the body did not remove LDL cholesterol as quickly as in well-nourished animals. In people with low blood levels of vitamin C, high-density lipoprotein (HDL) cholesterol (sometimes called the "good" cholesterol) is frequently below protective levels. A few studies have also found higher blood pressure in people with low levels of vitamin C in their blood. Because vitamin C assists vitamin E, it may also prevent heart disease by boosting vitamin E's effectiveness.

Beta-carotene may also benefit the heart, but the evidence is less convincing than that for the other antioxidant vitamins. One small preliminary study in men found that beta-carotene supplements decreased the risk of a repeat heart attack. That's important because the risk of a second heart attack is much higher than the risk of a first, and the chances of surviving it are even poorer. However, three large clinical trials recently concluded that beta-carotene offers no benefit to healthy people, while two suggested that high-dose supplements may even be harmful to smokers.

While antioxidants have claimed the limelight for some time, attention is now turning to several B vitamins for possible protection against heart disease. Vitamin B6 and vitamin B12 help return blood levels of the amino acid homocysteine to normal. Experts believe homocysteine damages blood vessels. They now consider a high blood level of homocysteine to be an important risk factor for heart disease—perhaps as important as elevated blood cholesterol levels.

How convenient that a diet rich in these heart-healthy vitamins is also rich in fiber and low in fat, saturated fat, and cholesterol. To reap the benefits of such a diet, focus on whole grains, yellow-orange and dark-green leafy vegetables, and citrus fruits. You can also include chicken, lean meats, fish, and skim milk.

CANCER

As with heart disease, antioxidant vitamins may also reduce the risk of cancer in several different ways. One way is by interfering with the growth of tumors. Antioxidants may keep the immune system operating at its peak so it can seek out and destroy tumor cells.

Another way antioxidants may protect against cancer is by preventing chemicals from being transformed into cancer-causing substances, or carcinogens, in the first place. For example, vitamin C can stop the transformation of nitrates—chemicals added to processed meats and found in cigarette smoke—into powerful carcinogens called nitrosamines. But nitrates discourage the growth of microorganisms in meats—and, therefore, perform an important function. So, instead of eliminating nitrates, manufacturers now add vitamin C to these foods to prevent their transformation into carcinogenic nitrosamines.

More than 40 studies have documented an association between eating foods rich in vitamin C and a decreased risk of cancer. Indeed, gastric cancer rarely occurs in people with high intakes of this nutrient. However, because diets rich in vitamin C are also rich in other nutrients, it's difficult to attribute benefits specifically to vitamin C. Unlike beta-carotene and vitamin E, which are found in relatively few foods, vitamin C is widely distributed among foods, from oranges and strawberries to tomatoes, green peppers, and potatoes. Its widespread presence in the diet makes it difficult to pinpoint the specific benefit of vitamin C. Other than gastric cancer, cervical cancer is the only type of cancer consistently associated with a low vitamin C intake. Vitamin C may work indirectly; it may be that vitamin C's most significant contribution to preventing cancer is in boosting immune system function.

It's been difficult to find a specific role for vitamin E as well. Although one study found that people with poor vitamin E nutrition had two to four times the risk of getting cancer or dying from it than people with good vitamin E nutrition, the results from most studies have been mixed. Some evidence hints at possible benefits from vitamin E for breast and lung cancers.

High beta-carotene intakes, on the other hand, appear to benefit cancers of the cervix, esophagus, stomach, intestines, bladder, and head and neck. Beta-carotene has been thought to be especially protective against lung cancer, particularly among smokers. Recent studies, however, question beta-carotene's protective role. Much of the support for beta-carotene's connection to lung and bladder cancers is from studies measuring consumption of foods rich in beta-carotene. More reliable research measures actual blood levels of the nutrients, which reflect nutrient intake from food as well as from supplements. Most important, two recent studies of smokers suggested an increase in lung cancer among those given beta-carotene supplements. Researchers are now urging caution for smokers taking beta-carotene.

The track record for vitamin A in protecting against cancer may be the most impressive of all the vitamins. Unlike beta-carotene, vitamin A is not an antioxidant, so its benefits relate to its possible roles in reversing tumor development and boosting immune function. In fact, in the early stages of vitamin A deficiency, changes that resemble the early stages of cancer occur in cells of the skin, mouth, lungs, and intestines. Vitamin A directs cells to produce new cells that are identical reproductions of the originals. (Tumors form when new cells that are different from the original cells begin to reproduce.) Drug companies have harnessed this role of vitamin A to produce powerful synthetic forms of the vitamin called retinoids. They have used them in the treatment of cancer, with some success for cancers of the lung, mouth, and cervix.

Vitamin D may also protect against cancer. In one study, people with the lowest intakes of vitamin D and calcium were those who developed colon and rectal cancers during a year-long period. It is not clear whether low vitamin D has a specific effect on the development of these cancers or whether its effect stems from aggravating a calcium deficiency. Vitamin D is necessary to absorb calcium, and a low calcium intake increases the risk of colon and rectal cancers.

A study in the United States that measured differences in rates of breast cancer between the Northeast and the South raised a possible link between vitamin D and breast cancer. The rates of breast cancer in the Northeast were almost twice the rates in the sunnier South. Dietary intakes of the vitamin did not differ between regions, but women in the South are exposed to more sunlight and thus make more vitamin D in their skin.

Folate, too, has shown some potential in fending off cancer. Folate supplements reversed an ominous change in cervical cells called cervical dysplasia—believed to be a forerunner of cervical cancer. Folate may influence cell development through DNA, the genetic material of cells.

DIABETES

Keeping blood sugar, or glucose, from getting too high is the goal of diabetes treatment. The majority of the complications from diabetes—from heart disease to cataracts—are caused by damage to tissues from high blood sugar. Antioxidants might protect the cells of the pancreas that produce insulin from free-radical damage. This damage might be responsible for type I diabetes—the kind that develops in childhood and depends on insulin injections to control blood sugar levels.

Vitamin C and vitamin E may offer some benefits for people with diabetes. The structure of vitamin C is similar to that of glucose. Because of this similarity, the vitamin may bind to proteins before glucose can. This may change the structure of some tissues and alter their functions. Vitamin C levels in the blood of a person with diabetes are as much as 80 to 85 percent lower than in people without the disease. Recent clinical trials suggest that supplementation with 100 to 600 milligrams a day may be beneficial.

By protecting cell membranes from oxidation, vitamin E may improve the effectiveness of insulin, which is responsible for removing glucose from the blood. Indeed, in one study of people with type II diabetes, blood sugar control improved after vitamin E supplements were administered at druglike doses of 90 times the RDA for adult men. Additional studies are necessary to evaluate the impact of vitamin E supplements in individuals who have type I diabetes and require insulin injections.

AGING

Rumors have long been rampant that vitamin E holds the secret to everlasting youth and virility. Though claims of increased virility haven't panned out, vitamin E's antioxidant properties have renewed interest in its anti-aging potential.

As we age, our organs and tissues begin to break down slowly with the wear and tear of continued use. This deterioration—caused, at least in part, by free-radical damage to cells—contributes to an erosion of vitality and health. As an antioxidant, vitamin E may be able to slow down or even prevent this destructive process by protecting cells from free-radical damage.

While nothing can really stop the aging process, vitamin E may be able to prevent or at least delay a number of conditions common among older people, such as Parkinson disease. The heart, brain, eyes, lungs, kidneys, and liver all might benefit from adequate vitamin E intake. It may not be the fountain of youth, but vitamin E, along with other antioxidants, may play a role in keeping you young at heart—literally.

IMMUNE FUNCTION

A healthy immune system fights off tumors as well as infection. It stands to reason, then, that a declining immune system leaves you vulnerable not only to colds, but to cancer as well. It can also sap you of your energy. Because immunity declines with age, adults over age 50 usually suffer from more infections, tumors, and lack of energy than younger adults, and thus are more likely to benefit from immune-boosting vitamins.

The immune system requires the production of large numbers of immune cells, or white blood cells, to mount attacks against bacteria or other foreign substances. These immune cells produce free radicals in response to the ensuing inflammation. So while other vitamins—such as folate and vitamins A, B6, and D—may have important roles in preserving immune function, antioxidant nutrients are the most important because they quash these free radicals.

Surprisingly, of the antioxidants, it is vitamin E—not vitamin C—that appears to have the most impact on immune function. Older people with high levels of vitamin E in their blood are less susceptible to diseases such as influenza and pneumonia than people of the same age with lower blood levels of vitamin E. In a study of older adults, vitamin E and beta-carotene supplements administered at two to three times the RDA strengthened the immunity that study participants received from a flu vaccine. However, a more recent study that looked at the effect of giving beta-carotene supplements alone to healthy older adults found no boost in immunity.

A recent study raised the possibility that beta-carotene might improve immune function in people infected with the human immunodeficiency virus (HIV). At doses of 180 milligrams (mg) of beta-carotene, or 30 times the recommended amount, the immune cells targeted by HIV—"helper" T cells—increased in number. It is still too early to predict if the body can sustain this benefit over a long period of time.

Vitamin C's possible effectiveness in preventing the common cold has been the subject of controversy for many years. Linus Pauling first suggested the vitamin could prevent colds over 30 years ago, but rigorous scientific studies have failed to confirm his belief. However, these studies did find that the symptoms of a cold may be less severe and may not last as long after taking vitamin C. (As an antioxidant, vitamin C protects specific immune cells called macrophages from the free radicals released when these cells battle bacteria or viruses. This protection lets the macrophages be more effective in combating infection.)

When the presence of bacteria, viruses, tumor cells, or other foreign substances in the system activates immune cells, they must multiply to challenge these foreign substances successfully. Vitamins that are important to cell reproduction, such as vitamin B6 and folate, play a vital role in this aspect of immune function. Vitamin B6 also helps produce antibodies—proteins that recognize and attack specific foreign substances. Research shows maximum benefit from vitamin B6 supplements at doses of 3 mg—only slightly higher than the 2-mg requirement for adult men.

Vitamin A's role in immune function is especially critical to children, whose need for this vitamin during growth is especially high. In developing countries where vitamin A deficiency is common, children often die from infections. A single vitamin A supplement given to children in Nepal resulted in a substantial reduction in deaths among those younger than five years of age.

The effect of vitamin A on immune function is far-reaching. Every aspect of immunity is dependent in some way on this vitamin, even though it is not functioning as an antioxidant in this case. So powerful are its effects that high doses of vitamin A are now being tested to stimulate normal immune responses into more aggressive activity. These tests use druglike synthetic forms of the vitamin, which are toxic at high doses. Do not attempt such supplementation without the supervision of a physician.

CATARACTS

The lens of the eye is exceedingly vulnerable to free-radical damage caused by sunlight. With age, the damage accumulates, and the lens becomes cloudy from the continuous bombardment of ultraviolet rays. Between the ages of 52 and 64, about five percent of adults have some form of cloudiness, or cataracts. Between ages 75 and 85, the number increases to 46 percent. As cataracts worsen, they reduce vision. Indeed, cataract formation is now one of the major causes of blindness in the elderly.

The antioxidant vitamins C and E protect against cataracts. Animals who come out only at night—and thus aren't exposed to light rays—have much lower concentrations of vitamin C in their lenses than animals who are active during the day. One study found that middle-aged adults who had high blood levels of two of three antioxidants—vitamin C, vitamin E, or beta-carotene—had a reduced risk of cataracts. In another study, adults aged 55 or older who took supplements of vitamins E and C reduced their risk of cataracts by 50 percent or more. And most recently, a study of 247 women aged 56 to 71 years old who had taken vitamin C supplements for more than ten years (at least 400 milligrams a day) found a 77 percent lower incidence of clouding of the lenses, an early stage in cataract development.

NEURAL TUBE DEFECTS

A neural tube defect is a birth defect of the developing nervous system of a fetus, causing the spine not to close properly. Spina bifida and anencephaly are examples of such birth defects. About 0.1 percent of American women of childbearing age are at risk of giving birth to a child with a neural tube defect.

Researchers from the United Kingdom first believed genetic predisposition was responsible for that country's unusually high rate of neural tube defects. But then multivitamin supplements showed promise in lowering the rate. Finally, researchers zeroed in on folate. Subsequent studies reinforced the link between increased folate consumption and prevention of neural tube defects. The protection afforded by folate was so striking in one study that researchers stopped the trial early so that the control group could reap the rewards of folate supplementation, too.

Because folate acts in the very early stages of pregnancy—usually before a woman realizes she is pregnant—it is important for any woman who might get pregnant to get adequate folate. The U.S. Public Health Service now recommends that all women in their childbearing years consume at least 400 micrograms (µg) of folate daily. This level can be hard to attain from food sources alone, so supplementation may be necessary. The Food and Drug Administration now requires that folate be included with the B vitamins and iron now added to enriched flour.

Although too much folate does not appear to have any major toxic effects, there is a danger associated with exceeding the 400-μg level without a physician's supervision. If you are a woman with a family history of neural tube defects and are planning a pregnancy, you might want to discuss with your doctor the possibility of taking a high-potency folate supplement. Excess folate can mask a vitamin B_{12} deficiency, and an undetected deficiency of vitamin B_{12} can permanently damage the nervous system.

OSTEOPOROSIS

Osteoporosis usually brings to mind the need for the mineral calcium, but vitamins are just as important in a behind-the-scenes way. This disease, which involves a loss of considerable amounts of bone, primarily affects white and Asian women of slight build during the years after menopause. There are many factors contributing to this disease, but experts recognize dietary intake of certain nutrients earlier in life as one of the most important. Dietary calcium is, indeed, the primary nutrient involved because it is so important to bone composition, but so are other nutrients, whose supporting roles cannot make up for inadequate calcium intake.

Among the vitamins that support healthy bone are vitamins A, C, D, and K. Vitamin D has a crucial role because it influences the amount of calcium absorbed from the diet and how well the body uses calcium. Reactions that occur in the liver and kidney activate vitamin D. A decline in kidney function with age can decrease the amount of active vitamin D. For people who have trouble activating the vitamin, calcium supplements will not prevent bone loss. Taking a vitamin D supplement or getting more sunlight to increase the vitamin in the skin will not be particularly helpful either. In this case, only taking the active form of the vitamin will help.

Some of the structures that support bone require vitamin A. This vitamin also helps regulate the rate at which bone breaks down and is replaced by new bone. Upsetting this balance could contribute to bone loss. Indeed, bones develop abnormally in children with severe vitamin A deficiency. Paradoxically, excessive vitamin A also promotes the breakdown of bone.

Connective tissue called collagen surrounds and supports bone. Vitamin C contributes to bone development by ensuring that collagen is strong.

For many years the role of vitamin K was not clear, but researchers have recently discovered that vitamin K plays a critical role in the making of several proteins needed to form bone. In research studies, vitamin K supplements reduced the amount of calcium lost from the body in the urine of women around or past menopausal age. Less calcium lost means more calcium retained by bone, and that means stronger bone.

CHAPTER 7

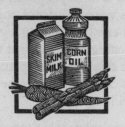

Vitamin Profiles

Vitamin A: Retinol

As far as vitamin A is concerned, the eyes have it. Vitamin A, or retinol, plays a vital role in vision.

HISTORY

As indicated by its position at the head of the vitamin alphabet, vitamin A was the first vitamin discovered. In the early 1900s, researchers recognized that a certain substance in animal fats and fish oils was necessary for the growth of young animals. Scientists originally called the substance fat-soluble A to signify its presence in animal fats. Later, they renamed it vitamin A.

FUNCTIONS

Vitamin A's most clearly defined role is the one it plays in vision. Metabolites of the vitamin combine with certain proteins to make visual pigments that help the eye adjust from bright to dim light. This process, however, uses up a lot of vitamin A. If it's not replaced, night blindness can result.

Moreover, a deficiency of vitamin A dries out the transparent coating of the eye (the cornea) and the "whites" of the eye (the conjunctiva). If not treated, this condition, called xerophthalmia, causes irreversible damage and blindness. Vitamin A deficiency is a major cause of blindness in the world.

Vitamin A is also important for normal growth and reproduction—especially proper development of bones and teeth. Animal studies show that vitamin A is essential for normal sperm formation, for growth of a healthy fetus, and perhaps for the synthesis of steroid hormones.

Another important, but misunderstood, role of vitamin A involves preserving healthy skin—inside and out. Taking extra vitamin A won't make your sagging skin suddenly beautiful, but a deficiency of it will cause skin problems. Furthermore, an adequate vitamin A intake ensures healthy mucous membranes of the gastrointestinal and respiratory tracts. In this way, vitamin A helps the body resist infection.

SOURCES OF VITAMIN A

Vitamin A is found in foods of both plant and animal origin. Retinol, also called preformed vitamin A, is the natural form found in animals. Carotenoids, found in plants, are a group of pigmented compounds, including provitamins, that the body can convert to vitamin A. Bright-orange beta-carotene is the most important carotenoid, because it yields more vitamin A than alpha- or gamma-carotenes.

Some carotenoids, such as lycopene, cannot be converted to vitamin A. Lycopene, the orange-red pigment that can be found in tomatoes and watermelon, is still of value, however, because it is an antioxidant that is even more potent than beta-carotene. (See Chapter 5 for more on antioxidants.)

Liver is the single best food source of vitamin A. However, many experts recommend limiting consumption to once or twice a month because of the toxic substances it can contain. Environmental pollutants tend to congregate in an animal's liver. Egg yolk, cheese, whole milk, butter, fortified skim milk, and margarine are also good sources of vitamin A. (All these foods except fortified skim milk are also high in total fat and saturated fat. And all except margarine are high in cholesterol.) Red palm oil, used for cooking in many tropical countries, and fish liver oils taken as supplements are also rich in vitamin A. One tablespoon of cod liver oil contains more than 12,000 international units (IU), more than twice the daily recommended intake for adults.

Because of the high fat and cholesterol content of these foods, as well as the potential for overdosing, it is recommended that you do not look to these sources to fulfill your need for vitamin A. (Recent studies suggest that vitamin A, as retinol, can be toxic at much lower doses than previously thought.) Instead, rely on the provitamin plant forms of carotenoids, which do not accumulate in your liver. Currently, Americans get about half their vitamin A as retinol from animal sources and half as carotenoids from plant sources.

Orange and yellow fruits and vegetables have high vitamin A activity because of the carotenoids they contain. Generally, the deeper the color of the fruit or vegetable, the higher the concentration of carotenoids it has. Carrots, for example, are especially good sources of beta-carotene and, therefore, are high in vitamin A value. Green vegetables, such as spinach, asparagus, and broccoli, also contain large amounts of carotenoids, but their intense green pigment, courtesy of chlorophyll, masks the tell-tale orange-yellow color. (See the table on pages 111–112 for a list of good food sources of vitamin A.)

DIETARY REQUIREMENTS FOR VITAMIN A

The Recommended Dietary Allowance (RDA) for vitamin A is 1,000 retinol equivalents (RE) for men and 800 RE for women. (The RDAs for vitamin A for children are listed in RDA Table 1, page 16–17.) Retinol equivalents are the preferred measure for vitamin A because this method takes into account both forms of the vitamin—retinol and carotenoids. One RE is equal to 3.33 international units (IU) of retinol or 10 IU of beta-carotene. Assuming you get the vitamin from both sources, the RDAs are equivalent to about 5,000 IU for men and 4,000 IU for women.

It's not necessary to obtain the RDA amount for vitamin A each day. Since vitamin A is not soluble in water, you do not excrete excess amounts of the vitamin. The liver stores vitamin A, and the body can tap into the reserves whenever dietary intake is too low. For most adults it takes months to deplete stored amounts. As long as you have a well-balanced diet that includes milk and large amounts of yellow and green vegetables, your overall intake should be sufficient to provide the vitamin A your body needs.

The tables on pages 114–115 identify the vitamin A content of two typical daily diets—one formulated for a woman and the other for a teenage boy.

DEFICIENCY OF VITAMIN A

Vitamin A deficiency is common in the United States among low-income groups. Children are especially vulnerable because they are still growing rapidly. People who eat very-low-fat diets and those who experience fat malabsorption from conditions such as celiac disease or infectious hepatitis can also become deficient in vitamin A. A zinc

Sources of Vitamin A

Food	Quantity	International Units (IU)
Sweet potatoes, baked (peeled after baking)	1 medium	28,805
Pumpkin, canned	½ cup	27,018
Sweet potatoes, candied	1 medium	25,188
Beef liver, cooked	2 ounces	20,230
Spinach, canned, drained	1 cup	18,781
Sweet potatoes, canned	1 cup	15,966
Spinach, cooked, fresh or frozen	1 cup	14,790
Carrot, raw	1 medium	12,767
Cantaloupe	½ medium	12,688
Peas and carrots, frozen (boiled, drained)	1 cup	12,418
Liverwurst, fresh	2 slices (¼-inch thick)	9,960
Apricot halves, dried	1 cup	9,412
Beef and vegetable stew	1 cup	8,984
Turnip greens, cooked	1 cup	7,917
Apricots, dried, cooked, unsweetened	1 cup	5,908
Vegetarian soups, ready to serve	1 cup	5,878
Cabbage, spoon or bok choy, cooked	1 cup	4,366
Collards, cooked	1 cup	3,491
Broccoli, cooked, drained	1 cup	3,481
Apricots, canned in heavy syrup	1 cup	3,173
Vegetable beef soup, ready to serve	1 cup	2,611

Sources of Vitamin A (continued)

Food	Quantity	International Units (IU)
Red pepper, cooked	½ cup	2,577
Watermelon, raw	1 wedge	1,764
Beef chili with beans	1 cup	1,511
Asparagus	1 cup	1,472
Tomatoes, canned (solids and liquid)	1 cup	1,450
Apricots, raw	3 medium	1,110
Macaroni and cheese (made with whole milk)	1 cup	1,071
Clams	1 dozen	855
Tomatoes, raw	1 medium	841
Lettuce, cos or romaine	1 cup	780
Tomato juice, canned	½ cup	674
Plums, canned with syrup	1 cup	668
Prunes, dried, medium	1 cup	649
Margarine	1 tablespoon	621
Peach halves, dried, cooked, unsweetened	1 cup	508
Milk, skim (fortified with vitamin A)	1 cup	500
Peaches, raw	1 medium	465
Butter	1 tablespoon	435
Milk, whole	1 cup	307
Endive, curly	½ cup	297
Corn, fresh or frozen	½ cup	203
Orange juice, unsweetened, fresh or frozen	½ cup	194
Tuna salad	1 cup	175
Corn	1 ear	167

deficiency can also trigger a vitamin A deficiency by making it difficult to use the body's own stores of the vitamin.

An early warning sign of vitamin A deficiency is the inability to see well in the dark, a condition called night blindness. If the deficiency is not corrected, the outer layers of the eyes become dry, thickened, and cloudy, leading to blindness if left untreated.

Vitamin A deficiency also causes dry and rough skin, which can result in a kind of "goose flesh" appearance. In addition, this deficiency can cause one to become more susceptible to infectious diseases. That's because a lack of vitamin A damages the linings of the gastrointestinal and respiratory tracts; as a result, they can't act as effective barriers against bacteria. Infections of the vagina and the urinary tract are also more likely.

USE AND MISUSE
OF VITAMIN A

Treatment for children with xerophthalmia starts with large doses of vitamin A, decreasing to smaller amounts after just a few days.

Diseases such as obstructive jaundice or cystic fibrosis cause poor absorption of dietary fat and the fat-soluble vitamins that fat carries. Consequently, even if people with these diseases consume adequate amounts of vitamin A, they may still develop a deficiency because of poor absorption. To overcome

Vitamin A Content in Two Daily Diets

Typical Day's Diet for a Woman (1,700 Calories)*		International Units (IU) of Vitamin A
Breakfast	4 ounces orange juice	270
	1 ounce enriched cornflakes	1,250
	1 slice whole-wheat toast	none
	1 pat fortified margarine	170
	1 cup low-fat milk	500
	Black coffee	none
Lunch	Sandwich: 2 slices whole-wheat bread, 1 slice Swiss cheese, 2 ounces turkey breast	490
	1 cup skim milk (fortified)	500
	½ cup coleslaw	60
Dinner	½ chicken breast, fried	70
	1 medium baked potato	none
	1 cup tossed green salad	180
	½ cup peas, cooked	480
	1 enriched dinner roll	none
	2 pats fortified margarine	340
	1 cup frozen yogurt	150
	Black coffee	none
Total		**4,460**
RDA		**4,000**

*This diet represents what is typical for a woman between the ages of 18 and 35, not what is recommended.

Vitamin A Content in Two Daily Diets

Typical Day's Diet for a Teenage Boy (3,000 Calories)*		International Units (IU) of Vitamin A
Breakfast	½ medium pink grapefruit	540
	2 scrambled eggs	620
	2 slices whole-wheat toast	none
	1 pat fortified margarine	170
	1 cup whole milk	310
Lunch	1 cheeseburger	360
	2 cups whole milk	620
	10 large french fries	none
	1 medium banana	230
Dinner	4 ounces round steak	25
	1 cup green beans	780
	1 cup mashed potatoes	40
	Lettuce and tomato salad	400
	2 slices whole-wheat bread	none
	1 pat fortified margarine	170
	1 cup whole milk	310
	4 chocolate chip cookies	50
Snacks	Cola drink	none
	½ cup ice cream	270
	½ of 14-inch cheese pizza	200
Total		**5,095**
RDA		**5,000**

*This diet represents what is typical for a teenage boy, not what is recommended.

this obstacle, doctors may prescribe large amounts of a water-soluble form of vitamin A.

A disease accompanied by prolonged fever, such as infectious hepatitis or rheumatic fever, can rapidly deplete the liver's reserves of vitamin A. As part of the treatment, a doctor may prescribe vitamin A in amounts greater than the RDA to prevent deficiency.

Vitamin A derivatives are used to treat skin disorders. Isotretinoin acne medicine (brand name: Accutane) is an oral medication used for severe cystic acne. Because of the possibility of such serious side effects as liver damage and elevated blood triglycerides, a doctor must closely monitor treatment with this medication. Any woman capable of becoming pregnant needs to use reliable birth control when taking this medicine because it can cause spontaneous abortion or serious birth defects. Pregnant women must avoid it altogether.

Tretinoin (brand name: Retin-A) is a topical medication primarily used for acne, with less potential for serious side effects than oral isotretinoin. It treats baldness when prescribed along with minoxidil. It also may reduce the appearance of wrinkles and reverse the effects of sun damage on the skin. Another vitamin A derivative, etretinate, may treat psoriasis.

Recent studies have shown that people with a high intake of foods rich in beta-carotene—the carotenoid with the greatest vitamin A value—are less likely to develop lung cancer. Even among smokers, lung cancer is less likely to occur in those people who eat a diet that includes lots of vegetables that contain beta-carotene.

Taking a beta-carotene supplement in pill form does not appear to have the same effect, however, perhaps because of other substances in these foods which offer protection as well. A recent study was halted nearly two years early because the data suggested that lung cancer increased in smokers taking high doses of beta-carotene.

Vitamin A is not an antioxidant, so the protective effects of beta-carotene that are due to its antioxidant properties (see Chapter 5) do not apply to retinol. But vitamin A may have other protective roles. Among them are a possible reversal of damaged DNA and a boost in immunity, both of which may help prevent cancer.

Large amounts of vitamin A are clearly toxic. One massive dose or large doses taken over an extended period of time can cause hair loss, joint pain, nausea, bone and muscle soreness, headaches, dry and flaky skin, diarrhea, rashes, enlarged liver and spleen, cessation of menstruation, and stunted growth. Doses of only five to ten times the RDA for vitamin A can cause toxicity when taken over a long period.

Two recent studies indicate that toxicity can occur at levels far lower than previously thought. Researchers report that daily doses of 25,000 IU over a period of time have caused lasting liver damage. And a recent study of pregnant women found a fivefold increase in the risk of giving birth to a baby with a birth defect for women taking daily doses of vitamin A that exceeded 10,000 IU.

The danger of toxicity may be compounded by "overage." This refers to the manufacturers' practice of including more than the labeled amount of some vitamins in supplements to ensure their stated potency throughout their shelf life. For example, the overage may be as high as 40 percent for vitamin A. This means that a supplement with a labeled dose of 25,000 IU may actually provide as much as 35,000 IU when first purchased.

In a few reported instances, vitamin A toxicity has occurred after eating large amounts of liver. (Polar bear liver is especially high in vitamin A; it contains as much as 560,000 IU per ounce!) Because the liver stores vitamin A, eating it daily is not wise.

While the liver stores retinol, excess carotenoids accumulate in the fat just beneath the skin. If you eat a lot of carotene-rich foods, you may notice a yellowing of your skin, especially on the palms of your hands and soles of your feet. This is generally considered to be harmless, though carotene-containing tanning pills used in Europe reportedly cause infertility in women.

Vitamin B₁: Thiamin

The 1930s heralded the discovery of many of the B vitamins. Thiamin was discovered in 1934, a year after riboflavin. Researchers discovered niacin in 1937 and vitamin B₆ in 1939.

The discovery of thiamin was the key that unlocked the mystery of a disease—a disease born of technology but called beriberi. The word means weakness in an East Indian dialect.

HISTORY

Beriberi, a debilitating, often fatal ailment, wasn't a serious health problem among the rice-eating peoples of Asia until the end of the 19th century when mills began to polish rice—a process that removes the outer brown layers of the grain, leaving behind smooth, white kernels. Rice stripped of this outer layer of bran loses much of its thiamin.

Not surprisingly, soon after this refining practice began, the incidence of beriberi rose to epidemic levels in Asia. A similar situation occurred in countries where wheat was a dietary staple when refined white flour began to replace whole-wheat flour. The increased prevalence of beriberi spurred efforts to find its cause and cure. Still, the search took almost 50 years and did not end until thiamin was discovered.

A medical officer in the Japanese navy, named K. Takaki, was the first to suspect the relationship between diet and beriberi. In the 1880s, Takaki sought the root of this disease, which afflicted large numbers of Japanese sailors on long voyages—a situation reminiscent of scurvy. To test his belief that diet was at fault, Takaki added meat and milk to the rice diet of the sailors. Only a few men came down with the malady—those who refused to eat the milk and meat.

Further evidence came from the Indonesian island of Java, where the Dutch physician Cristiaan Eijkman found that chickens fed polished rice exhibited symptoms similar to those of beriberi. When he fed the chickens unpolished rice, the symptoms soon disappeared. Eijkman then tried the same experiment on people and confirmed that unpolished rice could prevent and cure beriberi.

Still, it wasn't until 1910 that researchers began searching for the mystery substance in unpolished rice in earnest. Chemist Robert Williams analyzed liquid extracted from rice polishings, painstakingly testing each substance from it for its effect on polyneuritis, the chicken disease similar to beriberi. In 1934, Williams isolated the substance that would solve the beriberi riddle—the vitamin thiamin.

FUNCTIONS OF THIAMIN

Like other B-complex vitamins, thiamin acts as a biological catalyst, or coenzyme. As a coenzyme, thiamin participates in the long chain of reactions that provides energy for the body and heat. Thiamin helps the body manufacture fats and metabolize protein. It's also needed for normal functioning of the nervous system.

SOURCES OF THIAMIN

The term "enriched" on food labels means that three B vitamins (thiamin, niacin, and riboflavin) plus one mineral (iron) have been added to make up for the nutrients lost in processing. Enriched breads and cereals are, therefore, very good sources of thiamin. Pork, oysters, green peas, and lima beans are also good sources. Most other foods contain only very small amounts of thiamin. A variety of sources of the vitamin thiamin are listed on page 122.

Did you know that high cooking temperatures can easily destroy thiamin? As a water-soluble vitamin, thiamin also tends to leach out of food into the cooking water. In order to preserve thiamin, it's best to cook food over low temperatures in small amounts of water for short periods. Steaming and microwaving can help minimize losses of thiamin and preserve the natural flavors of the foods.

To help preserve their bright green color, some people add baking soda to vegetables when they cook them. This is not a good idea, however. Not only does the baking soda make the vegetables lose their shape and consistency, but it destroys the thiamin content as well. Sulfites, used as

Sources of Thiamin

Food	Quantity	Milligrams (mg)
Pistachio nuts	½ cup	0.54
Watermelon	1 slice	0.39
Filberts or hazelnuts	½ cup	0.34
Oatmeal, ready-to-serve	1 cup	0.28
Macaroni, cooked, enriched	1 cup	0.28
Cashews, roasted	½ cup	0.28
Peas, green, cooked	1 cup	0.28
Fish	3 ounces	0.27–0.57
Rice, enriched, cooked	1 cup	0.25
Sunflower seeds	1 tablespoon	0.21
Cantaloupe	½ medium	0.18
Pecan halves	½ cup	0.17
Sausage	3 links	0.15
Macadamia nuts	½ cup	0.14
Orange	1 medium	0.14
Potato, baked, with skin	1 medium	0.13
Bacon	3 slices	0.12
Bread, enriched white	1 slice	0.10
Liverwurst	2 slices	0.10
Lamb chop	3 ounces	0.09
Okra	½ cup	0.09
Yogurt, low-fat frozen	1 cup	0.08
Bread, whole-wheat	1 slice	0.07
Chicken, dark meat, no skin	3 ounces	0.06
Peanut butter	1 tablespoon	0.03
Orange juice, unsweetened	4 ounces	0.02

preservatives, also destroy thiamin. Your best bet for preserving a food's thiamin content is to use additives sparingly and keep the cooking time short.

DIETARY REQUIREMENTS FOR THIAMIN

The amount of thiamin your body requires depends on the number of calories you eat, particularly the calories you get from carbohydrates. You need 0.5 milligrams (mg) of thiamin for every 1,000 calories (assuming an average intake of carbohydrates). Thiamin intake should be at least 1.0 mg per day even if the total calorie intake is less than 2,000. By increasing your intake of carbohydrates, you also increase your need for thiamin. A pregnant or nursing woman, who needs more calories, also requires more thiamin than other women.

The RDA for thiamin is 1.5 mg for men and 1.1 mg for women until age 50. Unless older adults are very active, their calorie needs usually decrease. After age 50, the requirement decreases to 1.2 mg for men and 1.0 mg for women.

DEFICIENCY OF THIAMIN

Numbness, muscle weakness, loss of appetite, and disorders of the nervous system characterize the form of beriberi known as "dry beriberi." In contrast, "wet beriberi" features fluid accumulation, especially in the lower legs. This more severe form

Thiamin Content of Common Foods

Food	Quantity	Milligrams (mg)
Meat–Protein Group		
Ham	3 ounces	0.60
Pork chop	3 ounces	0.54
Pork roast	3 ounces	0.48
Bologna	2 slices	0.24
Dried beans or peas, cooked	1 cup	0.21
Beef liver	3 ounces	0.18
Peanuts	½ cup	0.18
Frankfurter	1	0.09
Chicken, white meat, no skin	3 ounces	0.06
Milk–Dairy Group		
Yogurt, low-fat	1 cup	0.10
Cottage cheese, low-fat	1 cup	0.05
Ice cream	1 cup	0.05
Bread–Cereal/Grain Group		
Breakfast cereals (enriched)		
Total cereal	1 ounce	1.75
Raisin Bran cereal	1 ounce	0.49
Wheaties cereal	1 ounce	0.37
Macaroni, noodles, or spaghetti, cooked, enriched	1 cup	0.28
Fruits–Vegetables Group		
Peas, cooked	½ cup	0.28
Baked potato	1 medium	0.15
Orange	1 medium	0.12
Orange juice, unsweetened	4 ounces	0.10

Thiamin Content of Common Foods
(continued)

Food	Quantity	Milligrams (mg)
French fries	10 pieces	0.10
Asparagus	½ cup	0.06
Carrot, raw	1 medium	0.06
Potato chips	15 pieces	0.06
Banana	1 medium	0.05
Green or snap beans	½ cup	0.04

of the disease interferes with the heart and the circulatory system, and can eventually cause heart failure.

Severe thiamin deficiency seldom occurs today in the Western world. However, alcoholics who eat little or no food for extended periods of time are susceptible to thiamin deficiency and may develop a pattern of neurologic symptoms known as Wernicke-Korsakoff syndrome.

Deficiency may also occur in people who make poor food choices through ignorance, neglect, or poverty. Diets deficient in thiamin are often deficient in other B vitamins as well.

USE AND MISUSE OF THIAMIN

You need doses of thiamin two to five times the RDA to treat a deficiency. Fortunately, large amounts of thiamin are not toxic.

Because thiamin plays a part in the reactions that supply the body with energy, "stress formula" supplements often tout it as a cure for stress and fatigue, but thiamin does not provide instant energy. It has no known effect on fatigue unless a true thiamin deficiency is causing the fatigue. Some doctors have used thiamin to treat mild depression. However, it is effective only when the depression itself results from inadequate thiamin intake.

Vitamin B2: Riboflavin

In the 1920s and 1930s, nutritionists were searching for a growth-promoting factor in food. Their search kept turning up yellow substances. Meanwhile, biochemists who were busy trying to solve the mysteries of metabolism kept encountering a yellow enzyme. The yellow substances in both the food and the enzyme were riboflavin.

HISTORY

Most nutritionists in the 1920s believed that there were only two unidentified essential nutrients—a fat-soluble A and a water-soluble B. Soon, however, they found there was a second water-soluble B compound waiting to be identified.

During the course of their work, nutritionists gradually isolated growth-producing substances from liver, eggs, milk, and grass. All of the substances were yellow. In 1933, L.E. Booher reported that she had also obtained a yellow growth-promoting substance from milk whey. In addition, she observed that the darker the color of the substance, the greater its potency. Booher's observation led nutritionists to discover that all the yellow growth-producing substances in foods were one and the same—riboflavin.

While nutritionists zeroed in on the yellow substance in food, biochemists studied a yellow enzyme found to be essential for the body's energy needs. Biochemists were eventually able to separate the enzyme into two parts: a colorless protein and a yellow organic compound that turned out to be the riboflavin itself.

FUNCTIONS OF RIBOFLAVIN

Riboflavin acts as a coenzyme—the nonprotein, active portion of an enzyme—by helping to metabolize carbohydrates, fats, and proteins to provide the body with energy. Riboflavin doesn't act alone, however; it works in concert with its B-complex relatives. Riboflavin also plays a role in the metabolism of other vitamins.

SOURCES OF RIBOFLAVIN

Milk is the best source of riboflavin in the American diet. A glass of milk provides one-fourth of the RDA of riboflavin for men and one-third of the RDA for women. Other dairy products, such as cheese, yogurt, and ice cream, are also good sources of riboflavin. Meats, especially liver and kidney, and some green leafy vegetables are other rich sources. Enriched breads and cereals often have riboflavin added to them. (See the table on page 129 for riboflavin sources.)

Heat and oxygen do not easily destroy riboflavin, but light does. Did you know that milk can lose one-half or more of its riboflavin content when exposed to light for four to six hours? To prevent this loss, do not store milk in clear glass or translucent plastic containers. Cardboard containers or colored plastic jugs are a better choice.

DIETARY REQUIREMENTS
FOR RIBOFLAVIN

The Recommended Dietary Allowance (RDA) for riboflavin is 0.6 mg for every 1,000 calories. This works out to be 1.7 mg each day for the average adult man and 1.3 mg for the average adult woman.

A pregnant woman needs an additional 0.3 mg. During a baby's first six months, a nursing mother needs an additional 0.5 mg daily; during the second six months, she needs only 0.4 mg more. Recommended levels decrease slightly to 1.4 mg for men and 1.2 mg for women older than 50 years of age as energy needs decrease.

DEFICIENCY OF RIBOFLAVIN

In riboflavin deficiency, the skin becomes greasy, scaly, and dry. There may be cracks, or fissures,

Sources of Riboflavin

Food	Quantity	Milligrams (mg)
Milk shake, thick	1 cup	0.50
Cottage cheese, low-fat	1 cup	0.41
Milk, whole	1 cup	0.39
Buttermilk, from whole milk	1 cup	0.38
Buttermilk, from skim milk	1 cup	0.37
Yogurt, low-fat frozen	1 cup	0.37
Pancakes	3 medium	0.36
Sweet potatoes	1 cup	0.33
Pretzels	1 cup	0.25
English muffin	1 medium	0.24
Cornbread	1 piece	0.24
Mushrooms	½ cup	0.24
Chicken, dark meat, no skin	3 ounces	0.21
Avocado	1 small	0.21
Almonds	½ cup	0.20
Almonds, whole, shelled	½ cup	0.20
Brussels sprouts	1 cup	0.17
Wild rice	1 cup	0.15
Corn chips	1 cup	0.13
Honeydew melon	½ cup	0.13
Sherbet	1 cup	0.13
Lima beans	1 cup	0.10
Dried peas, beans	1 cup	0.09
Tomatoes, canned	½ cup	0.07
Corn	½ cup	0.06
Turnip greens, cooked	½ cup	0.05

at the corners of the mouth, inflammation and soreness of the lips, and a smooth, reddish-purple tongue.

Because prolonged deficiency of riboflavin causes severe eye damage in animals, some say eye problems in people, such as cataracts, might be due to a lack of riboflavin. However, there is little evidence to support this idea.

Though hypersensitivity to light may be a sign of riboflavin deficiency, the condition can also be caused by a deficiency of several B vitamins. Since the B vitamins work together in a sequence of reactions, a deficiency of one vitamin is likely to affect the entire sequence.

USE AND MISUSE
OF RIBOFLAVIN

Riboflavin deficiency requires treatment with doses as high as two to five times the RDA. Therapeutic doses of riboflavin are not used to treat any other condition.

Large doses of riboflavin are not toxic. However, they will cause the urine to appear bright yellow.

Niacin

Niacin, a member of the B complex family, has found many uses in the treatment of disease, and it may have more, yet undiscovered roles.

Riboflavin Content of Common Foods

Food	Quantity	Milligrams (mg)
Meat–Protein Group		
Beef liver	3 ounces	3.48
Tuna, canned in water	3 ounces	0.57
Pork chop, cooked	3 ounces	0.27
Egg	1 whole	0.25
Mixed vegetables	1 cup	0.22
Ground beef	3 ounces	0.18
Roast beef	3 ounces	0.15
Ham	3 ounces	0.15
Chicken, white meat, no skin	3 ounces	0.09
Milk–Dairy Group		
Milk shake, thick	1 cup	0.50
Yogurt, low-fat	1 cup	0.44
Milk, skim	1 cup	0.34
Ice cream	1 cup	0.25
Cheese, natural	1 ounce	0.10
Cheese, processed	1 ounce	0.07
Bread–Cereal/Grain Group		
Breakfast cereals (enriched)	1 ounce	0.4–1.7
Macaroni, enriched, cooked	1 cup	0.14
Bread, white, enriched	1 slice	0.06
Oatmeal, cooked	1 cup	0.05
Bread, whole-wheat	1 slice	0.03
Rice, cooked	1 cup	0.02
Fruits–Vegetables Group		
Spinach, cooked	½ cup	0.16

Riboflavin Content of Common Foods (continued)

Food	Quantity	Milligrams (mg)
Banana	1 medium	0.11
Asparagus, cooked	½ cup	0.09
Broccoli, cooked	½ cup	0.08
Strawberries, raw	½ cup	0.05
Orange	1 medium	0.05
Carrot, raw	1 medium	0.04

Cardiologists prescribe megadoses of niacin to lower blood cholesterol and triglyceride levels in some people. Psychiatrists have thought that large doses of the vitamin might be useful in the treatment of schizophrenia, but scientific evidence supporting this use is lacking. In moderate doses, niacin can cure one disease—the one that led investigators to discover this vitamin.

HISTORY

In the early part of the 18th century, a disease characterized by red, rough skin began to appear in Europe. Almost 200 years later, the disease was still a scourge—at least for people in the southern United States. The disease, called pellagra, was almost epidemic in the South by the early part of the 1900s.

It was so common that many believed it was an infectious disease spread from person to person.

Others thought it was caused by eating spoiled corn. Some even believed it was spread by a type of fly because outbreaks of the malady were more severe in the spring during flies' hatching season.

Few people believed that pellagra was a simple dietary deficiency, even though corn-based diets apparently made people susceptible to the disease. One person who did was Dr. Joseph Goldberger. He proved the link between diet and the disease by experimenting with the diets of children in a Mississippi orphanage who suffered from pellagra and 11 volunteers from a Mississippi prison farm. In both groups, when Goldberger added lean meat, milk, eggs, or yeast, their symptoms vanished.

This was in 1915, yet many physicians remained skeptical until 1937 when Conrad Elvehjem and his coworkers at the University of Wisconsin cured dogs with symptoms similar to pellagra by giving them nicotinic acid—a form of niacin. Soon doctors were using nicotinic acid to cure pellagra in humans.

FUNCTIONS OF NIACIN

Niacin occurs in two forms—nicotinic acid and nicotinamide (also called niacinamide)—both found in food. Nicotinic acid converts to nicotinamide in the body.

Like the other B vitamins thiamin and riboflavin, niacin acts as a coenzyme, assisting other substances in the conversion of proteins, carbohydrates, and fats into energy.

SOURCES OF NIACIN

The niacin value of foods includes niacin itself—called preformed niacin—and the amino acid tryptophan, which converts to niacin in the body. Food composition tables, however, list only preformed niacin. Niacin equivalent is the term used to refer to either 1 mg of niacin or to 60 mg of tryptophan (it takes 60 mg of tryptophan to make 1 mg of niacin).

Most proteins contain tryptophan. In the average protein-rich American diet, tryptophan provides about 60 percent of the niacin you need. If a diet is adequate in protein, it will supply enough niacin equivalents from both sources to meet daily needs. The best sources of niacin are foods with a high protein content, such as meat, eggs, and peanuts. Other good sources of niacin equivalents, such as milk, actually provide more tryptophan than niacin. Mushrooms and greens are good vegetable sources. Niacin is also added to enriched breads and cereals.

DIETARY REQUIREMENTS FOR NIACIN

The RDA takes into account both preformed niacin and that available from tryptophan. Together they account for the recommendation of 6.6 mg of niacin for each 1,000 calories eaten. For

Sources of Niacin

Food	Quantity	Milligrams (mg)
Peanut halves, roasted, salted	1 cup	20.6
Product 19 cereal	1 ounce	20.0
Tuna, canned in water, drained	3½ ounces	12.2
Chicken, white meat, no skin	3½ ounces	9.5
Beef liver	3 ounces	9.1
Turkey, light or dark meat, no skin	3½ ounces	7.3
Lamb chops, cooked	3½ ounces	6.1
Beef round, bottom, broiled	4 ounces	5.3
Cheerios cereal	1 ounce	5.0
Ground beef	3 ounces	5.0
Chicken, dark meat, no skin	3½ ounces	4.9
Pork chops, cooked	3½ ounces	4.4
Ham, baked	3 ounces	3.5
Salmon, broiled or baked	3 ounces	3.4
Roast beef	3 ounces	3.4
Peanut butter	1 tablespoon	2.1
Chicken liver, cooked	2 ounces	1.2
Frankfurter, all beef, cooked	1	1.1
Dried beans or peas, cooked	1 cup	1.0
Cheese, blue	1 ounce	0.29
Yogurt	1 cup	0.29
Cottage cheese, creamed	1 cup	0.27

Food	Quantity	Milligrams (mg)
Milk, whole or skim	1 cup	0.21
Ice cream	1 cup	0.16
Egg	1 whole	0.03
Cheese, cheddar	1 ounce	0.02

women, this should total no less than 13 mg (niacin equivalents) and for men, no less than 18 mg (niacin equivalents). Pregnant and lactating women require slightly more.

DEFICIENCY OF NIACIN

The first symptoms of pellagra are weakness, loss of appetite, and some digestive disturbances. As the deficiency disease progresses, the skin becomes rough and red in areas exposed to sunlight, heat, or irritation. Later, open sores, diarrhea, dementia, and delirium may develop. Death results if the condition is left untreated.

This disease, now rarely seen in the United States, is still common in parts of the world where corn is the major cereal grain. Corn is deficient in tryptophan, and the niacin it contains is difficult to absorb. In Latin American countries, they combine cornmeal with the mineral lime when making tortillas; the alkalinity of the lime frees the niacin so that it can be absorbed.

USE AND MISUSE OF NIACIN

Treatment for niacin deficiency involves giving 25 to 50 mg of the vitamin daily.

Some practitioners still recommend megavitamin niacin therapy for mental illness and learning disorders in children, but no scientific studies support either use.

Large doses of nicotinic acid, in amounts from 500 mg to 3 or 4 grams (g) daily, are effective in lowering blood cholesterol and triglycerides levels. To reduce the risk of heart attack and stroke, this use of nicotinic acid is becoming increasingly popular. It is actually safer and more effective than many other cholesterol-lowering drugs.

Used in such large doses, however, nicotinic acid is no longer working as a vitamin, but as a drug, and side effects can occur. Doses of 75 mg or more cause blood-vessel dilation, which can result in tingling, itching, and flushing of the face, neck, and chest—a condition called nicotinic acid flush. The condition is uncomfortable, but not dangerous. A slow-release form of nicotinic acid can reduce skin flushing but carries the risk of liver toxicity.

In addition, large doses of nicotinic acid can cause indigestion, peptic ulcers, injury to the liver, and an increased blood level of both uric acid and glucose. This can lead to misdiagnosis of diabetes or gout.

Niacin Content in Two Daily Diets[*]

Typical Day's Diet for a Woman (1,700 Calories)[**]		Milligrams (mg) of Niacin
Breakfast	4 ounces orange juice	0.25
	1 ounce enriched cornflakes	0.1
	1 slice enriched white toast	0.8
	1 pat margarine	none
	1 cup skim milk	0.2
	Black coffee	none
Lunch	Sandwich: 2 slices whole-wheat bread, 1 slice Swiss cheese, 2 ounces turkey breast	7.1
	1 cup skim milk	0.2
	½ cup cole slaw	0.3
Dinner	4-ounce pork chop	4.4
	1 medium baked potato	1.3
	1 cup tossed green salad	0.1
	½ cup peas, cooked	1.2
	1 enriched dinner roll	1.2
	2 pats margarine	none
	½ cup low-fat frozen yogurt	1.6
	Black coffee	none
Total		**18.8**
RDA		**15.0**

[*]Values for preformed niacin. Totals would be higher if tryptophan contribution were included.

[**]This diet represents what is typical for an adult woman between the ages of 18 and 35, not what is recommended.

Niacin Content
in Two Daily Diets*

Typical Day's Diet for a Teenage Boy (3,000 Calories)**		Milligrams (mg) of Niacin
Breakfast	½ medium pink grapefruit	0.4
	2 scrambled eggs	0.2
	2 slices enriched white toast	1.7
	1 pat margarine	none
	1 cup whole milk	0.2
Lunch	1 cheeseburger (¼ lb.)	7.0
	2 cups whole milk	0.4
	10 large french fries	0.9
	1 medium banana	0.6
Dinner	4 ounces round steak	5.3
	1 cup green beans	0.3
	1 cup mashed potatoes	2.3
	Lettuce and tomato salad	0.4
	2 slices enriched white bread	1.7
	1 pat margarine	none
	1 cup whole milk	0.2
	4 chocolate chip cookies	1.2
Snacks	Cola drink	none
	½ cup ice cream	0.08
	¼ of 14-inch cheese pizza	4.2
Total		**27.1**
RDA		**20.0**

*Values for preformed niacin. Totals would be higher if tryptophan contribution were included.

**This diet represents what is typical for a teenage boy, not what is recommended.

High doses of the other form of niacin, niacinamide, do not cause any adverse reactions. However, niacinamide also does not lower blood cholesterol and triglyceride levels.

Some headache specialists prescribe niacin in daily doses of 150 mg to help treat migraines, in the hopes that the dilating effects of niacin will help stabilize the overdilating-constricting cycle of cerebral blood vessels.

Pantothenic Acid

Pantothenic acid is virtually everywhere. It occurs in all living cells and can be found, at least to some extent, in all foods. Appropriately, its name comes from the Greek word pantos, meaning "everywhere."

Although discovered more than 50 years ago, nutritionists have never become too excited over the vitamin because deficiency of the vitamin in humans is very rare. In fact, symptoms of pantothenic acid deficiency in people occur only after long periods of food restriction.

That hasn't stopped authors of some popular nutrition books from blaming pantothenic acid deficiency for arthritis, Addison disease, and allergies. Others tout the vitamin as improving mental processes, getting rid of gray hair, and ensuring normal births.

HISTORY

Unlike the discovery of other vitamins, when investigators discovered pantothenic acid in the 1930s, they weren't looking for the cause of a specific human disease. They were looking for a substance necessary for yeast to grow. Along the way, researchers noticed that diets lacking pantothenic acid caused certain disorders in animals, including a retarded growth rate, anemia, degenerated nerve tissue, decreased production of antibodies, ulcers, and malformed offspring.

Since many animal species proved to have a dietary requirement for pantothenic acid, scientists believed that people probably needed it, too. Experiments in the 1950s tested how a diet without pantothenic acid affected humans. After three or four weeks on a highly purified diet that lacked only pantothenic acid, volunteers complained of weakness and an overall "unwell" feeling. One person had burning cramps.

A few volunteers received a diet not only deficient in pantothenic acid, but also containing a compound that specifically interfered with the vitamin. These people developed symptoms faster than those in the other group and complained of insomnia, depression, gastrointestinal problems, leg cramps, and a burning sensation in the hands and feet.

In both groups, volunteers showed signs of reduced antibody production. In everyone, symp-

Pantothenic Acid Content of Common Foods

Food	Quantity	Milligrams (mg)
Meat–Protein Group		
Beef liver, raw	3 ounces	3.90
Beef kidney, raw	3 ounces	1.44
Liverwurst	1 ounce	0.82
Ham, cured	3 ounces	0.66
Egg, fresh, raw	1 whole	0.63
Pork chop, meat only, cooked	3 ounces	0.48
Salmon, canned	3 ounces	0.47
Ground beef	3 ounces	0.30
Round steak	3 ounces	0.30
Almonds, dried, shelled	3½ ounces	0.24
Milk–Dairy Group		
Yogurt, low-fat	1 cup	1.57
Milk, whole or skim	1 cup	0.81
Ice cream	1 cup	0.77
Cottage cheese, low-fat	1 cup	0.54
Blue cheese	1 ounce	0.49
Swiss cheese	1 ounce	0.12
Cheddar cheese	1 ounce	0.12
Bread–Cereal/Grain Group		
100% Bran cereal	½ cup	0.49
40% Bran Flakes cereal	¾ cup	0.21
Bread, whole-wheat	1 slice	0.17
Bread, rye	1 slice	0.13
Bread, white, enriched	1 slice	0.07

Pantothenic Acid Content
of Common Foods (continued)

Food	Quantity	Milligrams (mg)
Fruits–Vegetables Group		
Cauliflower, raw	1 cup	0.65
Grapefruit	½ medium	0.41
Orange	1 medium	0.33
Banana	1 medium	0.30
Tomato juice	4 ounces	0.30
Asparagus, fresh	1 cup	0.29

toms disappeared after adding back pantothenic acid, proving that pantothenic acid was indeed an essential vitamin for humans.

FUNCTIONS OF PANTOTHENIC ACID

Pantothenic acid, formerly called vitamin B3, is a part of important biological compounds. One of these, called coenzyme A, is involved in the release of energy from carbohydrates, fats, and proteins and in the synthesis of certain compounds. The other, acyl carrier protein (ACP), participates in the synthesis of fats.

SOURCES OF PANTOTHENIC ACID

All foods contain pantothenic acid in some amount. The best sources include an eclectic mix:

eggs, salmon, liver, kidney, peanuts, wheat bran, and yeast. Fresh vegetables are better sources than canned vegetables because the canning process reduces the amount of pantothenic acid available. (See the table on page 142–143.)

DIETARY REQUIREMENTS FOR PANTOTHENIC ACID

The estimated safe and adequate daily intake of pantothenic acid for adults is 4 to 7 mg. The average American gets about 10 to 20 mg in a typical diet. Bacteria living in the intestinal tract make some pantothenic acid, but no one knows yet if this contributes to the body's supply.

DEFICIENCY OF PANTOTHENIC ACID

Pantothenic acid deficiency is not likely to occur as long as people eat ordinary diets that consist of a variety of foods. Symptoms of deficiency, such as insomnia, leg cramps, or burning feet, have only occurred in experimental situations. Even then, severe symptoms occur only if people also take a drug that interferes with the vitamin.

USE AND MISUSE OF PANTOTHENIC ACID

Pantothenic acid isn't used to treat any health problem or condition other than its own deficiency.

A deficiency of pantothenic acid in black laboratory rats results in gray hair. This finding led some people to surmise that supplements of the vitamin could prevent graying of the hair. Unfortunately, this just isn't true. Pantothenic acid does not prevent or reverse graying.

Massive doses of pantothenic acid (as much as 10 to 20 g a day) have been reported to cause diarrhea in some people, but serious toxicity is not known to occur.

Vitamin B6: Pyridoxine

Nutritionists aren't sure whether Americans get enough vitamin B6 or not. Although there's no evidence of widespread deficiency, some nutritionists believe the usual intake of the vitamin is just barely enough, perhaps causing borderline deficiency.

HISTORY

Researchers discovered early on that vitamin B6 is not one substance but three: pyridoxine, pyridoxamine, and pyridoxal. All three substances have the same biological activity, and all three occur naturally in food.

FUNCTIONS OF PYRIDOXINE

Pyridoxine functions mainly by helping to metabolize protein and amino acids. Though not directly

Sources of Vitamin B6 (Pyridoxine)

Food	Quantity	Milligrams (mg)
Banana	1 medium	0.66
Corn Flakes cereal	1 cup	0.52
Instant breakfast drink	1 envelope	0.50
Brussels sprouts, cooked	1 cup	0.45
Halibut	3 ounces	0.43
Cheerios cereal	1 cup	0.41
Avocado	½ medium	0.36
Pork chop	3 ounces	0.33
Potato, baked, without skin	1 medium	0.28
Roast beef	3 ounces	0.27
Cantaloupe	¼ melon	0.26
Cottage cheese, low-fat	½ cup	0.18
Lamb chop	3 ounces	0.15
Tomato	1 medium	0.14
Brewer's yeast	1 tablespoon	0.14
Sunflower seeds	2 tablespoons	0.14
Yogurt, low-fat	8 ounces	0.10
Lima beans, fresh or frozen	½ cup	0.10
Wheat germ	2 tablespoons	0.10
Summer squash, fresh or frozen	½ cup	0.10
Ice cream	1 cup	0.07

involved in the release of energy, like some other B vitamins, pyridoxine helps remove the nitrogen from amino acids, making them available as sources of energy. Pyridoxine also helps manufacture other important compounds, such as antibodies, hemoglobin, and hormones.

Pyridoxine has a significant role in lowering dangerous homocysteine levels (see heart disease in Chapter 6). In fact, new research suggests that a deficiency of pyridoxine all by itself is a risk factor for heart disease.

SOURCES OF PYRIDOXINE

Vitamin B6 is in all foods, in one form or another. Plant foods are generally high in pyridoxine; pyridoxamine and pyridoxal are more common in foods of animal origin. All three forms of vitamin B6—pyridoxine, pyridoxamine, and pyridoxal—appear to have the same biological activity.

Whole wheat, salmon, nuts, wheat germ, brown rice, peas, and beans are good sources. Vegetables contain smaller amounts, but if eaten in large quantities, they can be an important source. Even though pyridoxine is lost during the milling of grains to make flour, manufacturers do not regularly add it back to enriched products, except some highly fortified cereals.

DIETARY REQUIREMENTS
FOR PYRIDOXINE

The amount of protein you eat determines your dietary requirement for pyridoxine because it functions in protein metabolism. The RDA for pyridoxine is 2.0 mg for men and 1.6 mg for

Vitamin B6 Content of Common Foods

Food	Quantity	Milligrams (mg)
Meat–Protein Group		
Beef liver	3 ounces	0.78
Chicken, white meat, no skin	3 ounces	0.48
Round steak	3 ounces	0.36
Tuna, canned in water	3 ounces	0.32
Chicken, dark meat, no skin	3 ounces	0.30
Salmon, canned	3 ounces	0.25
Milk–Dairy Group		
Cottage cheese	1 cup	0.15
Milk, whole or skim	1 cup	0.10
Cheddar cheese	1 ounce	0.02
Bread–Cereal/Grain Group		
Ready-to-eat breakfast cereals (enriched)		
Total cereal	1 cup	2.34
Special K cereal	1 cup	0.60
Bread, whole-wheat	1 slice	0.04
Fruits–Vegetables Group		
Banana	1 medium	0.66
Boiled potatoes	1 cup	0.42
Spinach, fresh or frozen	½ cup	0.14
Potato chips	10 chips	0.13
Asparagus	½ cup	0.02
Peanuts	2 tablespoons	0.05
Grapefruit	½ medium	0.12
Lima beans, fresh or frozen	½ cup	0.10
Tomato juice	4 ounces	0.10

women. Pregnant and nursing women require more. Children under ten years of age, however, require slightly less. Even with the large amount of protein that Americans eat, the RDA for pyridoxine is sufficient for most people. The problem is that many people are not even meeting the RDA for it.

DEFICIENCY OF PYRIDOXINE

The 1980 Nationwide Food Consumption Survey showed that pyridoxine intake was below 70 percent of the RDA in half of the people surveyed. A 1990 survey showed that intake of the vitamin was still inadequate for most men and women. Other studies show reduced blood levels of pyridoxine in some pregnant women, elderly adults, alcohol abusers, and people with disorders such as kidney disease and Down syndrome.

Some prescription medications, including birth control pills, steroids, and the antibiotics isoniazid and penicillamine, can increase the need for pyridoxine. If you take one of these medicines, discuss with your doctor whether you should also take a pyridoxine supplement.

USE AND MISUSE OF PYRIDOXINE

People who need more pyridoxine because of a medical condition are often treated with supplemental pyridoxine, in doses of 10 to 50 mg per day. Some people are born with metabolic errors that increase their need for the vitamin. Supplements of pyridoxine are also used for people with sickle-cell disease.

It is popular to recommend pyridoxine supplements for many disorders, including nausea from pregnancy, premenstrual symptoms, sensitivity to the flavor enhancer monosodium glutamate, and carpal tunnel syndrome. There is controversy about pyridoxine's usefulness in these situations, however, because supporting data are lacking and the potential danger from large doses does exist.

Despite being water-soluble, pyridoxine is toxic in high doses, causing reversible nerve damage to the extremities. For example, women taking doses of 500 mg—250 times the RDA—or more of pyridoxine for an extended period of time developed such tingling and numbness in their hands and feet that they were unable to walk. When they discontinued the supplement, the symptoms began to disappear.

Excessive pyridoxine may also increase excretion of oxalate in the urine, which may increase the risk of developing kidney stones.

Biotin

"Caution! Egg whites may be hazardous to your health." No, the Surgeon General has not decided to print that phrase on egg cartons, and no one is in any real danger. However, almost 70 years ago, raw egg whites caused a real problem for some experimental animals. And the cure for the animals' problem turned out to be a previously undiscovered essential nutrient for people.

HISTORY

In the 1930s, an investigator at the Lister Institute of Preventive Medicine in London, England, was experimenting with the diets of rats. After feeding the rodents raw egg whites for several weeks, he noticed they developed an eczemalike skin condition, lost their hair, became paralyzed, and began to hemorrhage under the skin.

Later, another team of investigators fed rats different foods to see which ones prevented or alleviated the "egg-white syndrome." Various foods, such as dried yeast, milk, and egg yolk, were successful in curing the rats' conditions. But what did all of these foods have in common?

It was 1940 before scientist Paul Gyorgy identified the common denominator as a vitamin. At first, thinking that it was an isolated substance, he named it vitamin H. Soon after, however, scientists realized it was actually another member of the B complex family. They soon did away with vitamin H and renamed the vitamin biotin.

FUNCTIONS OF BIOTIN

Biotin acts as a coenzyme in several metabolic reactions. It plays a role in the manufacture of

Biotin Content of Common Foods

Food	Quantity	Micrograms (µg)
Meat–Protein Group		
Beef liver, raw	3½ ounces	100
Oysters, raw	3½ ounces	10
Sardines, in oil	3½ ounces	5
Clams, raw	3½ ounces	2
Frankfurter	1	1
Milk–Dairy Group		
Whole milk	1 cup	8
Blue cheese	3½ ounces	7
Brie	3½ ounces	7
Skim milk	1 cup	5
Yogurt	1 cup	3
Cheddar	3½ ounces	3
Cottage cheese	3½ ounces	2
Bread–Cereal/Grain Group		
Raisin Bran cereal	¾ cup	3
Bran Flakes cereal	¾ cup	3
Wheat Chex cereal	⅔ cup	2
Fruits–Vegetables Group		
Cauliflower	1 cup	17
Banana	1 medium	4
Grapefruit	½ medium	3

body fats, the metabolism of carbohydrates, the breakdown of proteins to urea, and the conversion of amino acids from protein into blood sugar for energy.

SOURCES OF BIOTIN

Milk, liver, egg yolk, yeast, and dried peas and beans have been shown to be good sources of biotin. Nuts and mushrooms contain smaller amounts of the vitamin. Biotin is also made by bacteria in the intestine.

DIETARY REQUIREMENTS FOR BIOTIN

The safe and adequate intake of biotin is 30 to 100 micrograms (µg) per day. The typical varied diet of Americans provides about 100 to 300 µg. This amount, in addition to that which is produced by intestinal bacteria, is more than sufficient to meet the needs of healthy people.

DEFICIENCY OF BIOTIN

A deficiency of biotin occurs only in unusual circumstances. People on bizarre diets that include large amounts of raw egg whites have been shown to exhibit symptoms of a biotin deficiency. The deficiency was not the result of a lack of biotin, per se, but because raw egg whites contain a substance called avidin that ties up the vitamin, preventing its absorption. Cooking egg whites deactivates the avidin and makes the egg whites safe to eat.

A biotin deficiency can also result from prolonged use of antibiotic medications that destroy intestinal bacteria, but this only leads to true deficiency when combined with a diet that lacks sufficient biotin.

Some people are born with an inherited disorder that increases their need for biotin. In this situation, a supplement may be necessary to prevent a biotin deficiency from occurring.

USE AND MISUSE OF BIOTIN

Biotin supplements may be needed in the rare instances cited above. Recently, however, it has been touted as a vitamin that can strengthen nails. But the scientific proof to back up the claim is slim. Large doses of biotin have not been found to be toxic.

Folate

Folacin, folic acid, and folate all refer to the same B vitamin, which occurs in foods in all three forms. The term folate covers all three, and the term folate activity describes the actual biological potency, or vitamin value, of a food.

Folic acid is the simplest form of the vitamin. It's found in only small amounts in foods, but it's the form used in most vitamin supplements.

HISTORY

The discovery of folate was closely tied to the discovery of vitamin B12. These two vitamins work together in several important biological reactions.

A deficiency of either vitamin results in a condition known as megaloblastic or macrocytic (large-cell) anemia.

In 1930, researcher Lucy Wills and her colleagues reported that yeast contained a substance that could cure macrocytic anemia in pregnant women. But it wasn't until the early 1940s that folate was finally isolated and identified.

FUNCTIONS OF FOLATE

Folate functions as a coenzyme during many reactions in the body. It has an important role in making new cells, because it helps form the genetic material DNA (deoxyribonucleic acid) and RNA (ribonucleic acid). DNA carries and RNA transmits the genetic information that acts as the blueprint for cell production.

We especially need folate when new cells are manufactured. This function of folate helps to explain why the vitamin is necessary for normal growth and development, and why anemia occurs when there's not enough. The body makes large numbers of red blood cells each day to replace those it destroys. DNA is essential for this process; therefore, folate is as well.

SOURCES OF FOLATE

Green leafy vegetables, such as broccoli, spinach, and asparagus, are rich in folate. (Take care not to overcook vegetables, or the folate may be lost.) Seeds, liver, and dried peas and beans are other

Sources of Folate

Food	Quantity	Micrograms (µg)
Product 19 cereal	1 cup	400
Brewer's yeast	1 tablespoon	280
Asparagus	1 cup	242.5
Brussels sprouts	1 cup	156.9
Cocoa Krispies cereal	1 cup	133.1
Instant breakfast drink	1 envelope	99.9
Avocado	½ medium	80.3
Crispix cereal	¾ cup	75.0
Beets	½ cup	68.0
Orange juice, unsweetened	½ cup	54.5
Wheat germ	2 tablespoons	45.4
Romaine lettuce, chopped	1 cup	40.7
Orange	1 medium	39.7
Cantaloupe, diced	1 cup	39.2
Sweet potato	1 medium	29.9
Strawberries	1 cup	26.4
Yogurt, low-fat	8 ounces	22.0
Beer	12 ounces	21.4
Whole-wheat bread	1 slice	15.7
Grapefruit juice, unsweetened	½ cup	12.8
Milk, nonfat or whole	1 cup	12.7
Cucumber	1 small	10.1
Baked potato, without skin	1 medium	8.5

good sources. Orange juice is a good source of folate because it contains the most readily absorbed form of the vitamin. It also contains vitamin C, and vitamin C helps preserve folate.

DIETARY REQUIREMENTS
FOR FOLATE

The RDA for folate is 200 µg for adult men and 180 µg for adult women. Pregnant women require 400 µg because so many new cells are being made. The average American diet provides about 200 to 250 µg of the vitamin. Foods contain folate both in free form and bound to amino acids. To absorb folate, however, it must be freed. Vitamin B_{12} helps to free folate.

DEFICIENCY OF FOLATE

Folate deficiency can result from either inadequate intake or reduced absorption. It may also occur during periods of increased need, such as multiple pregnancies, cancer, or severe burns.

Some medications can interfere with the body's ability to use this vitamin. These medications include aspirin, oral contraceptives, and drugs used to treat convulsions, psoriasis, and cancer. In addition, abuse of alcohol can damage the intestine so that less folate is absorbed.

Symptoms of folate deficiency include diarrhea, weight loss, anemia, and a red, sore, and swollen tongue. The macrocytic anemia caused by folate deficiency is prevalent in underdeveloped countries among low-income pregnant women. Macrocytic anemia caused by folate deficiency rarely occurs in the United States because of the routine use of folate supplements during pregnancy.

Experts now emphasize the importance of folate supplementation in the very early stages of pregnancy because the vitamin plays an important role in early fetal development. Inadequate amounts during the first few weeks of pregnancy can cause birth defects of the spinal cord, known as neural tube defects. Because folate is so important at a time when many women might not even know they are pregnant, women planning to conceive—and any women capable of becoming pregnant—should be sure they are getting enough folate.

USE AND MISUSE OF FOLATE

Over-the-counter vitamin supplements generally contain about 400 µg of folic acid because they follow standards based on the previous RDAs. The most recent edition of the RDA halved the folate RDA. Why? Since deficiency was not common in the United States, the experts set the RDA within the range typical diets were providing—180 µg or 200 µg. With the new evidence of folate's importance to fetal development, and with even newer evidence of folate's protective role in heart disease, this may have been short-sighted. The upcoming RDAs may well return folate requirements to their original levels. And fortification of flour with folate—along with three B vitamins and iron—is now mandatory.

Doctors prescribe folate supplements if they diagnose a folate deficiency and have ruled out a vitamin B12 deficiency. Excessive intake of folate may actually mask a deficiency of vitamin B12 or an underlying case of pernicious anemia. Large doses of folate cause the blood to appear normal, which, in turn, may delay diagnosis and treatment of vitamin B12 deficiency, resulting in serious, irreversible damage to the nervous system. The longer the delay, the more serious the damage.

Under normal circumstances, large amounts of folate are not toxic. They can, however, interfere with the action of drugs taken to control seizures or with those drugs that are taken to treat cancer.

Vitamin B12: Cyanocobalamin/Cobalamin

Vitamin B12 is unique. It differs from other vitamins, even those of the B complex, in many ways. The vitamin has a chemical structure much more complex than that of any other vitamin. It's the only vitamin to contain an inorganic element (the mineral cobalt) as an integral part of its makeup. Only microorganisms can make B12. Plants and animals can't, although the vitamin does accumulate in animal products, which is where we get it.

A substance made in the stomach—called intrinsic factor—must be present to absorb vitamin B_{12} from the intestinal tract in significant amounts. Intrinsic factor combines with the vitamin B_{12} that is released from food during digestion. It carries the vitamin to the lower part of the small intestine, where, assisted by calcium, it attaches itself to special receptor cells. The vitamin B_{12} is then released from its carrier and enters these cells to be absorbed into the body. Without intrinsic factor, vitamin B_{12} misses its connection with the receptor cells and passes out of the body.

Some people have a condition known as pernicious anemia and can't make intrinsic factor. As a result, they can't absorb vitamin B_{12} even when there's plenty of the vitamin in their diets. Eventually, they show symptoms of a vitamin B_{12} deficiency. Pernicious anemia is a macrocytic, or large-cell, anemia similar to the anemia caused by folate deficiency.

HISTORY

The pursuit of vitamin B_{12} began in 1926, when two investigators found that patients who ate almost a pound of raw liver a day were effectively relieved of pernicious anemia. Scientists correctly speculated that liver contained a substance that prevents the disorder, but they wondered why victims of pernicious anemia needed so much of it.

William Castle suggested that liver contained an antipernicious anemia (APA) factor. He also believed that people who had the disease lacked a factor intrinsically necessary to use the APA factor. By eating about a pound of liver a day, these people could counteract the lack of the intrinsic factor and absorb the APA factor they needed.

For the next 20 years, scientists searched for the APA factor. Progress was slow until 1948, when testing began on an experimental "animal"—the microorganism *Lactobacillus lactis*. Instead of testing liver extracts on people, researchers tested them on the microorganisms. Since these microorganisms reproduce so quickly, many generations could be tested in a short period of time. In less than a year, two research groups—one in England and one in the United States—both managed to isolate pure vitamin B_{12}.

FUNCTIONS OF VITAMIN B_{12}

Vitamin B_{12} is essential to cells because it's needed to make DNA (deoxyribonucleic acid) and RNA (ribonucleic acid), which carry and transmit genetic information for every living cell. This information tells a cell how to function and must be passed along each time a cell divides. Rapidly dividing cells need a continuous supply of vitamin B_{12}. This vitamin works along with the vitamin folate in this important role.

Vitamin B_{12} also helps maintain normal bone marrow. And it functions in the production of a material called myelin, which covers and protects nerve fibers. Vitamin B_{12} also plays a central role in folate metabolism. It releases free folate from its bound form so it can be absorbed, and it helps in the transportation and storage of folate. A deficiency of vitamin B12 can create a folate deficiency even when dietary intake of folate is adequate. That is why a deficiency of either vitamin causes a similar type of anemia.

SOURCES OF VITAMIN B12

Vitamin B12 is found mostly in animal foods, such as liver, meat, clams, oysters, sardines, and salmon. Fermented bean products, such as tempeh, contain some vitamin B12. Manufacturers also add vitamin B12 to some cereals.

Bacteria in the intestines make some vitamin B12, but far less than the amount needed daily.

DIETARY REQUIREMENTS
FOR VITAMIN B12

The RDA for vitamin B12 is 2 µg daily for adults and 2.2 µg daily for women who are pregnant or breast-feeding. The average American diet provides 7 to 30 µg of the vitamin.

DEFICIENCY OF VITAMIN B12

When the supply of vitamin B12 in the body is low, it slows down the production of red blood cells (causing anemia) and the cells that line the intestine. This is similar to what happens as a result of insufficient folate. But unlike folate deficiency, a lack of vitamin B12 can also cause serious damage to the nervous system. If the condition persists for long, the damage is irreversible.

A deficiency of vitamin B12 caused by insufficient intake is not common. The average well-fed person has a supply of the vitamin stored in the liver that can last five years or longer. Dietary deficiency of vitamin B12 is usually seen only in strict vegetarians who don't eat foods of animal origin—not even milk or eggs.

Such a restricted diet is a particular problem for pregnant or breast-feeding women, since the baby can develop a vitamin B12 deficiency even if the mother remains healthy. For this reason, all vegetarian mothers should eat foods fortified with vitamin B12. However, vegetarians who regularly eat eggs or drink milk get all the vitamin B12 they need.

Pernicious anemia is usually an inherited disease in which a deficiency of vitamin B12 occurs despite adequate amounts in the diet. People with this disease cannot produce intrinsic factor, the substance needed to absorb vitamin B12. They need to receive injections of vitamin B12 so the vitamin can bypass the stomach and intrinsic factor and enter the bloodstream directly.

Pernicious anemia can also result from surgery. Because intrinsic factor originates in the stomach, partial or total removal of the stomach reduces absorption of vitamin B12. Moreover, removal of the end of the small intestine (ileum) also creates a

Sources of Vitamin B₁₂

Food	Quantity	Micrograms (µg)
Liver, beef	3½ ounces	70.4
Clams, canned	½ cup	24.7
Liver, chicken	3½ ounces	19.2
Oysters, raw	3½ ounces	19.0
Sardines	3½ ounces	8.7
Product 19 cereal	1 cup	6.0
Salmon, canned	3½ ounces	4.3
Grape-Nuts cereal	½ cup	3.0
Hamburger	3 ounces	2.3
Tuna, canned in water	3½ ounces	2.2
Lamb	3½ ounces	2.1
Haddock	3½ ounces	1.7
Beef steak	3 ounces	1.6
Veal, lean	3½ ounces	1.4
Yogurt, low-fat	8 ounces	1.4
Ham	3½ ounces	0.9
Milk, nonfat	1 cup	0.9
Cottage cheese, low-fat	½ cup	0.8
Pork sausage	3 links	0.7
Instant breakfast drink or breakfast bar	1 envelope or bar	0.6
Egg	1 whole	0.5
Crabmeat, canned	3½ ounces	0.5
Swiss cheese*	1 ounce	0.5
Buttermilk	8 ounces	0.5
Camembert cheese*	1 ounce	0.4
Cheddar cheese*	1 ounce	0.2

*As cheese ripens, the amount of B vitamins increases.

deficiency because that's where absorption of the vitamin takes place.

Stomach acid frees vitamin B_{12} from the proteins it is bound to in foods, but for the almost one half of adults who experience a decline in stomach acid as they age, this can be a problem. As many as 20 percent of people older than 65 may have low B_{12} blood levels. If undetected, the problem can cause nerve damage. An unexplained unsteady gait and loss of coordination are often the warning signs of this type of vitamin B_{12} deficiency.

USE AND MISUSE OF VITAMIN B_{12}

Physicians treat pernicious anemia with an injection of 50 to 100 µg of vitamin B_{12} three times a week until symptoms subside. These injections may be lifelong.

Some people believe giving injections of vitamin B_{12} to those without pernicious anemia can boost energy. More likely, they're a placebo. Use of B_{12} for this purpose is controversial.

There are no reports of vitamin B_{12} causing toxicity or adverse effects even when taken in large amounts. Taking the vitamin orally, however, will not help those people with undiagnosed pernicious anemia because they cannot absorb the nutrient.

Vitamin C: Ascorbic Acid

When you hear the words vitamin C, you may instinctively think of the common cold. For that you can thank Linus Pauling and his 1970 book, *Vitamin C and the Common Cold*. In it, Pauling recommended megadoses of vitamin C to reduce the frequency and severity of colds. The book triggered a sales boom for vitamin C that is still going strong. It also prompted nutritionists to begin a series of carefully designed studies of the vitamin and its functions.

Today, some people still swear by vitamin C. Nutritionists have found little proof of its effectiveness against catching the common cold, but there is evidence to suggest it can reduce the severity of a cold somewhat.

HISTORY

The story of vitamin C began centuries ago, with accounts of a disease called scurvy. The ailment causes muscle weakness, lethargy, poor wound healing, and bleeding from the gums and under the skin. As recounted in this book's introduction, scurvy was rampant around the world for centuries. Documents dating back before the time of Christ describe the disease. Ships' logs tell of its widespread occurrence among sailors in the 16th century. History books report that scurvy was a common problem among the troops during the American Civil War. And records of Antarctic explorers recount how Captain Robert Scott and his team succumbed to the malady in 1912.

Almost as old as reports of scurvy are reports of successful ways to treat the disease: eating green salads, fruits, vegetables, pickled cabbage, small onions, and an ale made of such things as wormwood, horseradish, and mustard seed. In the 1530s, French explorer Jacques Cartier told how the natives of Newfoundland cured the mysterious disease by giving his men an extract prepared from the green shoots of an evergreen tree.

However, the disease was still the "scourge of the navy" 200 years later, when the British physician James Lind singled out a cure for scurvy. Believing that acidic materials relieved symptoms of the illness, Lind tried six different substances on six groups of scurvy-stricken men. He gave them all the standard shipboard diet, but to one pair of men in each of the six groups he gave a different test substance. One pair received a solution of sulfuric acid each day; another, cider; and a third, sea water. The fourth pair received vinegar, and the fifth took a daily combination of garlic, mustard seed, balsam of Peru, and gum myrrh. The sixth pair in the experiment received two oranges and a lemon each day—lucky them.

Lind found that the men who ate citrus fruit improved rapidly; one returned to duty after only six days. The sailors who drank the cider showed slight improvement after two weeks, but none of the others improved.

Although Lind published the results of his experiment, 50 years passed before the British navy finally added lime juice to its sailors' diets. And it wasn't until 1932 that researchers isolated the vitamin itself. At the time, it carried the name hexuronic acid. Later, scientists renamed it ascorbic (meaning "without scurvy") acid.

FUNCTIONS OF VITAMIN C

A major function of vitamin C is its role as a cofactor in the formation and repair of collagen—the connective tissue that holds the body's cells and tissues together. Collagen is a primary component of blood vessels, skin, tendons, and ligaments. Vitamin C also promotes the normal development of bones and teeth. It's also needed for amino acid metabolism and the synthesis of hormones, including the thyroid hormone that controls the body's rate of metabolism. Vitamin C also aids the absorption of iron and calcium.

These days, vitamin C is heralded for its antioxidant status. It prevents other substances from combining with oxygen by tying up oxygen itself. In this role, vitamin C protects a number of enzymes involved in functions ranging from cholesterol metabolism to immune function.

Vitamin C is a useful food additive in many processed foods. When added to cured meats, vitamin C inhibits the formation of nitrosamines in the stomach—compounds known to cause cancer in laboratory animals.

SOURCES OF VITAMIN C

Of course, the famed citrus fruits—oranges, lemons, grapefruits, and limes—are excellent sources of vitamin C. Other often overlooked excellent sources of vitamin C are strawberries, kiwifruit, cantaloupe, and peppers. Potatoes also supply vitamin C. Though cooking destroys some of the vitamin, you can minimize the amount lost if the temperature is not too high and you don't cook them any longer than necessary. Even potato chips and french fries retain some of the vitamin C from the raw potato.

Rose hips from the rose plant—which are used to prepare rose hip tea—are rich in vitamin C. Fruit juices, fruit juice drinks, and drink mixes may be fortified with vitamin C at fairly high levels. (Refer to the table on pages 170–171 for sources of vitamin C.)

Vitamin C is easier to destroy than any other vitamin except folate. The amount of vitamin C in foods falls off rapidly during transport, processing, storage, and preparation. Bruising or cutting a fruit or vegetable destroys some of the vitamin, as do light, air, and heat. Still, if you cover and refrigerate orange juice, it will retain much of its vitamin C value, even after several days. To obtain maximum vitamin value, it's best to use

Sources of Vitamin C

Food	Quantity	Milligrams (mg)
Cantaloupe	½ medium	194.7
Currant juice, black	½ cup	194.4
Guava, fresh	1 medium	165.2
Honeydew melon	½ medium	160.0
Peppers, red, raw	1 pod	142.5
Kohlrabi, cooked	1 cup	86.8
Papayas, raw	1 cup (½-inch cubes)	86.5
Strawberries, frozen or fresh	1 cup	84.5
Green pepper, cooked (without stem or seeds)	1 medium	84.4
Cranapple juice	1 cup	78.4
Kiwifruit	1 medium	74.5
Brussels sprouts, cooked	1 cup	70.8
Tomato soup, canned, condensed (with equal amount milk)	1 cup	66.5
Grape juice, sweetened	1 cup	59.8
Mango	1 medium	57.3
Cauliflower, cooked (flowerbuds)	1 cup	56.3
Grapefruit sections, canned in syrup	1 cup	54.1
Gazpacho	1 cup	52.7
Mandarin orange sections	1 cup	50.3
Orange juice, fresh or canned	1 cup	48.4

Sources of Vitamin C (continued)

Food	Quantity	Milligrams (mg)
Beef and vegetable stew	1 cup	48.1
Watermelon, raw	1 wedge	46.3
Cranberry juice, sweetened	½ cup	44.8
Fruit cup, fresh (citrus, apple, grape)	1 cup	44.6
Asparagus, green, canned (solids and liquid)	1 cup	44.5
Cabbage, bok choy, cooked	1 cup	44.2
Gooseberries, raw	1 cup	41.6
Raspberries, red, frozen	1 cup	41.2
Spanish rice (homemade), meatless	1 cup	40.6
Turnip greens, cooked	1 cup	39.5
Cowpeas, cooked	1 cup	38.3
Broccoli, cooked	½ cup	36.9
Tomatoes, canned (solids and liquid)	1 cup	36.2
Grapefruit juice, fresh or canned	½ cup	36.1
Cole slaw with mayonnaise	1 cup	35.0
Sauerkraut, canned (solids and liquid)	1 cup	34.7
Tomato, raw	1 medium	34.4
Rutabaga	1 cup	32.0
Chard, Swiss, cooked, fresh or frozen	1 cup	31.5
Sweet potatoes, cooked	½ cup	31.4

Sources of Vitamin C (continued)

Food	Quantity	Milligrams (mg)
Raspberries, red, raw	1 cup	30.8
Lemon, fresh	1 medium	30.7
Cabbage, cooked (common varieties)	1 cup	30.2
Blackberries, raw	1 cup	30.2
Sweet potatoes, candied	1 medium	28.0
Tomato paste	¼ cup	27.7
Tangerine, raw	1 medium	26.9
Pineapple, raw, diced	2 slices	25.9
Winter squash, baked, mashed	1 cup	23.5
Spinach, cooked	1 cup	23.4
Cabbage, raw	1 cup	22.5
Loganberries	1 cup	22.5
Okra, cooked	½ cup	22.4
Tomato juice, canned	½ cup	22.2
Sweet potatoes, canned	1 cup	21.2
Cabbage, celery or Chinese, raw	1 cup	20.5
Fruit cobbler	1 cup	20.4
Parsnips, cooked	1 cup	20.2
Potatoes, hash brown	1 cup	20.0
Beef liver, cooked	3 ounces	19.6
Blueberries, raw	1 cup	18.8
Arugula	1 cup	18.2
Turnips, cooked, diced	1 cup	18.1
Grapes	1 cup	17.3

Sources of Vitamin C (continued)

Food	Quantity	Milligrams (mg)
Potato sticks	1 cup	17.0
Artichokes, cooked	1 cup	16.8
Peas, green, fresh or frozen	1 cup	15.8
Potato, baked	1 medium	15.7
Collards, cooked	1 cup	15.5
Spinach, canned (drained solids)	½ cup	15.3
Lemon juice, fresh	¼ cup	15.1
Cress, garden, raw	1 cup	14.6
Avocado, raw	1 medium	13.7
Pineapple juice, canned	1 cup	13.4
Spaghetti with meatballs and tomato sauce	1 cup	13.2
Potato, mashed (milk and butter added)	1 cup	13.0
Guacamole dip	2 tablespoons	12.0
Potatoes, boiled	1 cup	11.5
Beans, lima, fresh or frozen	½ cup	10.9
Tomatoes, sun-dried	½ cup	10.6
Cherries, sweet, raw	1 cup	10.2
Summer squash, cooked, diced	1 cup	9.9
Limeade, sweetened	1 cup	9.7
Lemonade concentrate, diluted, sweetened	1 cup	9.7
Beans, snap, green	½ cup	9.4
Peas, green, canned (solids and liquid)	½ cup	8.2

Sources of Vitamin C (continued)

Food	Quantity	Milligrams (mg)
Rhubarb, cooked (sugar added)	1 cup	7.9
Peaches, dried, uncooked	1 cup	7.7
Lettuce, cos or romaine	1 cup	7.2
Plum	1 medium	6.3
Parsley	1 tablespoon	5.0
Celery	½ cup	4.2
Papaya juice, canned	½ cup	3.8
Lobster salad	1 cup	3.4
Apricot halves, dried, uncooked	1 cup	3.1
Soybeans, boiled, drained	1 cup	2.9
Cucumber, raw, pared	½ cup	2.8
Lettuce, iceberg	1 cup	2.1

fresh, unprocessed fruits and vegetables whenever possible.

DIETARY REQUIREMENTS FOR VITAMIN C

The RDA for vitamin C is 60 mg daily for adults, with an additional 20 mg for pregnant women and an additional 40 mg for women who are breast-feeding.

The above RDAs are several times the amounts needed to treat deficiency symptoms. Even so, many people believe these levels are not high enough for optimal nutrition, which deals more with vitamin C's antioxidant properties than with prevention of a deficiency.

DEFICIENCY OF VITAMIN C

The classic vitamin C deficiency disease is scurvy. Early signs of the disease are bleeding gums and bleeding under the skin, causing tiny pinpoint bruises. The deficiency can progress to the point that it causes poor wound healing, anemia, and impaired bone growth.

The body normally stores about 1,500 mg of vitamin C at a time, and symptoms of a deficiency do not occur until the body pool is less than 300 mg. It would take several weeks on a diet containing no vitamin C for this drop to occur in an otherwise well-nourished person.

Since only 10 mg of vitamin C is needed daily in order to prevent scurvy, the disease is rarely seen in the United States today, except in infants who are not given supplemental vitamin C. But even without signs of scurvy, low intakes of vitamin C can compromise many body functions, including the ability to rid the body of cholesterol and the immune system's ability to fight off infection and disease.

People who smoke cigarettes and women who take oral contraceptives have lower than normal blood levels of vitamin C. The RDA level of vitamin C has been raised for smokers, who are estimated to

Vitamin C Content of Common Foods*

Food	Quantity	Milligrams (mg)
Fruits–Vegetables Group		
Orange, fresh	1 medium	69.7
Grapefruit, fresh	½ medium	50.1
Broccoli, raw	½ cup	41.0
Vegetable juice	½ cup	33.5
Cauliflower, chopped, raw	½ cup	23.2
Asparagus, cooked	½ cup	22.0
Scallions	¼ cup	18.0
Spinach, raw	1 cup	15.7
Onions, raw	½ cup	15.1
Corn flakes	1 cup	15.0
French fries	1 cup (about 25 pieces)	12.1
Banana	1 medium	10.4
Apple	1 medium	7.9
Corn, canned	½ cup	6.9
Potato chips	1 cup	6.2
Zucchini	½ cup	4.1

*Milk and milk products, cereal foods (unless fortified), and meats contain little or no ascorbic acid. Organ meats are exceptions—beef liver contains 23 mg of ascorbic acid in a three-ounce serving.

need as much as 100 percent more of the vitamin in their diets than nonsmokers.

VITAMIN C USE AND MISUSE

Vitamin C supplements easily cure scurvy. Doctors sometimes use vitamin C to acidify the urine when treating certain bladder or kidney disorders, and may prescribe vitamin C supplements before surgery to ensure a sufficient supply of the vitamin to promote wound healing.

Vitamin C is the most popular single vitamin supplement. Besides taking it to try to prevent colds, people take vitamin C in the hopes it will ease schizophrenia, senility, cancer, and other medical problems. For some disorders, it's hard to separate the true effects of the vitamin from the psychological effects—called the placebo effect.

Scientifically controlled studies testing the value of vitamin C in preventing or treating colds show only a slight benefit in reducing a cold's severity, similar to antihistamine's effect. For the most part, however, studies have not proved that megadoses of the vitamin prevent colds.

What about cancer treatment? A study testing the value of 10 g (10,000 mg) a day of vitamin C in cancer patients showed no effect on relieving symptoms or on prolonging survival. However, vitamin C may have a role in preventing cancer (see Chapter 6).

Large single doses of vitamin C are not toxic; the excess is simply excreted in the urine. However, large habitual intakes may cause problems. Some people develop stomach cramps and diarrhea when taking 1,000 mg (1 gram) or more of vitamin C a day.

Large doses of vitamin C may decrease the amount of copper that the body absorbs. It also increases the amount of iron that is absorbed—a problem for people who have hemochromatosis, or iron-overload disease, an inherited defect in their ability to control iron absorption.

It's suspected that some susceptible people might develop calcium oxalate kidney stones after taking large doses of vitamin C. The vitamin may promote stone formation.

Large doses of vitamin C can break down red blood cells in people with sickle-cell disease. Because individuals with this condition have an abnormal hemoglobin protein that's distorted by vitamin C, they should avoid taking large amounts of the vitamin.

Increased excretion of uric acid can also result from large doses of vitamin C. This can be a problem for people who suffer from gout. It can also lead to a misdiagnosis of the condition.

Chewable vitamin C tablets can erode tooth enamel if used over a long period of time. Large doses of vitamin C may also interfere with the action of some anticlotting medications.

Some nutritionists warn that if you take more than 1,000 mg per day of vitamin C, you risk developing rebound scurvy when you stop the supplements. Apparently your body develops a mechanism for breaking down and excreting the vitamin quickly, so that a deficiency may develop when you resume normal intake. To be safe, people taking large amounts of vitamin C should wean themselves gradually from it rather than stopping abruptly. The body can then become accustomed to lower intakes.

There have been cases of babies who developed scurvy after their mothers took large amounts of vitamin C during pregnancy. The babies developed an increased need for the vitamin due to their exposure to large amounts before birth.

Vitamin C is chemically similar to glucose. Physicians need to know if you are taking megadoses of vitamin C so that they won't misinterpret laboratory tests for the presence of glucose in the urine. This can also create problems for people with diabetes who need to monitor blood glucose levels. Large amounts of vitamin C can also cover up the presence of blood in the stool, distorting the results of tests designed to detect colon cancer.

Vitamin D: Cholecalciferol

Vitamin D is known as the sunshine vitamin—and for good reason. If you get enough sunshine, your body can make its own vitamin D.

HISTORY

Years ago, few children in tropical countries developed the malformed bones and teeth characteristic of rickets. Yet many children in temperate climates and large industrial cities did. Why the difference? The sun.

Skin contains the substance provitamin D, which starts to convert to vitamin D when exposed to sunlight. In tropical countries, sunlight shone on children year-round. Since these children had ample opportunity for exposure, their skin formed adequate amounts of vitamin D, and thus they didn't experience the symptoms of rickets.

Children in temperate zones, however, got little exposure to the sun during the winter months, and their skin could not make enough vitamin D. Neither could the skin of children in large, industrial cities because the smoke-filled air filtered out much of the sun's ultraviolet light.

In the early 1900s, rickets afflicted large numbers of children in this country. While searching for the cause, researchers fed various diets to experimental animals. Those diets that prevented calcium from depositing in the bones produced the soft bones that are characteristic of rickets. From this research, investigators concluded that rickets was actually a vitamin-deficiency disease.

However, researchers were perplexed when they discovered that ultraviolet light could also prevent the deficiency. In the 1920s, nutritionists were able to prevent or cure rickets by feeding children cod liver oil or food exposed to ultraviolet light. They also prevented rickets by exposing children to direct sunlight or the light from a sunlamp. The explanation for these findings didn't crystallize for several more years. Cod liver oil was effective against rickets because it contains vitamin D. Foods exposed to ultraviolet light were effective because the light changed a substance in plant foods into a form of the vitamin that the body can use—vitamin D_2.

Today, doctors seldom see cases of rickets in the United States. The few cases that do occur can usually be traced to poverty, neglect, or ignorance. The dramatic drop in rickets cases is primarily due to the increased availability of milk fortified with vitamin D. Choosing to fortify milk made sense because children usually drink lots of it. It's also the single best source of calcium in the American diet, and since vitamin D helps the body use calcium to build strong teeth and bones, milk was an appropriate food to select.

FUNCTIONS OF VITAMIN D

Vitamin D is necessary to help the body absorb the minerals calcium and phosphorus, which are needed for the proper growth and development of bones and teeth.

Whether it comes from food or is made in the skin, vitamin D must be activated before it's of use to the body. It first travels to the liver, where it undergoes a chemical change. Then it moves through the bloodstream to the kidneys, where it undergoes another change to become the active form of the vitamin. This active form—dihydroxy vitamin D—is the one that helps the body absorb calcium and phosphorus.

SOURCES OF VITAMIN D

Few foods contain significant amounts of vitamin D naturally. And the ones that do are not foods you want to overdo: butter, cream, egg yolk, and liver. But there are some good sources. All milk—including skim milk—is fortified with vitamin D at a level of 100 IU per cup. Some manufacturers also fortify cereals with vitamin D. Cod liver oil, as a supplement, contains over 1,200 IU of vitamin D per tablespoon.

Clouds, smog, clothing, and even window glass filter out ultraviolet rays. Housebound people, those with dark skin, and those who live in cloudy, northern climates are most likely to be deficient in vitamin D. These people must be sure to get vitamin D from foods.

A fair-skinned person can make a sufficient quantity of vitamin D with only 20 to 30 minutes of sun exposure a day. It would take three hours for a dark-skinned person to make an equal amount because skin pigment filters out ultraviolet rays.

You cannot overdose on vitamin D from sun exposure. Of course, you can get too much sun, increasing your risk of skin cancer. Unfortunately, because sunscreens filter out the ultraviolet rays that burn your skin, they block the manufacture of vitamin D as well. Exposing unprotected skin to the sun in the early morning or late afternoon solves both problems.

DIETARY REQUIREMENTS FOR VITAMIN D

Since 1980, we measure vitamin D in micrograms (µg) instead of International Units (IU). The RDA for children and for women who are pregnant or breast-feeding is 10 µg (400 IU). For other adults older than 24 years of age, the RDA is 5 µg (200 IU). One quart of fortified milk supplies 10 µg; one cup of milk contains 2.5 µg.

DEFICIENCY OF VITAMIN D

Vitamin D deficiency causes rickets in children. Because vitamin D is crucial to proper calcium absorption, the hallmark of rickets is the undermineralization of bones. One of its common signs is bowlegs. Another sign is beadlike swellings on the ribs—a condition called rachitic rosary. Teething is usually late in children with rickets, and the teeth that develop are susceptible to decay.

Though rickets is rare in the United States today, some cases do appear in low-income children, vegetarian children, and infants who were breast-fed for an extended period of time with no supplementation.

Vitamin D deficiency in adults is called osteomalacia. It involves the loss of calcium and protein

Sources of Vitamin D

Food	Quantity	Micrograms (μg)
Tuna salad	1 cup	7.5
Skim milk, fortified	1 cup	2.5
Milk, fortified	1 cup	2.5
Egg Beaters egg substitutes	½ cup	2.1
Eggnog	½ cup	1.5
Raisin Bran cereal	1 cup	1.4
Total cereal	1 cup	1.2
Product 19 cereal	1 cup	1.2
Yogurt, low-fat, flavored	1 cup	1.2
Special K cereal	1 cup	1.2
Kix cereal	1½ cups	1.2
Liver, pork, cooked	2½ ounces	0.8
Malted milkshake	10 ounces	0.8
Liver, beef, cooked	2½ ounces	0.8
Egg	1 large	0.6
Ice cream bar	1 bar	0.5
Swiss cheese	1 ounce	0.3
Beef liver, cooked	2½ ounces	0.2
Chicken liver, cooked	2½ ounces	0.2
Butter	1 tablespoon	0.1

from bones, due to insufficient vitamin D. Osteomalacia differs from osteoporosis in that bone loses only mineral. In osteoporosis, bone itself is lost. In developing countries, osteomalacia is prevalent in women who have low intakes of calcium and vitamin D and several closely spaced pregnancies that are followed by long periods of breast-feeding.

USE AND MISUSE OF VITAMIN D

Strict vegetarians who do not get enough sunlight should consider taking vitamin D supplements. Breast-fed babies routinely receive vitamin D supplements. Formula-fed infants, on the other hand, receive the recommended amount of vitamin D in commercial infant formula and do not require additional supplementation.

The standard treatment for rickets is a fairly high dose of vitamin D given under a doctor's supervision. Doctors give the active form of the vitamin in cases in which the conversion of vitamin D to the active dihydroxy form is inadequate.

Vitamin D is the most toxic of all the vitamins. As little as 2,000 IU a day can be toxic to children. Symptoms of overdose include diarrhea, nausea, headache, and elevated calcium levels in the blood. This condition, called hypercalcemia, can lead to calcium deposits in the kidneys, heart, and other tissues, causing irreversible damage.

The claim is sometimes made that natural sources of vitamin D, such as cod liver oil, are not toxic. This is not true. Toxicity symptoms have developed in children given large doses of cod liver oil.

Avoid supplements—natural or synthetic—in amounts over the RDA, unless prescribed by a doctor.

Vitamin E: Tocopherol

Perhaps no other vitamin has received more attention lately than vitamin E. Retail sales of vitamin E supplements are soaring. It has been suggested that vitamin E can increase physical endurance, enhance sexual potency, smooth scars, lower blood fat levels, and relieve hot flashes and other menopausal symptoms. Scientific evidence to support these claims is lacking, however.

What exactly is vitamin E? It's not a single compound, but several different compounds, all with vitamin E activity. One, alpha-tocopherol, has the greatest activity. Other compounds with vitamin E activity are beta-tocopherol, gamma-tocopherol, and delta-tocopherol.

HISTORY

Vitamin E's existence was first hinted at in 1922. Laboratory rats fed purified diets lost their reproductive ability; male rats became sterile, and female rats reabsorbed their fetuses or delivered deformed or stillborn offspring. When foods such as lettuce, wheat, meat, or butter were added to the animals' diets, an unknown factor was supplied that prevented these reproductive problems. Isolated in 1936, the discoverers named it tocopherol, from the Greek meaning "to bring forth offspring." Later the substance became known as vitamin E.

Researchers noticed that deficiency symptoms varied from one species to another. In rabbits, for example, vitamin E deficiency resulted in a degenerative muscle disease. Because these symptoms were similar to those seen in humans with muscular dystrophy, researchers hoped vitamin E could cure this crippling condition. Hopes were also high that the vitamin might help human cases of infertility and sterility. Since 1938, however, studies in humans have failed to confirm any of these benefits.

FUNCTIONS OF VITAMIN E

Vitamin E functions as an antioxidant in the cells and tissues of the body. That means it combines with oxygen to prevent other body substances from doing so. It protects polyunsaturated fats and other oxygen-sensitive compounds such as vitamin A from being destroyed by damaging oxidation reactions.

Vitamin E's antioxidant properties are also important to cell membranes. For example, vitamin E protects lung cells that are in constant contact with oxygen and white blood cells that help the body fight disease. A deficiency of vitamin E weakens the immune system, increasing susceptibility to infection.

But the benefits of vitamin E's antioxidant role may go much further. Evidence is starting to build that vitamin E can protect against heart disease and may slow the deterioration associated with aging. Critics scoffed at such claims in the past, but an understanding of the importance of vitamin E's antioxidant role may be beginning to pay off. (See Chapters 5 and 6 for more about the role of vitamin E in disease prevention.)

Vitamin E also acts as an antioxidant in foods. It helps keep vegetable oils from being oxidized and turning rancid. Likewise, it protects vitamin A from being oxidized in its food sources. This makes vitamin E a useful food preservative.

SOURCES OF VITAMIN E

Oils and margarines from corn, cottonseed, soybean, safflower, and wheat germ are all good sources of vitamin E. Generally, the more polyunsaturated an oil is, the more vitamin E it contains. Fruits, vegetables, and whole grains have smaller amounts. Refining grains reduces their vitamin E content, as does commercial processing and storage of food. Cooking foods at high temperatures also destroys vitamin E, so a polyunsaturated oil is useless as a vitamin E source if it's used for frying. Fresh and lightly processed foods, and those that aren't overcooked, are your best sources.

Loss of vitamin E from cooking and storage makes it difficult to get an adequate amount of the vitamin in the diet. Moreover, the current emphasis on greater intake of oils containing monounsaturated fats, such as olive oil or canola oil, rather than vitamin E-containing polyunsaturated fats, further decreases our intake of vitamin E. Monounsaturated fats have other benefits for the heart, though, so you shouldn't stop using olive and canola oils. It is important to find other sources of vitamin E. Besides, the less polyunsaturated fats you eat, the less vitamin E you need, so your requirements may be lower if you switch to olive or canola oils.

DIETARY REQUIREMENTS
FOR VITAMIN E

The RDA for vitamin E is 10 mg of d-alpha-tocopherol for adult men and 8 mg for women. One milligram of d-alpha-tocopherol is equal to 1.5 IU, so the RDA is equal to 15 IU and 12 IU for men and women, respectively. Food and supplement labels usually list amounts of vitamin E in milligrams rather than international units.

DEFICIENCY OF VITAMIN E

No obvious symptoms accompany a vitamin E deficiency, making it hard to detect. A brownish pigmentation of the skin, often called age spots or lipofuscin, may signal the problem, but only a blood test can confirm if vitamin E levels are actually too low.

When diseases of the liver, gall bladder, or pancreas reduce intestinal absorption, a mild defi-

Sources of Vitamin E

Food	Quantity	Milligrams (mg)
Just Right with Fiber cereal	1 cup	30.2
Wheat germ oil	1 tablespoon	24.6
Total cereal	1 cup	23.4
Hazelnuts	½ cup	16.1
Sunflower seeds	2 tablespoons	9.0
Sunflower oil	1 tablespoon	8.2
Peanuts	½ cup	6.6
Brazil nuts	½ cup	5.3
Cottonseed oil	1 tablespoon	5.2
Corn	1 ear	4.8
Safflower oil	1 tablespoon	4.7
Almonds	½ cup	4.0
Corn oil	1 tablespoon	2.8
Canola oil	1 tablespoon	2.8
Asparagus, fresh or frozen	1 cup	2.6
Soybean oil	1 tablespoon	2.0
Olive oil	1 tablespoon	1.6
Walnuts	½ cup	1.3
Brussels sprouts, fresh or frozen	1 cup	1.3
Wheat germ	2 tablespoons	1.1
Sweet potato	1 medium	1.1
Broccoli, fresh or frozen	1 cup	1.0
Pear	1 medium	0.9
Tomato	1 medium	0.8
Brown rice	1 cup	0.8
Plum	1 large	0.7
Oatmeal	1 cup	0.6

Sources of Vitamin E (continued)

Food	Quantity	Milligrams (mg)
Apple	1 medium	0.5
Whole-wheat flour	⅓ cup	0.4
Walnut oil	1 tablespoon	0.4
Grapefruit	½ medium	0.4
Egg	1 large	0.4
Raspberries	½ cup	0.3

ciency of vitamin E can result. A diet of processed foods that's very low in fat might also cause a deficiency.

Vitamin E deficiency may occur in newborn babies, especially those born prematurely, because the mother doesn't transfer much vitamin E to the developing fetus until the last few weeks of pregnancy. The deficiency can cause hemolytic anemia, a condition in which the red blood cells are so fragile they rupture.

USE AND MISUSE OF VITAMIN E

Premature babies receive vitamin E to reduce or prevent oxygen damage to the retina of the eye. Vitamin E therapy treats claudication—pains in the calf muscles that occur at night or during exercise. A more controversial use of vitamin E supplements is for the treatment of painful, benign breast lumps (fibrocystic breast disease). There is no evidence, however, that vitamin E can treat fertility problems and muscle degeneration in humans as it does in animals.

Ongoing animal studies suggest that vitamin E may help prevent lung damage caused by air pollution. It appears that vitamin E can reduce the activity of such common air pollutants as ozone and nitrogen dioxide.

Vitamin E applied to cuts may very well increase the healing rate because it minimizes oxidation reactions in the wound. The value of vitamin E in preventing the stretch marks of pregnancy is legendary, but this benefit has not been proved scientifically.

Many women report that vitamin E helps reduce hot flashes and other symptoms of menopause. These are considered anecdotal reports.

Though vitamin E can slow down the oxidation of fats that occurs in aging, experimental studies have not shown it to increase the life span of animals. Neither has it been shown to control such signs of aging as wrinkled skin or gray hair. However, the vitamin may indeed delay or prevent some diseases or a loss of function related to aging (see Chapter 6). While vitamin E may not make you live longer, it may help you live better as you get older.

Vitamin E seems to be fairly safe when taken in amounts of 400 IU daily for a long time.

Amounts larger than this might delay blood clotting, possibly causing an increased risk of the bleeding type of stroke. People on anticoagulant therapy (blood thinners) should not take megadoses of vitamin E for this reason.

Vitamin K: Phylloquinone and Menaquinone

The *K* in vitamin K seems strange, but it came from the Danish word koagulation, meaning "blood clotting," which precisely reflects the function of vitamin K in the human body.

HISTORY

The importance of a dietary factor in blood clotting was first recognized by Danish scientist Henrik Dam. In 1929, he reported that chicks fed diets lacking a particular dietary factor hemorrhaged. Their blood was slow to form the clots needed to control bleeding. The missing dietary factor was vitamin K.

FUNCTION OF VITAMIN K

The proteins used in blood clotting require vitamin K. When there isn't enough of the vitamin, blood takes longer to clot, which can increase the amount of blood lost. Vitamin K also helps make a protein that may help regulate blood calcium levels. Calcium, usually associated with keeping bones strong, is also necessary for blood clotting.

Sources of Vitamin K

The best food sources of vitamin K are green leafy vegetables such as cabbage, turnip greens, broccoli, lettuce, and spinach. Beef liver is another good source; chicken liver, pork liver, milk, and eggs contain smaller amounts of the vitamin. Liver, however, may also contain environmental toxins, so other sources may be better choices to meet the RDA for vitamin K.

We get only about half of the vitamin K we need from the foods we eat. The other half comes from the bacteria that live in our digestive tracts and produce vitamin K. The extent to which we are able to use bacterially produced vitamin K, however, is still somewhat uncertain.

Dietary Requirements for Vitamin K

For a long time, we simply didn't know enough about vitamin K to establish requirements for it. The first recommendation for the vitamin wasn't established until the 1989 edition of the RDAs. The requirement varies by age. For men, the requirement ranges from 45 to 80 µg as age increases from 11 to more than 50 years. For women, the requirement ranges from 45 to 65 µg. A typical well-balanced diet in the United States supplies approximately 300 to 500 µg of vitamin K—certainly more than enough to meet average dietary needs.

DEFICIENCY OF VITAMIN K

Liver or gall bladder disease, or any disease of the intestinal tract that interferes with absorption of fats, can cause a deficiency of vitamin K. Use of mineral oil or some of the medications that are prescribed to lower cholesterol interfere with vitamin K absorption, and this can lead to a deficiency as well.

Long-term use of oral antibiotics kills off the bacteria in the intestines that manufacture the vitamin. This can lead to a deficiency, especially if coupled with a diet that provides insufficient amounts of vitamin K.

Newborn babies, especially those born prematurely, are born with little vitamin K. For the first couple of days after birth, the baby's intestinal tract has no bacteria to make the vitamin either. Because the lack of vitamin K could lead to bleeding problems, newborns are routinely given a vitamin K supplement.

VITAMIN K USE AND MISUSE

People who cannot absorb vitamin K and sometimes those who are on long-term antibiotic therapy take vitamin K supplements. When there's a known deficiency, vitamin K is given before any surgery is performed.

Anticoagulants (blood thinners, such as dicumarol) are used in the treatment of heart disease and other diseases that cause the blood to clot too easily. Blood thinners interfere with the action of vitamin K and slow down the clotting process. People taking anticoagulants may inadvertently reduce the action of the drug by eating vitamin K–rich foods.

Large doses of vitamin K have been reported to cause bleeding. Water-soluble forms of vitamin K have occasionally caused toxicity (red-cell breakdown, jaundice, and brain damage) when given to infants or pregnant women.

CHAPTER 8

Vitaminlike Substances

There are other substances in food that function much like vitamins. They do not really fit the definition of vitamins, however, either because our bodies can make them or because we require them in larger amounts than we do vitamins. These substances occur so widely in foods that a deficiency is unlikely.

CHOLINE

Choline is a substance found in most animal tissues. It can exist by itself or as part of another substance. For example, it can be found in lecithin, a waxy material in the protective myelin sheath that surrounds nerve fibers. It can also exist as part of the neurotransmitter acetylcholine, a substance essential for the transmission of impulses through the nervous system.

When experimental animals had their pancreases removed, researchers discovered that the resulting lack of choline caused the condition hepatic cirrhosis, or fatty liver. When present, choline prevents the degenerative fatty changes that would otherwise occur. Could choline supplements do the same in humans? No one knows. Other equally controversial issues involve the use of choline to lower cholesterol levels and improve memory.

Researchers have had limited success treating certain conditions with large doses of choline and lecithin. One of these conditions is Alzheimer disease. Another is tardive dyskinesia, a syndrome marked by involuntary movements of the face and jaw resulting from long-term use of psychiatric medications.

Egg yolks, liver, beef, and soybeans are good sources of choline. Under normal circumstances, choline and lecithin supplements are not necessary because the body manufactures choline. (The American Academy of Pediatrics recommends that infant formula supply at least 7 mg of choline per 100 calories—the same amount present in human breast milk.)

BIOFLAVONOIDS

Citrus fruits and their skins are the secret hiding places of bioflavonoids. In the 1930s, nutritionists believed bioflavonoids could reverse the effects of vitamin C deficiency. This idea was later proved wrong; there is no evidence that bioflavonoids are essential to normal functioning. They may, however, prove to have some disease-preventing powers.

INOSITOL

Liver, wheat germ, citrus fruits, and meats are rich sources of inositol. The body can make inositol, concentrating it in hair and muscles. Perhaps because of this concentration in hair, inositol was once rumored to be effective against baldness. However, there's no scientific evidence for such a claim.

Of the nine compounds that are related to inositol, the only one that is considered important to plants and animals is myoinositol. Researchers don't yet completely understand myoinositol's function, but it is believed to aid in the metabolism of fats. Inositol is also useful in restoring nerve function to people with nerve damage resulting from diabetes.

LIPOIC ACID

Lipoic acid functions as a coenzyme along with the vitamin thiamin. Yeast and liver are good sources of this substance, which the body can also make.

CARNITINE (VITAMIN B-T)

Carnitine plays a role in fat and energy metabolism in the body. Recently, carnitine received publicity for its potential usefulness in fighting heart disease. However, scientists need to study it further to establish what value, if any, it has for heart patients.

Carnitine is found mostly in foods of animal origin and in lesser amounts in foods of plant origin; therefore, a vegetarian diet is apt to be low in carnitine.

Under normal circumstances the body makes this substance, so dietary sources are of little concern. Some people, however, may have an inherited inability to make sufficient amounts of carnitine and, therefore, need to be sure they have dietary sources of carnitine.

Symptoms of carnitine deficiency include muscle weakness, low blood sugar levels, and high blood ammonia levels. Carnitine supplements, however, reduce the symptoms only in some people. The most appropriate treatment for these symptoms and conditions is, unfortunately, not obvious.

COENZYME Q

Coenzyme Q, also called ubiquinone, is a chemical relative of vitamin E. Coenzyme Q is made by the body and plays a role in energy metabolism. Current research is examining the benefit of coenzyme Q supplements in the treatment of certain types of heart disease, but answers are still not definitive.

PARA-AMINOBENZOIC ACID (PABA)

Para-aminobenzoic acid (PABA) is part of the B vitamin folate and, therefore, isn't considered a separate vitamin. PABA is best known for its use in sunscreens. When applied to skin, PABA can help protect against sunburn. Taken orally, however, PABA does not have the same protective effect. Large doses taken over extended periods can cause nausea and vomiting. Oral use is not recommended.

CHAPTER 9

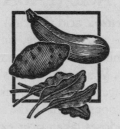

The Story of Minerals

Minerals, sometimes referred to as inorganic elements, make up about four percent—or about five pounds—of the body's weight. Even ancient peoples recognized the value and usefulness of minerals:

- Chinese writings from as early as 3000 B.C. recommended seaweed and burnt sponge to treat goiter, a deficiency of the mineral iodine. Seaweed and sponges are rich in iodine.
- In ancient Greece, people soaked hot iron swords in water and then used the iron-enriched water to treat anemia.
- As many as 30 references to salt—sodium chloride—can be found in the Bible, including its use in purifying ceremonies and as an offering to God.

- A Greek slave said to be "worth his weight in salt" actually commanded this price—payment in salt.
- At banquets, important people sat at the table closest to the salt cellar. This was considered a position of honor.
- The word salary is from the Latin word for salt, *saleria*.

Despite all these early references to minerals, many centuries passed before researchers clarified the role that minerals play in the body. In 1799, the French chemist Antoine Lavoisier—often called "the father of nutrition"—predicted correctly that scientists would isolate "elements" from the earth.

In 1804, another Frenchman, Theodore de Saussure, proved that the mineral makeup of soil influenced the mineral content of plants grown on that soil. Research during the second half of the 19th century concentrated mostly on trace minerals—those needed only in tiny amounts. In the early 20th century, as scientists isolated and identified vitamins, they also demonstrated that many minerals were essential to better health and nutrition.

Today, we are aware of 50 minerals in the body. Of these, 17 are definitely essential. The others are accidental contaminants or are waiting for us to discover their true importance. Recently, for example, researchers linked boron to mineral metabolism and bone development. Even small amounts of arsenic may prove useful to the body; its role has been linked to the metabolism of the amino acid methionine.

WHAT ARE MINERALS?

Minerals are different from vitamins; they are not organic substances made by plants or animals. They're actually inorganic elements found in soil. Plants absorb minerals directly from the soil, and animals get their supply indirectly, either by eating the plants or by eating other animals that have eaten the plants.

Minerals are grouped into two categories, depending on the amount found normally in the body. Macrominerals are those found in significant amounts—about five grams or more—in the body. They include calcium, phosphorus, magnesium, chlorine, sodium, potassium, and sulfur. Calcium and phosphorus are present in the largest amounts—about one pound.

Microminerals consist of the trace elements found in smaller amounts in the body. The daily requirements for these minerals are only a few milligrams or less. They include the essential minerals iron, iodine, zinc, fluoride, copper, chromium, manganese, selenium, molybdenum, and cobalt.

Research suggests that other trace minerals, such as nickel, tin, silicon, and vanadium, are essential for animals. They may prove to be necessary for humans as well.

Trace contaminants is a better term to describe cadmium, aluminum, and lead. Although they exist in the body, experts do not consider them essential. In the future, that status may change, but at present, avoid exposure to contaminants such as lead, cadmium, mercury, and arsenic.

The National Research Council has established Recommended Dietary Allowances (RDAs) for seven minerals: calcium, iron, phosphorus, magnesium, zinc, iodine, and selenium. Much less information is available about other minerals, making precise recommendations impossible. So, instead, the experts established ranges of "safe and adequate daily intakes" for sodium, potassium, chlorine, copper, fluoride, chromium, manganese, and molybdenum. (See page 20 for Table 2, "Estimated Safe and Adequate Daily Dietary Intakes of Additional Selected Vitamins and Minerals.")

WHAT MINERALS DO

Did you know that every cell in the body contains minerals? In fact, almost everything the body does involves minerals in some way or another. Their main functions are to help maintain the structure of living tissue and to regulate important body processes.

In their structural role, minerals contribute strength and firmness to bones and teeth. They're also part of essential body compounds. For example, iron is a part of hemoglobin (the oxygen-carrying substance in red blood cells) and is also a part of a number of different enzymes; iodine is a part of the thyroid hormone; and cobalt is a part of vitamin B_{12}.

In their role as regulators, minerals act as cofactors in enzyme-controlled body reactions. In other words, they keep enzyme reactions running up to speed. Iron, zinc, and copper are parts of enzymes. If the diet doesn't supply enough of these minerals, the body can't make enough enzymes.

Free mineral ions—particles with either a positive or negative electrical charge—have many important functions. These ions are important for maintenance of normal acid–base balance, transmission of nerve impulses, regulation of normal cell membrane function, and regulation of muscle response to nerve stimuli.

Some minerals have druglike effects. For example, fluoride prevents tooth decay, and chromium can help control blood sugar in people with diabetes.

MINERAL DEFICIENCIES

Nutrition surveys often find that intake of certain minerals, such as calcium, iron, and zinc, are lower than recommended. Part of the reason could be that refined and processed foods have fewer minerals. One way to remedy the loss is to replace those minerals lost in processing—a process called enrichment. In the 1920s, health authorities successfully prevented iodine-deficiency goiter by adding iodine to salt. And manufacturers currently add iron to cereals and breads that have the mineral stripped during processing. Many companies add calcium to fruit juices, breakfast cereals, and breads, too.

MINERAL TOXICITY

Excessive mineral supplements can be harmful. Large doses can cause abnormal fluid accumulations in vital organs, interfere with the functions of other minerals, and irritate the intestines, which may cause nausea and bleeding. A real danger is the replacement of one mineral with a similar one in an enzyme. The impostor enzyme doesn't function as the real one does, or it does not function at all.

A WORD ABOUT WATER

In the body, metabolic reactions involving vitamins and minerals take place in water. Thus, water is essential for the maintenance of normal body function. Water makes up about 60 percent of an adult's body and an even greater percentage of a child's body. Men have slightly more water in their bodies than women do, and younger people have more than older people. About 70 percent of lean body tissue, or muscle, is actually water.

Water carries nutrients into cells and transports wastes out of them. It acts as a solvent for compounds such as vitamins, minerals, glucose, and amino acids (the building blocks of protein). It lubricates joints, acts as a shock absorber inside the eyes and spinal cord, and helps the body maintain its temperature.

Most people drink about 2½ quarts of water daily. Normally, this comes from many sources: liquids (milk, tap water, noncaffeinated soft drinks, soups), animal foods (meat, fish, eggs), and fruits and vegetables. For example, cucumbers are about 96 percent water; lettuce, 94 percent; watermelon, 93 percent; broccoli, 91 percent; and oranges, 84 percent.

Beverages such as coffee, tea, caffeine-containing soft drinks, and alcoholic drinks do not add to our total water intake. The caffeine and alcohol they contain are diuretics, causing the body to lose more water than is added. Water is also lost in urine, stool, sweat, and the air we exhale.

People who are healthy generally excrete at least one quart of urine a day to rid the body of wastes. During waking hours, this means urinating about every four hours. Less frequent urination is a sign you're not consuming enough fluids.

Thirst partially controls the water content of the body, but often thirst lags behind the body's needs. That makes it even more important to pay attention to your thirst. When you thirst for water, you're usually already behind in fluid intake. So indulge yourself (unless your doctor has advised you to do otherwise). Drinking too much water poses no danger to healthy people; they just excrete the excess, producing a more dilute urine.

ELECTROLYTES

When found in body tissues, minerals occur mainly as mineral salts. When these mineral salts dissolve in water, they may separate into ions—electrically charged particles called electrolytes. Sodium and potassium are the body's major electrolytes. They are extremely important. The movement of nutrients and wastes, respectively, into and out of cells is controlled primarily by the level and types of electrolytes.

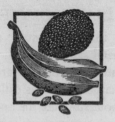

CHAPTER 10

Minerals and Disease

Minerals are not getting the same attention vitamins have been getting lately—not because they don't deserve it, though. Minerals can protect you from some of the same diseases that vitamins can. And some minerals work cooperatively with vitamins: Selenium and vitamin E, calcium and vitamin D, and zinc and vitamin A are just a few examples of vitamin and mineral teamwork.

Many minerals have unique effects that cannot be mimicked by vitamins. But minerals have the potential to be more toxic than vitamins. For many trace minerals, there is a fine line between not enough and too much. Most of the benefits attributed to minerals come from consuming the normal amounts found in foods. Unless you are correcting a deficiency under a doctor's supervision, taking more than twice the recommended amount of a mineral may do more harm than good.

HEART DISEASE

Several essential minerals may have an effect—and not necessarily a good one—on heart disease risk. Some minerals protect the heart by acting as antioxidants, some benefit the circulatory system by other means, and some may do harm when overdone.

SELENIUM

Selenium is an antioxidant thought to protect against heart disease. Unlike vitamin antioxidants, which act directly on free radicals, mineral antioxidants work with enzyme proteins. Taking a mineral supplement may ensure that these enzymes live up to their potential.

But the benefits of selenium are not unlimited. You won't receive any further advantage if your intake is higher than the level at which the enzymes are working at maximum capacity. This limited benefit is probably a good thing, considering that high doses of some minerals can be toxic.

The idea that selenium can protect the heart comes from studies of a particular type of heart disease in China called Keshan disease. Keshan disease involves deterioration of heart muscle in children and pregnant women. The disease is much more common in areas of China where the selenium content of the soil is poor.

Could there be a connection between Keshan disease and the selenium content of foods found in various regions? Keshan disease does not exist in the United States. Comparisons of soil selenium levels and rates of heart disease have not turned up consistent results. That may be because we eat foods from many regions of the country, not just locally grown produce. Or perhaps another factor combines with low selenium intake to trigger the disease.

Selenium protects the heart in other ways, too. The mineral controls the levels of hormonelike substances called prostaglandins. One of these substances promotes the ability for blood vessels to constrict and clots to form. Working as part of an antioxidant enzyme, selenium controls how much of this prostaglandin is formed. Selenium also favors production of another prostaglandin, which has the opposite effect. When there is insufficient selenium, too much of the first type of prostaglandin forms, which could lead to clogged arteries and heart disease.

CHROMIUM

Other minerals may also affect heart disease risk, even though they do not function as antioxidants. Investigators are looking at the potential for chromium supplements to lower blood cholesterol levels. Autopsies show that the blood chromium levels in people who died from heart disease are much lower than in people who died from accidents. People who live in countries where heart disease is common also have less chromium in their arteries than people from countries where heart disease is rare.

A recent study looked at people with high blood cholesterol levels who took 200 micrograms (μg) of chromium picolinate for six weeks. It lowered their total cholesterol approximately 19 percent and low-density lipoprotein (LDL) cholesterol by approximately 21 percent. Moreover, chromium lowered the blood level of bad LDL cholesterol without lowering the blood level of good high-density lipoprotein (HDL) cholesterol.

IRON

Recently, scientists renewed fears that too much iron might increase the risk of heart attack. A single study from Finland found that heart attacks occurred more often in men with high blood levels of the storage form of iron, ferritin. This study unleashed a rash of publicity about too much iron in our diets and in supplements. It suggested that women might be at lower risk for heart attacks because they consume less iron than men. However, researchers have yet to test the effects of iron on heart attacks in women.

There is concern about iron and a hereditary disease called hemochromatosis, or iron overload. One of the consequences of this insidious condition is heart disease. Most people do not absorb more iron than they need regardless of how much is in their diets because they have controls to prevent excessive absorption. But people who have this inherited defect, mostly men, do not have these normal controls.

Even people who haven't inherited the defect can override their bodies' controls by consuming large amounts of alcohol. Indeed, in the Finnish study, high ferritin levels were associated with increased alcohol consumption.

Until other investigators duplicate these results, a conservative approach toward iron is prudent. Yet it is unwise to avoid dietary iron, because a deficiency of this mineral has serious implications. Lowered resistance to infection could be life threatening, especially for children. It might also interfere with their ability to learn.

HYPERTENSION AND STROKE

High blood pressure, or hypertension, increases the risk of heart disease and stroke. Mineral protection comes from calcium, magnesium, and potassium, all of which promote low blood pressure. Hypertension is less frequent in regions of the country with hard water, which is higher in calcium and magnesium. Soft water usually contains more sodium.

People who eat diets rich in fruits, dark green leafy vegetables, and whole grains rarely suffer from high blood pressure. These foods contribute substantial amounts of potassium and magnesium to the diet. Consumption of calcium-rich milk is also directly related to a reduced risk of hypertension.

In addition to promoting lower blood pressure, dietary potassium may also protect against stroke. A study in southern California looked at the consumption of potassium and other minerals in adults between the ages of 50 and 79. The study found that the risk of dying from stroke over a 12-year period was two and a half times greater for the men who consumed the lowest amount of potassium, and it was five times greater for the women who consumed the lowest amounts. The effect of potassium intake on preventing stroke deaths was stronger than that of either calcium or magnesium.

CANCER

For a long time, the only mineral thought to offer protection against cancer was selenium. Calcium is now believed to offer that protection, too.

Early studies of selenium were confusing. Some found reduced rates of cancers in people living in areas with selenium-rich soil, whereas others showed higher rates of cancers. In one study in Finland, cancer risk was six times greater for people with the lowest levels of selenium in their blood, with an even higher risk for those whose vitamin E level also was low.

215

Whether selenium promotes cancer may depend on which carcinogens are present. As part of an antioxidant enzyme, selenium stimulates the system in the liver that is responsible for detoxifying chemicals. This system takes some carcinogens out of action, but it also triggers others. Because of this dual effect, it's important not to consume too much or too little of this mineral.

The possibility that calcium may offer protection against colon and rectal cancers has generated excitement among researchers. They're finding low rates of colon cancer where calcium intakes are high. In the Northeast, for example, where calcium intakes are the lowest in the United States, many more people die from these cancers than in other regions. Fewer people die from colon cancer in the western United States, where calcium intakes are the highest.

Recently, researchers confirmed that people getting more calcium (1,500 mg in this case) produced less bile acid than those getting little calcium. Bile acids are believed to stimulate tumor growth in the colon; therefore, excessive bile acid production could mean a greater risk of colon cancer.

Eating a diet rich in calcium might not be enough, however. A high fat intake might offset benefits from increased calcium intake. For this reason, turn to low-fat sources of calcium such as skim milk, yogurt, dried beans, dark green leafy vegetables, and tofu (coagulated with calcium) when trying to increase your calcium intake.

DIABETES

With age, some people find it more and more difficult to control blood sugar levels. This difficulty is usually linked to a loss in potency of the hormone insulin rather than to a deficiency of it. Deficiencies of several minerals may contribute to the problem as well.

Chromium assists insulin in removing sugar from the blood, but blood chromium levels decline with age, particularly in people who consume a diet of mostly processed foods. (Processing removes chromium from foods such as whole grains, which are a particularly rich source of chromium before being refined.) At the same time, foods rich in refined sugars such as sweets, presweetened breakfast cereals, and baked goods increase the need for this nutrient.

In one study of older people with non–insulin-dependent diabetes, blood sugar returned to normal when chromium supplements were taken. Older people with mildly elevated blood sugar levels are the most likely to respond to these supplements.

Magnesium supplements may also benefit blood sugar levels in older adults. Magnesium levels are lower in the blood of people with diabetes compared with healthy people, and like chromium, blood magnesium levels decline with age. In a study of older people with non–insulin-dependent diabetes, insulin's action on blood sugar improved with magnesium supplements.

The best sources of magnesium are spinach, other greens, and nuts. Since these aren't necessarily everyday foods, you might have to make an effort to get enough magnesium in your diet.

IMMUNE FUNCTION

If you've suffered a cold or the flu lately, you are one of millions who can appreciate how important a properly functioning immune system is. But it does more than you may think. Your immune system not only fights off viruses and bacterial infections, it also destroys cancer cells in the early stages of the disease. To ensure optimal immune function, several minerals, including iron, zinc, copper, and selenium, are also needed.

Iron-deficiency anemia is the most common nutritional deficiency disease in the world. Women during their child-bearing years and children are the most susceptible. Many people with iron-deficiency anemia die from infection because of weakened immune systems. Iron's role in maintaining immunity covers every aspect of how the system works. Iron is a vital component of a number of substances that are lethal to bacteria and found in saliva, tears, and human breast milk. Iron is also needed to help produce antibodies and to maintain your white blood cell count. Iron promotes the activity of "natural killer" immune cells, which are responsible for destroying cancer cells.

Although you need to make sure you are getting sufficient iron to keep your immune system active, too much iron can compromise your immune system. Bacteria and other organisms gobble up any excess iron and use it to help them thrive.

A robust immune system also calls for adequate zinc, though researchers aren't quite sure of its role. Zinc may help the functioning of two immune system organs: the thymic gland and the spleen. Zinc blood levels decline with age in some people, and when they do, a loss of immune function seems to follow. People with low blood levels of zinc suffer from more infection-related diseases than people with normal levels.

A few studies show improved immune function in elderly adults after taking zinc supplements, but other studies show no benefit. One study found that zinc supplements brought immune function in older adults back to levels seen in younger adults. As with iron, however, you must be careful not to take too much zinc. Levels twice the RDA boost immune function in men, but levels ten times the RDA actually depress it. Moreover, high doses of zinc can cause a copper deficiency.

Though copper may be another key mineral for the immune system, we know even less about its role than we do about the roles of iron and zinc. We do know that groups of people who experience clinical copper deficiency—preterm infants, children with genetic copper defects and hospital patients experiencing inadequate tube feedings— all suffer from depressed immune function, and all show improved immune response after taking copper supplements. Copper deficiency is rare, but intakes that are only marginally adequate are all too common.

OSTEOPOROSIS

Osteoporosis is a disease in which bone loss is so extensive that a bone can spontaneously fracture without any stress. These fractures are dangerous because they occur without warning and can cause falls or other accidents.

A calcium supplement will almost certainly be needed after menopause to help offset the bone loss caused by declining estrogen levels. Experts recommend that postmenopausal women take in 1,500 mg of calcium a day during the most susceptible time period—five to ten years after menopause.

Taking in a sufficient amount of magnesium is necessary to be sure the body is using calcium efficiently. Studies show that calcium supplements are not as effective in increasing bone density in people who are deficient in magnesium. In other words, calcium cannot correct bone loss if there is a magnesium deficiency. (The same is also true for vitamin D.)

Copper's contribution to bone strength receives little attention. The mineral network that supports bone depends on reactions involving copper. A weakness in this network weakens the entire structure. For example, preterm infants, who frequently develop copper deficiencies, suffer bone loss similar to that of adults with osteoporosis, despite their young ages. Though copper deficiency is rare in adults, many people may be getting suboptimal amounts. The consequences of a suboptimal intake are unknown.

CHAPTER 11

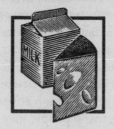

Mineral Profiles

Calcium

FUNCTIONS OF CALCIUM

Building strong bones and teeth is the most familiar function of calcium. Indeed, those bones and teeth contain 99 percent of all the calcium in your body. The remaining one percent circulates in blood or resides in the body's soft tissues. This one percent, however, plays many extremely important roles. It participates in blood clotting, contraction and relaxation of muscles, transmission of nerve impulses, activation of enzymes, and hormone secretion.

Because maintaining a normal blood calcium level is so important to vital functions such as heart rhythm, the body has a way to ensure a constant level of calcium in the blood, no matter how much your diet provides. The secret reservoir of calcium happens to be your bones, which release calcium into the blood as needed. But if this happens too rapidly, your bones suffer the consequences.

SOURCES OF CALCIUM

Milk, yogurt, cheese, and other dairy products are rich sources of calcium. Dried beans and peas and green vegetables such as broccoli, kale, bok choy, and chard are also good sources. Spinach, however, is not a good source; the calcium in spinach is not well absorbed because spinach contains a substance called oxalic acid that attaches to calcium, preventing its absorption.

Phytic acid, a substance found in whole grains and dried beans and peas, also combines with calcium and other minerals, preventing their absorption. This presents a problem only for people who consume extremely large amounts of these foods and do not drink milk. For those people, a calcium supplement might be necessary to prevent a deficiency.

Recently, fruit juices, cereals, and even bread are sporting added calcium. Fruit juices contain acids, such as citric acid, that boost the amount of calcium absorbed. For someone who does not, or cannot, drink milk, orange juice fortified with calcium can be a nutritious alternative. Mineral water may also contribute some calcium to the diet, as does hard water.

DIETARY REQUIREMENTS
FOR CALCIUM

The Recommended Dietary Allowance (RDA) for adults over age 25 is 800 milligrams (mg) of calcium. For women who are pregnant or breast-feeding, the RDA is now 1,200 mg. This is also the requirement for children more than 11 years of age, adolescents, and adults up to age 25.

But the RDAs are outdated. In 1994, the National Institutes of Health set higher standards for optimal calcium intake to help prevent or post-pone osteoporosis: 1,000 mg per day for women aged 25 to 50; 1,500 mg per day for postmeno-pausal women (1,000 mg per day if on hormone replacement therapy); 1,000 mg per day for men aged 25 to 65; 1,500 mg per day for men and women over age 65. These daily levels may be dif-ficult to meet from foods alone.

One quart of milk contains approximately 1,000 mg of calcium. Two cups of milk or its equivalent (as described in the Food Guide Pyramid in Chapter 1) contributes half an adult's daily requirement for calcium. Foods such as dark-green vegetables, breads, cereals, and dried beans provide the rest. If you cannot meet these levels through foods, you'll need a calcium supplement.

DEFICIENCY OF CALCIUM

A deficiency of calcium can stunt the development of bones and teeth. A lack of vitamin D, which is

Calcium Content of Common Foods

Food	Quantity	Milligrams (mg)
Meat–Protein Group		
Sardines, canned, drained	4 ounces	428
Salmon, pink, canned	4 ounces	239
Chicken, roasted, white meat, no skin	3 ounces	140
Navy beans	1 cup	127
Tofu (bean curd)	4 ounces	119
Almonds, roasted	¼ cup	69
Hamburger with bun	4 ounces	68
Peanuts, roasted	¼ cup	64
Milk–Dairy Group		
Yogurt, low-fat	1 cup	372
Milk, skim	1 cup	302
Milk, whole	1 cup	291
Swiss cheese	1 ounce	272
Ice cream	1 cup	169
American cheese	1 ounce	142
Cream cheese	1 tablespoon	8
Bread–Cereal/Grain Group		
Farina	1 cup	56
Bread, whole-wheat	1 slice	23
Bread, white, enriched	1 slice	21
Rice, white, cooked	1 cup	16
Fruits–Vegetables Group		
Turnip greens	1 cup	197
Figs, dried	½ cup	144
Broccoli	1 cup	94
Green beans	1 cup	61

Calcium Content of Common Foods
(continued)

Food	Quantity	Milligrams (mg)
Cabbage, raw	1 cup	33
Olives, green	10	24
Apple	1 medium	10
Other		
Soup, chicken noodle	1 cup	31

needed for calcium's absorption and use, can have a similar effect. Without it, there's a softening of bones, called rickets in children and osteomalacia in adults.

Bones suffer the brunt of insufficient calcium because they defer their needs to other functions that demand a higher priority. Blood clotting and muscle contraction are critical functions of calcium that must be sustained to preserve life. If muscle contractions go awry, your heart can stop. So when the blood contains too little calcium, bones give up their calcium for these functions. If this happens too often, your bones become porous and weak.

The result of such weakening is osteoporosis, or adult bone loss. If you lose one third or more of your bone mass, fractures can spontaneously occur. One in four postmenopausal women develops osteoporosis; in men, the condition is less common because they have a larger bone mass to work with and generally take in more calcium. Low calcium intake during childhood, teen, and early adult years can set the stage for osteoporosis in later life.

CALCIUM USE AND MISUSE

Doctors correct a calcium deficiency with calcium supplements, which often have vitamin D added to ensure calcium absorption. Doctors also prescribe calcium supplements to postmenopausal women to prevent osteoporosis, since it can be difficult to get the recommended amount of calcium. Some use the recommended amount of calcium as an adjunct to estrogen replacement therapy.

Recent research indicates that calcium supplements may benefit people who have high blood pressure. The supplements may also be useful in preventing a condition that sometimes occurs in pregnancy, called toxemia. In addition, studies show that people with higher intakes of calcium may be less likely to develop colon cancer (see Chapter 10 for more information).

The belief that large doses of calcium supplements will increase the risk of kidney stones is unfounded. Recent research showed that men who consumed more than 1,000 mg of calcium daily were only half as likely to get kidney stones as those who consumed less than 600 mg. This indicates that a high-calcium diet could actually protect against kidney stones rather than increase risk.

Calcium carbonate is the most common form of calcium found in supplements. This is the type of calcium in crushed oyster shells and some antacids. However, it is only 40 percent calcium. The label indicates this with a statement, such as: "Each tablet provides 1,250 mg of calcium carbonate, which yields 500 mg of elemental calcium."

Some people tout bone meal and dolomite as "natural" sources of calcium, but because they can be contaminated with lead, arsenic, or other toxic metals, their use is not recommended. (See the Supplement Product Profiles in Chapter 12 for an evaluation of specific calcium supplements.)

Phosphorus

Besides calcium, phosphorus is vital for strong bones and teeth. Phosphorus also plays an important role in energy storage and release. It's found in DNA (deoxyribonucleic acid) and RNA (ribonucleic acid), the genetic materials that serve as the blueprints for the formation of new cells. Phosphorus is necessary for normal milk secretion and a variety of metabolic reactions as well.

The RDA for phosphorus is 800 mg per day for adults older than 25 years of age. For pregnant and nursing women, however, the RDA increases to 1,200 mg. For most age groups, the RDA for phosphorus is the same as for calcium. The ideal

Phosphorus Content of Common Foods

Food	Quantity	Milligrams (mg)
Meat–Protein Group		
Sardines, Atlantic, canned	3 ounces	412
Peanuts, roasted, salted	½ cup	375
Pork and beans	1 cup	296
Kidney beans, canned	1 cup	254
Almonds, roasted	¼ cup	205
Roast chicken, white meat, no skin	3 ounces	185
Pistachio nuts	¼ cup	161
Tuna, canned in water	3 ounces	156
Beef, rib roast	3 ounces	138
Luncheon meat	2 slices	92
Frankfurter	1	39
Milk–Dairy Group		
Milk, skim	1 cup	247
Milk, whole	1 cup	228
Bread–Cereal/Grain Group		
Pancake, whole-wheat	1 medium	96
Rice, white, enriched, cooked	1 cup	68
Bread, whole-wheat	1 slice	65
Bread, white, enriched	1 slice	24
Fruits–Vegetables Group		
Broccoli	1 cup	101
Potato, baked with skin	1	70
Figs, dried	½ cup	68
Bean sprouts, cooked	½ cup	58
Cauliflower, cooked	1 cup	43

Phosphorus Content of Common Foods
(continued)

Food	Quantity	Milligrams (mg)
Corn, sweet, yellow, fresh	½ cup	38
Beans, green, cooked	½ cup	16
Grapefruit	½ medium	12
Apple	1 medium	10
Peppers, sweet, raw, green, chopped	½ cup	10

ratio of calcium to phosphorus is one to one. Milk contains phosphorus and calcium in approximately this ratio.

Good sources of phosphorus are also good sources of protein—for example, such foods as milk and other dairy products, eggs, meat, fish, poultry, nuts, and whole grains are good sources of both. Even sodas and food additives supply some phosphorous. As a result, it's not a problem for most Americans to get enough phosphorus. Perhaps getting too much is.

Although phosphorus deficiency has been reported in some infants fed cow's milk and in some people taking large amounts of antacids, a deficiency is unlikely. As a matter of fact, Americans consume as much as four times their recommended dietary allowance. American diets are heavy in high-protein foods (such as meat, fish, or poultry), carbonated beverages, and ready-to-eat convenience foods—all of which increase the body's supply of phosphorus.

Some nutrition experts believe that these excessive phosphorus intakes, when coupled with low intakes of calcium, may be a key factor in whether people develop osteoporosis, because high levels of phosphorus may interfere with calcium absorption. Your best bet is to consume phosphorus-rich foods or drinks in moderation.

Magnesium

Although the body has less than two ounces of magnesium, it's a vital mineral. Magnesium is another vital part of the mineral structure of bones and teeth. As with calcium, bones act as a reservoir for magnesium so that it will be available when needed.

Magnesium plays a role in protein synthesis, muscle relaxation, and energy release. It also triggers important metabolic reactions, including calcium metabolism. The parathyroid hormone needs magnesium to function normally; this regulates blood calcium levels.

Magnesium is found in most foods, particularly green leafy vegetables. This is because magnesium is part of chlorophyll, the pigment in plants that makes them green and fosters photosynthesis. Other good sources of magnesium are dairy products, breads and cereals, nuts, chocolate, and dried

Magnesium Content of Common Foods

Food	Quantity	Milligrams (mg)
Meat–Protein Group		
Navy beans, cooked	1 cup	108
Black-eyed peas, cooked	1 cup	91
Beans, lima, boiled	½ cup	41
Tuna, canned in water	4 ounces	32
Beef, chuck roast	3 ounces	23
Chicken breast, no skin	½	20
Egg, hard-boiled	1 large	5
Milk–Dairy Group		
Yogurt, nonfat	1 cup	47
Milk, whole	1 cup	33
Ice cream, vanilla, plain	½ cup	9
Cheddar cheese	1 ounce	8
Bread–Cereal/Grain Group		
Oatmeal	1 cup	57
Granola, ready-to-eat	½ cup	55
Noodles, egg	1 cup	30
Bread, whole-wheat	1 slice	27
Rice, white, cooked	⅔ cup	13
Fruits–Vegetables Group		
Figs, dried	½ cup	59
Broccoli, cooked	1 cup	37
Avocado	½ medium	34
Asparagus, fresh	½ cup	12
Strawberries, whole, fresh	⅔ cup	10
Cauliflower, cooked	½ cup	8
Apple	1 medium	7
Mushrooms, raw	½ cup	4

peas and beans. Hard water also contains significant amounts of magnesium—one of the minerals that makes it "hard."

The RDA for magnesium is 350 mg a day for men and 280 mg a day for women. Pregnant women need 20 mg per day more. Breast-feeding women require an extra 75 mg per day for the first six months to replenish the magnesium lost in breast milk. An additional 60 mg per day is enough during the second six months.

Magnesium deficiency can occur after prolonged vomiting or diarrhea, alcohol abuse, or long-term use of diuretics. A high intake of calcium can increase magnesium excretion, which can lead to problems such as nervousness and tremors. Magnesium deficiency also causes muscles to remain contracted, leading to a loss of muscle control. It may also be the cause of hallucinations in people undergoing alcohol withdrawal.

Although a true dietary deficiency of magnesium is unusual, some experts believe suboptimal intakes may be common, with long-term consequences for bone health. Moreover, research suggests that people who regularly drink hard water, which is high in magnesium, have a lower incidence of sudden death from heart failure than do people who regularly drink soft water.

Magnesium may also benefit blood pressure. Pregnant women and people taking diuretics may be able to lower their blood pressure with supplemental magnesium. Consult with your physician if you think you might benefit.

Magnesium toxicity, on the other hand, is also a potential problem because magnesium is present in so many over-the-counter preparations. Recently, the government revealed 14 deaths from magnesium toxicity over the past two and a half decades; they involved people who misused magnesium-containing antacids and laxatives, taking much more than label directions indicate. The risk is greatest for those who absorb more magnesium than usual and those who cannot effectively excrete an excess. This group includes older people and those with long-standing diabetes or kidney disease. People who have had intestinal surgery or who are taking medication to slow intestinal activity are also at higher risk of magnesium toxicity.

Chlorine

Chlorine is an important regulator of body systems, such as water balance, acid–base balance, and fluid pressure. For example, this mineral is part of hydrochloric acid, needed in the stomach for digestion. The acidity it creates ensures proper absorption of food and reduces the growth of harmful bacteria.

There is no RDA for chlorine. The recommended minimum safe intake is 750 mg. Regular table salt is 60 percent chlorine, as chloride. This source, along with the salt that occurs naturally in foods, provides all the chlorine that's needed. Even a diet restricted in sodium can supply adequate amounts of chlorine.

A chlorine deficiency is not likely because chlorine is so prevalent in foods, but it can happen under certain circumstances. For example, several years ago some infant formula was processed without chlorine. Children fed this formula as their sole food source developed chlorine deficiencies.

Sodium

FUNCTION OF SODIUM

Sodium plays a critical role in regulating water balance in the body. It's also important for regulating acid–base balance, transmitting nerve impulses, maintaining muscle activity and cell membrane function, and absorbing and transporting certain nutrients. Sodium is also a part of body fluids such as sweat and tears.

SOURCES OF SODIUM

There's sodium in almost all the foods you eat; it's there either naturally or is added in processing. Celery, carrots, greens, beets, eggs, and milk, for example, are naturally high in sodium. But no matter how high the natural sodium level of some foods, the level found in processed foods is always higher. Foods such as pickles, luncheon meats, canned vegetables, soups, and frozen dinners are extremely high in sodium because processing adds so much salt (sodium chloride).

Unfortunately, you can't always tell if food is high in sodium simply by tasting it. For example, cheese, cold breakfast cereal, ice cream, and prepared puddings are often high in sodium, even though they don't taste salty.

Even substances such as toothpaste and mouthwash contain sodium. So does the drinking water in many areas. Artificially softened water adds about 150 mg per quart of water—not a lot unless you are following a severely sodium-restricted diet. If so, run a separate line that bypasses the water softener to your kitchen sink cold water faucet. Your cooking and drinking water will then contain only the sodium naturally present in the water. You'll also preserve the calcium and magnesium in your water, since hard water is rich in these nutrients.

How can you tell how much sodium is in the foods you buy? Check the label. Though sodium has been on the label since 1986, specific guidelines for declaring sodium content and making health claims were only established in 1994.

Manufacturers may now use the following terms:

- sodium free—less than 5 mg of sodium per serving

- very low sodium—less than 35 mg per serving (for dehydrated soup mixes, less than 35 mg per 50 g serving after reconstituting)
- low sodium—less than 140 mg per serving
- reduced sodium—at least 25 percent less sodium than a comparable food (For example, potato chips would have to be compared with a similar salty snack.)
- unsalted—no salt added during processing (The salted version of the food it resembles and substitutes for must normally be processed with salt. An unsalted product has to state it is not sodium free if it contains sodium in forms other than sodium chloride.)
- salt free—must be sodium free

These rules apply to single foods only. For packaged main dishes, such as frozen dinners or entrées, the amounts of sodium are expressed per 100 g. Because of this, these products might be labeled low sodium but still have more sodium than the amounts given above.

DIETARY REQUIREMENTS OF SODIUM

Most of the sodium you eat comes from sodium chloride—common table salt. About 40 percent of table salt is sodium. On average, Americans eat about 4 to 5 g (4,000 to 5,000 mg) of sodium per day. (Your intake may be higher if your diet includes a lot of processed foods.) But you only need one tenth of that—about 500 mg of sodium—to meet your body's actual need for this mineral. Experts recommend that total daily sodium not exceed 2,400 mg.

DEFICIENCY OF SODIUM

Because the body has a large sodium reserve and, under normal circumstances, people eat plenty of sodium-containing foods, a deficiency is not likely. However, salt depletion can temporarily occur through profuse sweating if you exercise strenuously for a prolonged time in warm weather or hot climates. Even in this situation, salt that's lost is easily replaced by eating salty foods. Salt tablets are not necessary and can be dangerous.

SODIUM USE AND MISUSE

High blood pressure rarely appears in cultures with low salt intakes. Is that a coincidence? Most researchers think not. Yet for all the population studies that link high salt intake with high blood pressure, it's never been proven that salt causes blood pressure to rise.

A new study in chimps—as biologically close to humans as you can get—proved that salt could raise blood pressure and could lower it when removed. The Australian researchers used salt levels that mimicked human levels. They also eliminated calcium and potassium as factors by supplementing their diets with these minerals. The chimp study also confirmed the popular theory that some people may be "salt sensitive." These

Sodium Content of Common Foods

Food	Quantity	Milligrams (mg)
Meat–Protein Group		
Beef, ground	4 ounces	95
Pork, roasted	3 ounces	79
Peanut butter	1 tablespoon	76
Turkey, no skin, light or dark meat	3 ounces	66
Egg, whole	1 large	63
Chicken, white meat, without skin	3 ounces	60
Kidney beans, dried	1 cup	4
Milk–Dairy Group		
Cheese, cheddar	1 ounce	176
Milk, whole	1 cup	120
Ice cream, 10% fat	1 cup	105
Butter, salted	1 tablespoon	76
Bread–Cereal/Grain Group		
Bread, white	1 slice	127
Brewer's yeast, dried	1 tablespoon	10
Fruits–Vegetables Group		
Sauerkraut	1 cup	1,560
Pickle, dill	1	993
Olives, green	5	480
Tomato juice	½ cup	438
Raisins, seedless	½ cup	9
Asparagus, cooked	1 cup	7
Zucchini, cooked	1 cup	5
Potato, baked, without skin	1 medium	5
Apple	1 medium	0

Sodium Content of Common Foods
(continued)

Food	Quantity	Milligrams (mg)
Others		
Soy sauce	2 tablespoons	2,057
Baking powder, sodium aluminum sulfate	1 tablespoon	1,140
Potato chips	1 cup	195

individuals may be more susceptible than others to developing high blood pressure because of salt intake.

Because a tendency toward salt sensitivity might be inherited, you'd be wise to cut back on the salt in your diet and check your blood pressure regularly if you have a family history of hypertension. Because Americans as a group consume a lot of salt and high blood pressure is widespread, a low-salt diet might be a wise choice for everyone (unless otherwise directed by a doctor).

Doctors generally advise people diagnosed with high blood pressure to reduce their salt intake. But because not everybody is salt sensitive, not everyone will benefit from salt restriction. The only way to know for sure is to try it. Moreover, experts say a low-sodium diet improves the response to some medications, such as diuretics, making them more effective in treating high blood pressure.

Potassium

The body normally contains about 9 g of potassium. Most of it is found inside body cells. Potassium plays an important role in maintaining water balance and acid–base balance. Its presence is crucial in the transmission of nerve impulses from nerves to muscles. It also acts as a catalyst in carbohydrate and protein metabolism. Because potassium is a constant part of muscle, measurements of potassium content can estimate body composition.

Studies are increasingly suggesting that a high intake of potassium-rich foods reduces blood pressure and the risk of stroke.

Theoretically, when potassium intake is high, the body excretes more sodium, lowering blood pressure. Vegetarians, for example, have lower blood pressure than nonvegetarians. Though it is difficult to rule out all other factors, vegetarians do eat diets rich in fruits and vegetables, and thus rich in potassium.

Some diuretics commonly prescribed to treat high blood pressure cause the body to lose potassium. If you take such a diuretic, you can compensate for the loss by eating foods rich in potassium. While almost all whole foods contain some potassium, particularly good sources include milk, meat, potatoes, tomatoes, prunes, bananas, oranges, and dried peas and beans. As a group, fruits and vegetables reign supreme in the potassium-supply category. Processed foods, on the other hand, lose much of their potassium.

Potassium combined with chloride is effective at restoring potassium losses from the body and can satisfy a taste for table salt. In fact, many salt substitutes are compounds of potassium chloride. People with kidney disease, however, should avoid them.

Because potassium is found in so many foods, dietary deficiency is unlikely. However, uncontrolled diabetes or a prolonged, excessive water loss (as from sweating) may result in potassium depletion. Rapid weight loss—from liquid diets or fasting—can also deplete the body of potassium. Muscle weakness is an early sign that potassium depletion is occurring. Potassium depletion is a very serious situation. Not only can it interfere with muscle action and fluid balance, but it can lead to abnormal heart rhythm, possibly triggering a heart attack.

The safe minimum level of intake for potassium is 2,000 mg per day for adults. Some nutritionists think 3,000 mg per day would benefit those with high blood pressure.

Potassium supplements are not usually recommended. Physicians may prescribe them to prevent potassium depletion in people taking certain types of diuretics, however.

Potassium Content of Common Foods

Food	Quantity	Milligrams (mg)
Meat–Protein Group		
Lima beans, cooked	1 cup	955
Pinto beans, cooked	1 cup	800
Kidney beans, canned	1 cup	713
Peas, split, cooked	1 cup	710
Sirloin steak, lean	6 ounces	674
Peanuts, dried, unsalted	½ cup	491
Sole/flounder, baked	3 ounces	394
Milk–Dairy Group		
Yogurt	1 cup	624
Milk, whole	1 cup	370
Cheese, cheddar	1 ounce	28
Bread–Cereal/Grain Group		
Brewer's yeast	1 tablespoon	224
Wheat germ	2 tablespoons	134
Bread, whole-wheat	1 slice	78
Fruits–Vegetables Group		
Cantaloupe melon	½ medium	1,426
Bok choy, cooked	1 cup	631
Spinach, cooked	1 cup	566
Watermelon	1 slice	559
Beets, cooked	1 cup	518
Potato, baked, with skin	1 medium	510
Zucchini, cooked	1 cup	455
Banana	1 medium	451
Winter squash, baked	1 cup	407
Asparagus	1 cup	392
Broccoli	1 cup	331

Potassium Content of Common Foods
(continued)

Food	Quantity	Milligrams (mg)
Apricots	3 small	314
Cauliflower	1 cup	250
Orange	1 medium	237
Orange juice	½ cup	236
Celery	½ cup	172
Peach	1 medium	171

Sulfur

Sulfur is found throughout the body, especially in the skin, hair, and nails. The mineral aids in the storage and release of energy. It's a component of the genetic material of cells, and it helps promote enzyme reactions and blood clotting. Sulfur is part of two B vitamins—biotin and thiamin. Sulfur also combines with certain toxic materials so they can then be excreted safely from the body through the urine.

Although there is no RDA for sulfur, it's not because it plays an unimportant role. When protein intake is adequate, sulfur intake is adequate as well. That's because sulfur-containing amino acids (the building blocks of protein) supply the body with the amount of sulfur it needs. However, taking in adequate amounts of sulfur from other sources preserves these amino acids for their other vital functions.

A wide variety of foods contain sulfur. Cheese, eggs, fish, poultry, grains, nuts, and dried peas and beans are all rich sources.

Iron

FUNCTION OF IRON

Most of the body's iron resides in the hemoglobin of red blood cells—the pigment that makes these blood cells appear red. Hemoglobin carries oxygen to cells and transports carbon dioxide from cells. Iron is also essential to enzymes involved in energy release, cholesterol metabolism, immune function, and connective-tissue production.

SOURCES OF IRON

Good sources of iron include liver and other meats, whole grains, shellfish, green leafy vegetables, and nuts. Iron is one of the nutrients added to enriched cereals and bread. According to recent research, soybean hulls (not the whole soybean) contain a very absorbable form of iron. In the future, these hulls may fortify other foods with iron.

Cooking in iron pots adds iron to the foods prepared in them. This is especially true of acidic foods such as tomatoes. Take note that milk is a poor source of iron, however, and should not be relied on to fulfill iron requirements for infants and children.

DIETARY REQUIREMENTS FOR IRON

The RDA for iron is 10 mg per day for adult men and postmenopausal women and 15 mg per day for menstruating women. Women who are pregnant or breast-feeding require more iron. Iron requirements are also greater during periods of growth and development.

DEFICIENCY OF IRON

The typical American diet provides about 6 mg of iron for every 1,000 calories. This presents a problem for women who often eat fewer than 2,000 calories a day. Men, on the other hand, who often eat 2,500 calories a day or more, are much more likely to meet their RDA, which is lower anyway. Women lose iron in their menstrual flow each month, which adds to the concern of iron deficiency.

Absorption of iron is notoriously poor—only about ten percent of what's eaten. The iron in meat, heme iron, is absorbed better than the non-heme iron found in vegetables. (The soy hulls mentioned earlier are an exception.) Meat, fish, poultry, and vitamin C all increase iron absorption. Coffee, tea, whole soybeans, and whole grains, on the other hand, all reduce the amount of iron absorbed from foods eaten at the same meal.

Iron deficiency is the most common cause of anemia. Headache, shortness of breath, weakness, fatigue, heart palpitations, and sore tongue are some of the symptoms of anemia. For people who are anemic, even mild exercise can cause chest pain. Mild iron deficiency, even without anemia, may cause learning problems in school children.

Pica, an abnormal desire to eat nonfood substances such as clay, chalk, ashes, or laundry starch (none of which contains iron), sometimes accompanies iron deficiency. That's because the eating of such nonfoods may interfere with iron absorption and may be a factor contributing to the anemia.

Long-term use of aspirin can cause bleeding in the lining of the stomach and may lead to iron deficiency because of blood loss. Aspirin coated with a special material reduces irritation to the stomach lining. Drinking plenty of water when you take aspirin can also help.

Young children fed mostly milk can develop a milk-induced anemia. Milk contains little iron and in very large quantities may actually promote irritation and bleeding in the stomach. Anemia can result from this loss of blood.

The normal acidity of the stomach helps promote iron absorption in the intestine. A deficiency may

Iron Content of Common Foods

Food	Quantity	Milligrams (mg)
Meat–Protein Group		
Liver, beef	2½ ounces	4.8
Liver, chicken	½ cup	4.5
Soybeans, cooked	½ cup	4.4
Peas, dried, cooked	2½ cups	2.0
Beef, lamb	3 ounces	1.8–2.4
Chicken breast	1 whole	1.7
Pork, veal	3 ounces	0.9–3.3
Fish	3 ounces	0.6–1.5
Bread–Cereal/Grain Group		
Farina	1 cup	10.0
Bread, whole-grain	2 slices	1.7
Spaghetti, noodles, or macaroni, cooked	1 cup	1.5–2.0
Bread, enriched	2 slices	1.4
Cereals, enriched, ready-to-eat	1 cup	1.0–18.0
Fruits–Vegetables Group		
Spinach, cooked	1 cup	2.9
Figs, dried	½ cup	2.2
Potato, baked with skin	1 medium	1.7
Turnip greens, cooked	1 cup	1.2
Cherries, fresh	1 cup	0.6
Honeydew melon	½ medium	0.4
Grapes	1 cup	0.4
Raisins	2 tablespoons	0.4

result from chronic use of antacids, however, which decreases the acidity of the stomach, and reduces the amount of iron absorbed.

An estimated eight percent of women and one percent of men in the United States exhibit symptoms of iron deficiency. (More people are estimated to have inadequate iron reserves.) There's been an improvement in the iron status of infants, however, due in part to the greater use of iron-fortified formula.

IRON USE AND MISUSE

To treat an iron deficiency, you need iron supplements in conjunction with an iron-rich diet. Iron is available in both a ferrous and ferric form. Iron in the ferrous forms is better absorbed than ferric iron. When you read labels of iron supplements, you should note that the number of milligrams for each tablet refers both to the iron it contains and the carrier to which it's bound. For example, the label may state, "Each tablet provides 200 mg of ferrous fumarate, which yields 67 mg of elemental iron." The amount of elemental iron is what you should consider.

Some people don't tolerate iron supplements well and may develop side effects such as heartburn, nausea, stomachache, constipation, or diarrhea. Taking the supplement with food can eliminate or minimize these symptoms. You can also gradually work up to the desired dose or divide the high dose into several small doses. Do not worry if your stool appears dark or black. It's just some of the unabsorbed iron.

In healthy people, the intestines control the amount of iron that's absorbed. The body increases its rate of iron absorption if reserves are low. And when the body becomes saturated with iron, the rate of absorption decreases. If the intestines do not or cannot properly perform this regulatory function—as can happen from excessive and prolonged alcohol intake—the body can absorb toxic quantities.

A certain percentage of the population suffers from hemochromatosis, a hereditary disease in which the body absorbs too much iron and deposits it in body tissues. Unfortunately, symptoms of this condition only appear after significant and irreversible damage occurs. They include weakness, weight loss, change in skin color, abdominal pain, loss of sex drive, and the onset of diabetes. Heart, liver, and joints may become impaired as well. Men are affected by this disease more often than women. The treatment for this disease involves the removal of excess iron in the body.

Iron poisoning is the most common accidental poisoning in young children. Excess iron can be fatal. All supplements should be kept out of the reach of children.

Iodine

FUNCTIONS OF IODINE

Almost half the body's iodine is found in the thyroid gland. Iodine is an important component of thyroid hormones, which control energy metabolism in the body as well as body temperature, reproduction, and growth.

SOURCES OF IODINE

Saltwater seafood is a primary source of iodine. Iodized salt, in use since 1924, is another rich source. One teaspoon of iodized salt provides 260 micrograms (μg) of iodine, nearly twice the RDA. The amount of iodine in vegetables and grains varies according to how much is present in the soil where they are grown. In certain regions of the world, this amount is less than optimal.

In the United States, the need for iodized salt is not as great as it was 50 years ago. Thanks to refrigerated trucks, most of the country gets produce from coastal regions where soil is rich in iodine. Iodine deficiency is a concern only in isolated areas where all the food eaten is locally grown.

Dairy equipment is sometimes disinfected with iodine-containing compounds, and dairy cattle are fed iodine-containing feed. Both contribute to an increasing amount of iodine in milk and dairy products. Iodine is also in dough conditioners used by bakeries, in food colorings, and even in polluted air, providing perhaps the lone benefit of air pollution.

DEFICIENCY OF IODINE

A deficiency of iodine can cause the thyroid gland to enlarge greatly—a condition known as goiter. The thyroid gland, which is normally about the size of a lima bean, can sometimes become as large as a person's head. A deficiency of thyroid hormones can result in mental and physical sluggishness, slowed heart rate, weight gain, constipation, and increased sleep needs (14 to 16 hours a day). In pregnancy, the results of iodine deficiency are more serious. The baby of an iodine-deficient mother may have retarded physical and mental development—a condition known as cretinism.

Certain substances known as goitrogens induce goiter when iodine intake is low. Cabbage, brussels sprouts, cauliflower, turnips, and peanuts contain these substances. However, since heat destroys goitrogens, the potential dangers exist only if large amounts of these foods are eaten raw.

IODINE USE AND MISUSE

Because Americans are taking in several times the RDA for iodine, they rarely need supplements. Some experts even question whether iodized table salt is still necessary. As salt intake declines, this source becomes less important.

Some people who are overweight mistakenly blame their overweight condition on an underactive thyroid gland. In the hopes of speeding up their metabolism, they may start taking a supplement or eating sea salt or seaweed. But in very large amounts, iodine can be poisonous.

Some people are sensitive to this mineral and may break out in a rash if their iodine intake is excessive. The rash, which resembles acne, disappears when the iodine is reduced.

Zinc

FUNCTIONS OF ZINC

Most zinc resides in our bones. The rest of this trace mineral turns up in skin, hair, and nails. In men, the prostate gland contains more zinc than any other organ. Zinc is a part of more than 70 different enzyme systems that aid the metabolism of carbohydrates, fats, and proteins. One of these enzymes, superoxide dismutase, serves as an antioxidant in cells. Zinc is part of the hormone insulin, and it plays an important role in the transport of vitamin A from its storage site in the liver so that it can be used in the body.

SOURCES OF ZINC

Oysters contain more zinc than any other food. Meat, poultry, eggs, and liver are also rich sources. Two servings of animal protein daily provide most of the zinc a healthy person needs. Whole grains contain fair amounts of zinc, but they also harbor phytates, substances that combine with the zinc and prevent its absorption. Yeast counteracts the action of phytates, so eating whole-grain breads still affords good nutrition.

DIETARY REQUIREMENTS
FOR ZINC

The RDA for zinc is 15 mg daily for adult men and 12 mg daily for adult women. Pregnant or breast-feeding women need larger amounts. Experts estimate that the average American diet provides about 10 mg per day.

DEFICIENCY OF ZINC

Zinc deficiency has serious effects, including:

- retarded growth and sexual development
- delayed wound healing
- a low sperm count
- depressed immune system (making infections more likely)
- reduced appetite
- altered sense of taste and smell

Low zinc intakes may be a factor in toxemia—a condition that sometimes occurs in pregnancy and may contribute to a lower birth weight for the baby.

Many experts suspect that marginal zinc intakes are common in the United States. As many as 90 percent of elderly Americans may take in suboptimal amounts of zinc. Why? The decreased consumption of meat, which has become a fairly common health practice in the Amercan diet, results in reduced zinc intake. Low-calorie diets also tend to be low in zinc.

Vegetarian diets, especially vegan diets that do not contain any animal products, may promote a zinc deficit. If vegetarians eat whole-grain breads made with yeast, they absorb zinc better, because yeast breaks down the phytates in whole grains. Unleavened bread, such as pita and flat bread, contains intact phytates that tie up zinc, preventing its absorption. Strict vegetarians should be sure to consult their doctors about the use of a zinc supplement. (A multimineral supplement that contains iron might not provide the zinc you expect, however, because iron interferes with zinc absorption.)

Infections, injuries, or other physical sources of stress can cause zinc loss in the urine. Pica—eating nonfood substances such as clay, chalk, or ashes—can contribute to reduced zinc absorption.

ZINC USE AND MISUSE

These days, zinc is a popular supplement. Many people suffer a loss of smell and taste due to aging, cancer treatments, or serious infections. In some people, zinc supplements are legitimately useful in restoring these senses. Zinc also improves healing in people with bedsores and other wounds.

Zinc Content of Common Foods

Food	Quantity	Milligrams (mg)
Meat–Protein Group		
Oysters, Eastern, raw	6	76.3
Beef, chuck	3 ounces	4.4
Chicken, white meat, no skin	3 ounces	1.4
Peas, split, cooked	½ cup	1.0
Soybeans, cooked	½ cup	1.0
Salmon, steak, broiled	4 ounces	0.8
Peanut butter	2 tablespoons	0.8
Egg, whole	1 large	0.6
Milk–Dairy Group		
Milk, whole	1 cup	0.9
Cheese, American	1 ounce	0.8
Bread–Cereal/Grain Group		
Bran flakes	1 cup	2.0
Rice, brown	⅔ cup	0.8
Bread, whole-grain	1 slice	0.6
Egg noodles, enriched, cooked	½ cup	0.5
Bread, white, enriched	1 slice	0.2
Fruits–Vegetables Group		
Potato, baked, with skin	1 medium	0.4
Broccoli, cooked	½ cup	0.3
Carrot, raw	1 medium	0.2
Pineapple, fresh or canned	1 cup	0.1
Tomato, raw	1 medium	0.1
Orange	1 medium	0.1

Restoring zinc to optimal levels certainly aids these conditions, but whether zinc in excess of needs has any real effect is debatable.

People with sickle-cell disease may lose a lot of zinc in their urine. Zinc supplements can be helpful in restoring deficiencies. Zinc supplements may also help reduce perspiration odor and treat acne. The effectiveness of these treatments is still in question.

A rare inherited disease called acrodermatitis enteropathica impairs zinc absorption. Zinc supplementation can control the symptoms, which include eczema, hair loss, retarded growth, and emotional problems.

People who suffer from a rare inherited disorder called Wilson disease need zinc to treat the abnormally large copper accumulations that occur in their bodies.

Excessive zinc supplementation—more than 50 mg per day—can cause copper deficiency and anemia. Large amounts of zinc can cause vomiting, diarrhea, fever, kidney failure, and even death. In the past, when certain foods and drinks were served in galvanized containers, the zinc coatings leached into the food, poisoning people. However, the chance of such toxicity occurring is low.

Because of high zinc levels in the prostate gland, doctors use zinc therapy to treat and manage certain prostate disorders. Whether such zinc therapy is beneficial is still unclear. However, there is no hard evidence that a zinc deficiency causes these disorders, nor is there evidence that zinc therapy can be beneficial.

Fluoride

Fluoride is an essential trace mineral found in bones, teeth, and body fluids. If fluoride is available when bones and teeth develop, it's incorporated into their structures, making teeth more resistant to decay and bones more resistant to osteoporosis. Fluoride also maintains the structure of bones and teeth after they are formed.

There is no RDA for fluoride, but there is a suggested safe and adequate range of intake of 1.5 to 4.0 mg daily.

Water is the most common source of fluoride in the diet. Fish and tea are surprisingly good sources as well. A cup of tea provides about 0.2 mg of fluoride.

Research shows that people who live in areas where the drinking water contains less than one part per million of fluoride have more dental decay and osteoporosis. In many areas of the country, water is fluoridated to a level of one part per million—the optimal level. Studies clearly show that children raised in such areas have 50 percent fewer cavities than children who do not drink fluoridated water.

In areas where the natural fluoride concentration in the water is high (two to eight parts per million), the enamel on children's teeth may become mottled (spotted)—a condition called fluorosis. The condition doesn't seem to be harmful; in fact, mottled teeth are very resistant to decay.

There is strong opposition to fluoridation of drinking water in some areas. Opponents claim that fluoridated water increases the incidence of cancer, birth defects, and other health problems. However, there is no established evidence to indicate that drinking water containing one part per million of fluoride is harmful. Indeed, fluoridation is one of the most thoroughly studied community health measures in recent history. The U.S. Public Health Service, the World Health Organization, the National Cancer Institute, and the U.S. Centers for Disease Control have all refuted claims linking fluoridation to public health risks. The only effect optimally fluoridated water seems to have on lifelong users is a decreased incidence of tooth decay and osteoporosis.

Copper

Copper helps the body absorb and use iron. It's part of several enzymes that help form hemoglobin (the oxygen-carrying pigment in red blood cells) and collagen (a connective-tissue protein found in skin and tendons). Some of the best sources of copper include shellfish, liver, dried peas and beans, nuts, cocoa, raisins, fruits, and vegetables.

There is no RDA for copper, but the suggested safe and adequate range of intake is 1.5 to 3.0 mg. The average American diet provides about 2.0 mg per day.

A dietary deficiency of copper is very rare but has occurred in severely malnourished children, disrupting their growth and metabolism. It can also occur in infants born prematurely because copper isn't usually transferred from the mother to the fetus until the last few weeks of pregnancy.

An excessive intake of copper, which has been reported to occur after water was stored in copper tanks, may cause headaches, dizziness, nausea, and vomiting.

Children who inherit the gene for Wilson disease cannot get rid of excess copper. It accumulates in certain organs in their bodies, especially the eyes, brain, liver, and kidneys. It's treated with a copper-free diet and medication designed to bind with the copper, rendering it harmless.

Chromium

Chromium is part of the glucose tolerance factor (GTF) that regulates the actions of insulin—the hormone necessary for glucose metabolism. In chromium-deficient people, insulin doesn't function properly. In such cases, chromium supplements can improve the body's ability to handle glucose. Experts believe a suboptimal chromium deficit is widespread, particularly among older people, and may explain why the incidence of glucose intolerance increases with age.

A diet rich in refined carbohydrates such as sugar increases the need for chromium. And the more refined and processed foods are, the less chromium they contain. Americans' high intake of sugary, processed foods could well be contributing to a minor chromium crisis.

Brewer's yeast and wheat germ are rich in chromium. Other sources include whole grains, meats, cheese and other dairy products, seafood, broccoli, and eggs.

Chromium picolinate supplements have become increasingly popular. And though they may improve some people's chromium nutrition, they will not magically melt away pounds as some advertisements imply.

There is no RDA for chromium. However, a suggested safe and adequate range of intake is 0.05 to 0.2 mg per day. If you have diabetes or glucose intolerance, consult with a physician before taking supplements. Although they might benefit your condition, they might also alter your need for medication.

Manganese

About 20 mg of manganese is in the body. Manganese helps ensure proper bone formation and connective-tissue growth. It activates many enzymes that regulate metabolism. It may also play a role as an antioxidant, as part of the enzyme superoxide dismutase.

Good sources of manganese include nuts, whole grains, and dried peas and beans. There is no RDA for manganese. However, a suggested safe and adequate range of intake is 2.0 to 5.0 mg per day. Deficiencies have not been reported. Miners who have been exposed to large amounts of manganese dust over long periods of time show symptoms of brain disease, however.

Selenium

Selenium is found in all body tissues, with the highest concentrations in the kidneys, liver, spleen, pancreas, and testicles.

Selenium functions as an antioxidant as part of the enzyme glutathione peroxidase. It helps prevent cell damage from free radicals that form when oxygen attacks, or oxidizes, fats and other compounds. Severe deficiency of selenium affects heart function, but a deficiency is hard to detect because vitamin E can substitute for selenium in some of its functions, thus masking the classic symptoms.

A super source of selenium is the Brazil nut. More down-to-earth sources include meat and fish. The amount found in grains depends on the selenium content of the soil in which they were grown.

The RDA for selenium is 55 µg for adult women and 70 µg for adult men. A typical American diet generally provides this amount.

Because selenium works as an antioxidant along with vitamin E, some studies suggest that the mineral may have anticancer properties (see Chapter 5). This idea arose from research on cancer rates that are high in areas of the world where the soil contains little selenium.

A recent Harvard University study, however, found no such protective effect when it looked at 1,000 women who were followed at six different cancer sites. In a surprising twist, the study actually found an increased risk for cancer among the women with the highest selenium intakes.

Too much selenium can be toxic because this mineral can substitute for sulfur in the proteins of some important enzymes, altering their functions. So if you take selenium supplements, they should contain no more than the RDA. Selenium taken as seleno-amino acid is much less toxic because the selenium substitution has already been made.

Molybdenum

This hard-to-pronounce mineral (muh LIB duh num) functions as part of the enzyme systems involved in carbohydrate, fat, and protein metabolism.

Good sources of molybdenum are liver, wheat germ, whole grains, and dried peas and beans. The molybdenum content of food varies according to what was in the soil from which it came. No RDA exists for molybdenum, but a safe and adequate range of intake is 0.075 to 0.25 mg daily—easily acquired from the average diet.

Reports indicate that excessive intakes of molybdenum trigger goutlike symptoms and other toxic effects. Do not take supplements of this mineral unless a doctor advises you to do so.

Cobalt

As part of vitamin B12, cobalt plays a major role in the body's metabolic processes. There is no RDA for cobalt because it is usually obtained from vitamin B12.

Other Trace Minerals

While we do not yet know enough about some of the trace elements to establish requirements for them, evidence is accumulating that some of them may be essential for humans.

There is a case for a mineral being declared essential when its presence in the diet promotes growth or other responses related to health. Another piece of evidence occurs when the absence of the element in the diet causes blood levels to decrease. Perhaps the most convincing of all is when the mineral is found in the tissues of newborn infants. The placenta normally serves as a barrier to protect the fetus from environmental contaminants. If a mineral transcends this barrier, it is probably because the fetus needs it.

Evidence is growing that nickel, silicon, arsenic, and boron will soon be classified as essential for humans. Nickel is present in all tissues of the body. It is firmly attached to DNA and a protein that binds to it in the blood. Silicon has been shown to stimulate bone growth in animals, and boron is involved in human bone growth. Even arsenic might be essential, based on its importance for metabolism of the amino acid methionine.

CHAPTER 12

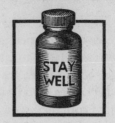

Supplement Product Profiles

A lthough we make it clear throughout this book that there's no substitute for a healthy diet, we also know that nutritional needs can change with time and circumstance. We live in a time when we are unsure of the optimal amounts of vitamins and minerals needed to prevent disease. The levels for some nutrients may be too high to get from diet alone, and so a supplement may be needed.

Food should supply the basic levels of nutrients. Supplements should only be used to provide any additional amounts you may be lacking. By relying on food for most of your nutritional needs, you get the benefits of the other components of foods—namely, phytochemicals. Supplements cannot offer you those benefits.

Until we know exactly how much of each nutrient is ideal, be sure to keep dosages at reasonable levels to prevent toxicity.

To guide you in your choice of supplements, we've profiled more than 90 of the mainstream vitamin, mineral, and combination products commonly available in the United States. In each profile, you will find the product name, the manufacturer, the dosage form (capsules, tablets, liquid), the ingredients, and their amounts. Other information, such as warnings or possible side effects, is included as it applies.

The dosage levels are expressed as a percentage of the U.S. RDA because this conforms to the current labeling regulations for dietary supplements. This may change when new regulations take effect. Specific comments, however, are based on the current 1989 RDAs and not on the older U.S. RDAs.

CONSUMER GUIDE™ does not recommend that people who are in good health use supplements as a way to replace a balanced diet. If you're in doubt as to your vitamin or mineral status, check with your doctor or a registered dietitian. After a thorough evaluation of your diet, eating habits, state of health, and other factors that may affect your nutritional needs, he or she can help you determine whether supplements are necessary and which ones might be beneficial.

ALLBEE C-800
(multivitamin supplement)

Manufacturer: A.H. Robins Company

Dosage form: Tablets

Ingredients:

vitamin C	800 mg
thiamin (B$_1$)	15 mg
riboflavin (B$_2$)	17 mg
niacin	100 mg
vitamin B$_6$	25 mg
pantothenic acid	25 mg
vitamin E	45 IU
vitamin B$_{12}$	12 μg

Comments:

- This product contains more than 100 percent of the adult RDAs for the nutrients included.
- This product has more than three times the upper limit of the recommended intake for pantothenic acid.
- Vitamin C, thiamin, and riboflavin are given in megadoses (ten or more times the RDA).

ALLBEE C-800 PLUS IRON
(multivitamin supplement with iron)

Manufacturer: A.H. Robins Company

Dosage form: Tablets

Ingredients:

vitamin C	800 mg
thiamin (B1)	15 mg
riboflavin (B2)	17 mg
niacin	100 mg
vitamin B6	25 mg
pantothenic acid	25 mg
vitamin E	45 IU
folic acid	0.4 mg
vitamin B12	12 µg
iron	27 mg

Comments:

- This product contains more than 100 percent of the RDAs for adult men and women for all of the nutrients that it contains. It also has more than three times the upper limit of the recommended intake for pantothenic acid.
- Vitamin C, thiamin, and riboflavin are given in megadoses (ten or more times the RDA).
- Iron interacts with antacids and oral tetracycline antibiotics, reducing their absorption.
- Accidental iron poisoning is a possibility, especially with young children. Be sure to keep all supplements stored out of their reach.

ALLBEE WITH C
(vitamin C supplement with B vitamins)

Manufacturer: A.H. Robins Company
Dosage form: Caplets

Ingredients:

vitamin C	300 mg
thiamin (B₁)	15 mg
riboflavin (B₂)	10.2 mg
niacin	50 mg
vitamin B₆	5 mg
pantothenic acid	10 mg

Comment:

• This product contains more than 100 percent of the RDAs for adult men and women for all of the nutrients that it contains.

AVAIL
(calcium supplement plus multivitamins/minerals)

Manufacturer: Menley & James
Dosage form: Tablets
Ingredients:

vitamin A	5,000 IU
vitamin D	400 IU
thiamin (B₁)	2.25 mg
riboflavin (B₂)	2.55 mg
niacin	20 mg
vitamin C	90 mg
vitamin B₆	3 mg
vitamin B₁₂	9 µg
folic acid	0.4 mg
vitamin E	30 IU
iron	18 mg
magnesium	100 mg

calcium	400 mg
zinc	22.5 mg
iodine	150 µg
chromium	15 µg
selenium	15 µg

Comments:
- This product contains more than 100 percent of the RDA for vitamins C, B1, B2, B6, and B12 and the mineral zinc.
- Accidental iron poisoning is a possibility, especially with young children. To avoid accidental poisoning, be sure to keep all supplements stored out of their reach.

BETA-CAROTENE
(vitamin supplement)

Manufacturer: Nature's Bounty, Inc.
Dosage form: Softgels
Ingredient:
  beta-carotene (provitamin A)   25,000 IU

Comments:
- There is currently no RDA for beta-carotene. The intake recommended by many health professionals is 6 mg (10,000 IU). This product provides 15 mg, or 2½ times the recommended amount.
- Ample provitamin A can be provided by beta-carotene-rich deep-yellow or dark-orange vegetables and fruits and green, leafy vegetables.

BUGS BUNNY COMPLETE
(multivitamin/mineral children's chewable supplement)

Manufacturer: Miles Laboratories, Inc.
Dosage form: Chewable tablets
Ingredients:

vitamin A	5,000 IU
vitamin D	400 IU
vitamin E	30 IU
vitamin C	60 mg
folic acid	0.4 mg
thiamin (B_1)	1.5 mg
riboflavin (B_2)	1.7 mg
niacin	20 mg
vitamin B_6	2 mg
vitamin B_{12}	6 μg
biotin	40 μg
pantothenic acid	10 mg
iron	18 mg
calcium	100 mg
copper	2 mg
phosphorus	100 mg
iodine	150 μg
magnesium	20 mg
zinc	15 mg

Comments:

• Dosage levels for most of the nutrients are at 100 percent of the adult RDAs. Despite the name, the vitamin levels are greater than most RDAs for children.

- Calcium and magnesium levels are well below recommended amounts.
- This product contains no manganese, selenium, chromium, or molybdenum.
- This product contains phenylalanine and should not be used by those with phenylketonuria.
- Iron is well above the level recommended for children.
- Iron interacts with antacids and oral tetracycline antibiotics, reducing absorption of these drugs.
- Accidental iron poisoning is a possibility, especially with young children. Be sure to keep all supplements, especially those that are designed to be attractive to children, stored out of their reach.
- This product is sugar free.

BUGS BUNNY PLUS IRON
(multivitamin children's chewable supplement)

Manufacturer: Miles Laboratories, Inc.
Dosage form: Chewable tablets
Ingredients:

vitamin A	2,500 IU
vitamin D	400 IU
vitamin E	15 IU
vitamin C	60 mg
folic acid	0.3 mg

thiamin (B$_1$)	1.05 mg
riboflavin (B$_2$)	1.2 mg
niacin	13.5 mg
vitamin B$_6$	1.05 mg
vitamin B$_{12}$	4.5 µg
iron	15 mg

Comments:

- Dosage levels are reasonable for most of the nutrients provided.
- Calcium and magnesium are well below recommended amounts.
- This product contains phenylalanine and should not be used by those with phenylketonuria.
- Iron interacts with antacids and oral tetracycline antibiotics, reducing their absorption.
- Accidental iron poisoning is a possibility, especially with young children. Store all supplements out of their reach.
- This product is sugar free.

BUGS BUNNY
WITH EXTRA C
(multivitamin children's
chewable supplement)

Manufacturer: Miles Laboratories, Inc.
Dosage form: Chewable tablets
Ingredients:

vitamin A	2,500 IU
vitamin D	400 IU

vitamin E	15 IU
vitamin C	250 mg
folic acid	0.3 mg
thiamin (B_1)	1.05 mg
riboflavin (B_2)	1.2 mg
niacin	13.5 mg
vitamin B_6	1.05 mg
vitamin B_{12}	4.5 μg

Comments:
- Dosage levels are reasonable for most of the nutrients provided.
- This product is sugar free.

CALTRATE 600
(calcium supplement)

Manufacturer: Lederle Laboratories
Dosage form: Tablets
Ingredient:

elemental calcium	600 mg

Comments:
- The calcium is provided as calcium carbonate (1,500 mg).
- This product has no sugar, salt, or lactose.

CALTRATE 600 + D
(calcium supplement with vitamin D)

Manufacturer: Lederle Laboratories
Dosage form: Tablets

Ingredients:

elemental calcium	600 mg
vitamin D	200 IU

Comments:

- The calcium is provided as calcium carbonate (1,500 mg).
- The vitamin D may not be needed if you are taking a multivitamin supplement that contains vitamin D. The vitamin is important to the process of calcium deposition in bones.
- This product does not contain sugar, salt, or lactose.

CALTRATE PLUS
(multivitamin/mineral supplement)

Manufacturer: Lederle Laboratories
Dosage form: Tablets
Ingredients:

elemental calcium	600 mg
vitamin D	200 IU
magnesium	40 mg
zinc	7.5 mg
copper	1 mg
manganese	1.8 mg
boron	250 μg

Comment:

- The calcium is provided as calcium carbonate (1,500 mg).

CENTRUM
ADVANCED FORMULA
(multivitamin/mineral supplement)

Manufacturer: Lederle Laboratories
Dosage form: Tablets
Ingredients:

vitamin A	5,000 IU
vitamin E	30 IU
vitamin C	60 mg
folic acid	0.4 mg
thiamin (B_1)	1.5 mg
riboflavin (B_2)	1.7 mg
niacinamide	20 mg
vitamin B_6	2 mg
vitamin B_{12}	6 µg
vitamin D	400 IU
biotin	30 µg
pantothenic acid	10 mg
calcium	162 mg
phosphorus	109 mg
iodine	150 µg
iron	18 mg
magnesium	100 mg
copper	2 mg
manganese	3.5 mg
potassium	80 mg
chloride	72 mg
chromium	65 µg

molybdenum	160 µg
selenium	20 µg
zinc	15 mg
vitamin K	25 µg
nickel	5 µg
tin	10 µg
silicon	2 mg
vanadium	10 µg
boron	150 µg

Comments:

- This product contains more than 100 percent of the adult RDA for vitamin B_{12}, vitamin E, and iron.
- This product has reasonable amounts of vitamins A, C, and B_6 and most minerals.
- The levels of calcium, magnesium, potassium, and selenium are below recommended intake levels.
- This product also includes trace minerals for which a need has not been demonstrated.
- Accidental iron poisoning is a possibility, especially with young children. Be sure to keep all supplements stored out of their reach.

CENTRUM
Advanced Formula
(multivitamin/mineral
supplement)

Manufacturer: Lederle Laboratories
Dosage form: Liquid

Ingredients:

vitamin A	2,500 IU
vitamin E	30 IU
vitamin C	60 mg
thiamin (B1)	1.5 mg
riboflavin (B2)	1.7 mg
niacinamide	20 mg
vitamin B6	2 mg
vitamin B12	6 µg
vitamin D	400 IU
biotin	300 µg
pantothenic acid	10 mg
iodine	150 µg
iron	9 mg
manganese	2.5 mg
chromium	25 µg
molybdenum	25 µg
zinc	3 mg

Comments:

- Don't be fooled. Though it has the same name, this liquid form of Centrum Advanced Formula has an entirely different formulation from the tablets.
- This supplement contains more than 100 percent of the adult RDA for both vitamin B12 and vitamin E.
- This product has reasonable amounts of vitamins A, C, and B6.
- It contains no folate, calcium, magnesium, copper, potassium, or selenium. Molybdenum is below the recommended intake level.

CENTRUM JR. WITH IRON
(multivitamin/mineral children's chewable supplement)

Manufacturer: Lederle Laboratories
Dosage form: Chewable tablets
Ingredients:

vitamin A	5,000 IU
vitamin E	30 IU
vitamin C	60 mg
thiamin (B_1)	1.5 mg
riboflavin (B_2)	1.7 mg
niacinamide	20 mg
folic acid	0.4 mg
vitamin B_6	2 mg
vitamin B_{12}	6 µg
vitamin D	400 IU
biotin	45 µg
pantothenic acid	10 mg
vitamin K	10 µg
iodine	150 µg
iron	18 mg
calcium	108 mg
phosphorus	50 mg
magnesium	40 mg
manganese	1 mg
chromium	20 µg
copper	2 mg
molybdenum	20 µg
zinc	15 mg

Comments:
- For children 2 to 4 years of age, this supplement contains more than 100 percent of the RDA for all the nutrients it contains, except vitamin D.
- This product contains no potassium or selenium. Molybdenum is below recommended intake level.

CITRACAL
(calcium supplement)

Manufacturer: Mission Pharmaceuticals
Dosage form: Tablets
Ingredient:

calcium	200 mg

Comment:
- The calcium in this supplement is provided as calcium citrate (950 mg).

DAYALETS
(multivitamin supplement)

Manufacturer: Abbott Laboratories
Dosage form: Tablets
Ingredients:

vitamin A	5,000 IU
vitamin D	400 IU
vitamin E	30 IU
vitamin C	60 mg
folic acid	0.4 mg
thiamin (B$_1$)	1.5 mg

riboflavin (B2)	1.7 mg
niacin	20 mg
vitamin B6	2 mg
vitamin B12	6 µg

Comments:
- Levels of vitamins are reasonable.
- This product is sugar free.

DAYALETS PLUS IRON
(multivitamin supplement plus iron)

Manufacturer: Abbott Laboratories
Dosage form: Tablets
Ingredients:

vitamin A	5,000 IU
vitamin D	400 IU
vitamin E	30 IU
vitamin C	60 mg
iron	18 mg
folic acid	0.4 mg
thiamin (B1)	1.5 mg
riboflavin (B2)	1.7 mg
niacin	20 mg
vitamin B6	2 mg
vitamin B12	6 µg

Comments:
- Accidental iron poisoning is a possibility, especially with young children. Be sure to keep all supplements stored out of their reach.
- This product is sugar free.

ENER-B
(vitamin B12 supplement)

Manufacturer: Nature's Bounty, Inc.
Dosage form: Intranasal gel
Ingredient:
  vitamin B12   400 µg
Comments:
- Each applicator delivers $\frac{1}{10}$ cc of gel into the nose.
- Each application contains a megadose of vitamin B12 (ten or more times the adult RDA).
- The name is gimmicky. Vitamin B12 does NOT provide energy.

FEMIRON
(iron supplement)

Manufacturer: Menley & James
Dosage form: Tablets
Ingredient:
  Iron   20 mg
Comments:
- This supplement contains more than 100 percent of the adult RDA for iron.
- This supplement should not be used by alcoholics or by anyone who has liver or pancreatic disease.
- This product could irritate the stomach and intestines if not taken with food.

- A darkened stool may result from use of this supplement.
- Iron interacts with antacids and oral tetracycline, reducing absorption of these drugs.
- Accidental iron poisoning is a possibility, especially with young children. Be sure to keep all supplements stored out of their reach.

FEMIRON MULTIVITAMINS AND IRON
(iron supplement plus multivitamins)

Manufacturer: Menley & James
Dosage form: Tablets
Ingredients:

iron	20 mg
vitamin A	5,000 IU
vitamin D	400 IU
thiamin (B_1)	1.5 mg
riboflavin (B_2)	1.7 mg
niacin	20 mg
vitamin C	60 mg
vitamin B_6	2 mg
vitamin B_{12}	6 µg
pantothenic acid	10 mg
folic acid	0.4 mg
vitamin E	15 IU

Comments:
- Amounts of vitamins included in this supplement are at reasonable levels.

- This supplement contains more than 100 percent of the adult RDA for iron.
- This product does not contain vitamin K or biotin.
- This product should not be used by alcoholics or individuals with chronic liver or pancreatic disease.
- This product could depress zinc absorption.
- This product could irritate the linings of the stomach and intestines if not taken with some food.
- A darkened stool may result from use of this supplement.
- Iron interacts with antacids and oral tetracycline antibiotics, reducing absorption and efficacy of these drugs.
- Accidental iron poisoning is a possibility, especially with young children. Be sure to keep all supplements stored out of their reach.

FEOSOL
(iron supplement)

Manufacturer: SmithKline Beecham
Dosage form: Capsules
Ingredient:
  elemental iron   50 mg
Comments:
- The supplement contains 500 percent of the RDA for iron for men and more than 300 percent of the RDA for iron for women.

- Capsules contain FD&C Red No. 40. The safety of this food colorant is in question.
- This product may cause gastrointestinal discomfort and nausea. These side effects may be minimized by taking the supplement with meals.
- Other side effects include constipation or diarrhea.
- This product could depress zinc absorption.
- Iron interacts with antacids and oral tetracycline antibiotics, reducing the absorption of these drugs.
- Accidental iron poisoning is a possibility, especially with young children. Be sure to keep all supplements stored out of their reach.

FEOSOL ELIXIR
(iron supplement)

Manufacturer: SmithKline Beecham
Dosage form: Liquid
Ingredient:
  elemental iron   44 mg
Comments:
- This supplement contains more than 400 percent of the adult RDA for iron.
- This product contains 5 percent alcohol.
- This product may cause gastrointestinal discomfort and nausea. These side effects may be minimized by taking the supplement along with meals.

- Other side effects include constipation or diarrhea and temporary staining of the teeth.
- The amount of iron in this product might depress zinc absorption.
- Iron interacts with antacids and oral tetracycline antibiotics, reducing absorption of these drugs.
- Accidental iron poisoning is a possibility, especially with young children. Be sure to keep all supplements stored out of their reach.

FERGON
(iron supplement)

Manufacturer: Bayer Corp.
Dosage form: Tablets
Ingredient:
  elemental iron   36 mg
Comments:

- The iron in this product provides more than 300 percent of the RDA for iron for men and more than 200 percent for women.
- Iron is provided in the form of ferrous gluconate (320 mg).
- This product may cause nausea, abdominal cramps, constipation, or diarrhea.
- The amount of iron in this product might depress zinc absorption.
- Iron interacts with antacids and oral tetracycline antibiotics, reducing proper absorption of these drugs.

- To prevent iron poisoning, store all supplements out of children's reach.

FERRO-SEQUELS
(iron supplement)

Manufacturer: Lederle Laboratories
Dosage form: Timed-release tablets
Ingredient:

elemental iron	50 mg

Comments:

- Iron is provided as ferrous fumarate (150 mg).
- This product contains 100 mg of docusate sodium to prevent constipation.
- This product contains lactose and sodium but qualifies as "low sodium."
- It is formulated to release iron slowly.
- Iron interacts with antacids and oral tetracycline antibiotics, reducing their absorption.
- To prevent iron poisoning, store all supplements out of children's reach.

FLINTSTONES
(multivitamin children's chewable supplement)

Manufacturer: Bayer Corp.
Dosage form: Chewable tablets
Ingredients:

vitamin A	2,500 IU
vitamin D	400 IU
vitamin E	15 IU

vitamin C	60 mg
folic acid	0.3 mg
thiamin (B$_1$)	1.05 mg
riboflavin (B$_2$)	1.2 mg
niacin	13.5 mg
vitamin B$_6$	1.05 mg
vitamin B$_{12}$	4.5 μg

Comments:

- For children 2 to 4 years of age, this product contains more than 100 percent of the RDA for vitamins C and E, folic acid, thiamin, riboflavin, niacin, and vitamin B$_6$. It contains more than 400 percent of the RDA for vitamin B$_{12}$.
- For children older than age 4, this product contains more than 100 percent of the RDA for folic acid and vitamins B$_{12}$, C, and E.
- This product does not include vitamin K, biotin, or pantothenic acid.
- This product should not be used by children who have phenylketonuria.

FLINTSTONES WITH EXTRA C
(multivitamin children's chewable supplement)

Manufacturer: Bayer Corp.
Dosage form: Chewable tablets
Ingredients:

vitamin A	2,500 IU
vitamin D	400 IU

vitamin E	15 IU
vitamin C	250 mg
folic acid	0.3 mg
thiamin (B_1)	1.05 mg
riboflavin (B_2)	1.2 mg
niacin	13.5 mg
vitamin B_6	1.05 mg
vitamin B_{12}	4.5 µg

Comments:

- For children 2 to 4 years of age, this product contains more than 100 percent of the RDA for vitamin E, folic acid, thiamin, riboflavin, niacin, and vitamin B_6, more than 500 percent of the RDA for vitamin C, and more than 400 percent of the RDA for vitamin B_{12}.
- For older children, this product contains more than 100 percent of the RDA for folic acid and vitamins E and B_{12}. It contains more than 500 percent of the RDA for vitamin C.
- This product does not include vitamin K, biotin, and pantothenic acid.
- This product should not be used by children who have phenylketonuria.

FLINTSTONES WITH IRON
(multivitamin children's chewable supplement with iron)

Manufacturer: Bayer Corp.
Dosage form: Chewable tablets

Ingredients:

vitamin A	2,500 IU
vitamin D	400 IU
vitamin E	15 IU
vitamin C	60 mg
folic acid	0.3 mg
thiamin (B$_1$)	1.05 mg
riboflavin (B$_2$)	1.2 mg
niacin	13.5 mg
vitamin B$_6$	1.05 mg
vitamin B$_{12}$	4.5 μg
iron	15 mg

Comments:

- For children aged 2 to 4 years, this product contains more than 100 percent of the RDA for vitamins E, B$_6$, and C; folic acid; thiamin; riboflavin; niacin; and iron; and more than 400 percent of the RDA for vitamin B$_{12}$.
- This product does not contain vitamin K, biotin, or pantothenic acid.
- This product should not be used by children who have phenylketonuria.
- To prevent iron poisoning, store all supplements out of children's reach.

FLINTSTONES COMPLETE
(multivitamin/mineral children's chewable supplement)

Manufacturer: Bayer Corp.
Dosage form: Chewable tablets

───────────────── ◉ ─────────────────

Ingredients:

vitamin A	5,000 IU
vitamin D	400 IU
vitamin E	30 IU
vitamin C	60 mg
folic acid	0.4 mg
thiamin (B_1)	1.5 mg
riboflavin (B_2)	1.7 mg
niacin	20 mg
vitamin B_6	2 mg
vitamin B_{12}	6 μg
biotin	40 μg
pantothenic acid	10 mg
iodine	150 μg
iron	10 mg
calcium	100 mg
phosphorus	100 mg
magnesium	20 mg
copper	2 mg
zinc	15 mg

Comments:

- For children 2 to 4 years of age, this supplement contains more than 100 percent of the RDA for vitamin C, thiamin, riboflavin, niacin, and vitamin B_6 and 500 percent or more of the RDA for folic acid, vitamin E, and vitamin B_{12}.

- For children older than 4 years of age, this product contains more than 100 percent of the RDA for vitamin C, folic acid, vitamin E, and vitamin B_{12}.

- This product contains sorbitol and aspartame.
- This product should not be used by children who have phenylketonuria.

GARFIELD
(multivitamin/mineral children's chewable supplement)

Manufacturer: Menley & James
Dosage form: Chewable tablets
Ingredients:

vitamin A	5,000 IU
vitamin D	400 IU
vitamin E	30 IU
vitamin C	60 mg
folic acid	0.4 mg
thiamin (B1)	1.5 mg
riboflavin (B2)	1.7 mg
niacin	20 mg
vitamin B6	2 mg
vitamin B12	6 µg
biotin	40 µg
pantothenic acid	10 mg
iodine	150 µg
iron	18 mg
calcium	100 mg
phosphorus	100 mg
magnesium	20 mg
copper	2 mg
zinc	15 mg

Comments:

- For children 2 to 4 years of age, this supplement contains more than 100 percent of the RDA for vitamin C, thiamin, riboflavin, niacin, B_6, and iron. It contains 500 percent or more of the RDA for folic acid, vitamin E, and vitamin B_{12}.
- For children older than 4 years of age, this product contains more than 100 percent of the RDA for vitamin C, folic acid, vitamin E, vitamin B_{12}, and iron.
- This product contains sorbitol and aspartame.
- This product should not be used by children who have phenylketonuria.

GERITOL
(iron and multivitamin tonic)

Manufacturer: SmithKline Beecham
Dosage form: Liquid
Ingredients:

iron	18 mg
thiamin (B_1)	2.5 mg
riboflavin (B_2)	2.5 mg
niacin	50 mg
pantothenic acid	2 mg
vitamin B_6	0.5 mg
choline	50 mg
methionine	25 mg

Comments:

- This product contains more than 100 percent of the adult RDA for thiamin, riboflavin, and iron. It contains more than 300 times the adult RDA for niacin.

- Vitamin B6 is at about one-third the level of the adult RDA for this vitamin. The level of pantothenic acid is below the recommended range.
- This product does not contain vitamin B12.
- The usefulness of added choline and methionine is questionable.
- The product contains alcohol, which may accelerate the absorption of iron.
- This supplement should not be used by alcoholics or individuals with chronic liver or pancreatic disease. Those with inherited iron storage disease also should not use this product.
- This product may cause darkening of the stool.
- Iron interacts with antacids and oral tetracycline antibiotics, reducing the absorption of these drugs.
- Accidental iron poisoning is a possibility, especially with young children. Be sure to keep all supplements stored out of their reach.

GERITOL COMPLETE
(multivitamin/mineral supplement)

Manufacturer: SmithKline Beecham
Dosage form: Tablets

Ingredients:

vitamin A	
(as beta-carotene)	6,000 IU
vitamin E	30 IU
vitamin C	30 mg
folic acid	0.4 mg
thiamin (B₁)	1.5 mg
riboflavin (B₂)	1.7 mg
niacin	20 mg
vitamin B₆	2 mg
vitamin B₁₂	6 µg
vitamin D	400 IU
biotin	45 µg
pantothenic acid	10 mg
vitamin K	25 µg
calcium	162 mg
phosphorus	125 mg
iodine	150 µg
iron	50 mg
magnesium	100 mg
copper	2 mg
manganese	2.5 mg
potassium	37.5 mg
chloride	34.1 mg
chromium	15 µg
molybdenum	15 µg
selenium	15 µg
zinc	15 mg
nickel	5 µg
silicon	80 µg
tin	10 µg
vanadium	10 µg

Comments:

- This product contains more than 400 percent of the adult RDA for iron. It also contains more than 100 percent of the adult RDA for vitamin A, vitamin E, folic acid, vitamin B_{12}, and vitamin D. It also contains more than the recommended intake for pantothenic acid.
- This supplement should not be used by alcoholics or by individuals who have chronic liver or pancreatic disease.
- This product contains FD&C Red No. 40. The safety of this food colorant is in question.
- Accidental iron poisoning is a possibility, especially with young children. Be sure to keep all supplements stored out of their reach.

GERITOL EXTEND
(multivitamin/mineral supplement for adults 50+)

Manufacturer: SmithKline Beecham
Dosage form: Caplets
Ingredients:

vitamin A	3,333 IU
vitamin E	15 IU
vitamin C	60 mg
folic acid	0.2 mg
thiamin (B_1)	1.2 mg
riboflavin (B_2)	1.4 mg
niacin	15 mg
vitamin B_6	2 mg

vitamin B_{12}	2 µg
vitamin D	200 IU
vitamin K	80 µg
calcium	130 mg
phosphorus	100 mg
iodine	150 µg
iron	10 mg
magnesium	35 mg
selenium	70 µg
zinc	15 mg

Comments:

- This product contains more than 100 percent of the adult RDA for vitamin E and folic acid.
- This product does not contain pantothenic acid or biotin.
- It contains FD&C Red No. 40. The safety of this food colorant is in question. It also contains yellow dye No. 6—tartrazine—to which some people are allergic.
- To prevent iron poisoning, store all supplements out of children's reach.

GEVRABON
(multivitamin/mineral supplement)

Manufacturer: Lederle Laboratories
Dosage form: Liquid
Ingredients:

| thiamin (B_1) | 5 mg |
| riboflavin (B_2) | 2.5 mg |

niacin	50 mg
vitamin B$_6$	1 mg
vitamin B$_{12}$	1 µg
pantothenic acid	10 mg
iodine	100 µg
iron	15 mg
magnesium	2 mg
zinc	2 mg
choline	100 mg
manganese	2 mg

Comments:

- This product provides more than 100 percent of the adult RDA for thiamin, riboflavin, and niacin and above the recommended range of intake for pantothenic acid.
- This product contains most of the B vitamins. Folic acid is not included.
- Except for iron, this product contains only small amounts of some minerals.
- The usefulness of choline is questionable.
- This supplement contains 18 percent alcohol.
- Accidental iron poisoning is a possibility, especially with young children. Be sure to keep all supplements stored out of their reach.

GOOD SENSE CENTURY
(multivitamin/mineral supplement)

Manufacturer: Perrigo
Dosage form: Tablets

Ingredients:

vitamin A	5,000 IU
vitamin E	30 IU
vitamin C	60 mg
folic acid	0.4 mg
thiamin (B$_1$)	1.5 mg
riboflavin (B$_2$)	1.7 mg
niacinamide	20 mg
vitamin B$_6$	2 mg
vitamin B$_{12}$	6 µg
vitamin D	400 IU
biotin	30 µg
pantothenic acid	10 mg
calcium	162 mg
phosphorus	109 mg
iodine	150 µg
iron	18 mg
magnesium	100 mg
copper ·	2 mg
manganese	3.5 mg
potassium	80 mg
chloride	72 mg
chromium	65 µg
molybdenum	160 µg
selenium	20 µg
zinc	15 mg
vitamin K	25 µg

Comments:

- This product contains more than 100 percent of the adult RDA for vitamins B$_{12}$ and E and iron.

- This product has reasonable amounts of vitamins A, C, and B6 and most minerals.
- The levels of calcium, magnesium, potassium, and selenium are below recommended intake levels.
- Accidental iron poisoning is a possibility, especially with young children. Be sure to keep all supplements stored out of their reach.

HALLS VITAMIN C DROPS
(vitamin C supplement)

Manufacturer: Warner-Lambert
Dosage form: Drops
Ingredient:

vitamin C	60 mg

Comments:
- This product provides 100 percent of the adult RDA for vitamin C.
- This product contains sugar.

ICAPS PLUS
(antioxidant supplement)

Manufacturer: La Haye Laboratories
Dosage form: Tablets
Ingredients:

vitamin A (as beta-carotene)	6,000 IU
vitamin E	60 IU
vitamin C	200 mg
riboflavin (B2)	20 mg

301

copper	2 mg
manganese	5 mg
selenium	20 μg
zinc	40 mg

Comments:

- This product contains more than 100 percent of the RDA for vitamin A, vitamin C, vitamin E, and riboflavin.
- This supplement contains more than 100 percent of the RDA for zinc.
- Copper, manganese, and selenium are within recommended levels.

MYADEC PROFESSIONAL FORMULA
(multivitamin/mineral supplement)

Manufacturer: Parke-Davis
Dosage form: Tablets
Ingredients:

vitamin A	5,000 IU
vitamin D	400 IU
vitamin E	30 IU
vitamin C	60 mg
folic acid	0.4 mg
thiamin (B_1)	1.7 mg
riboflavin (B_2)	2.0 mg
niacin	20 mg
vitamin B_6	3 mg
vitamin B_{12}	6 μg

pantothenic acid	10 mg
vitamin K	25 µg
biotin	30 µg
iodine	150 µg
iron	18 mg
magnesium	100 mg
copper	2 mg
zinc	15 mg
manganese	2.5 mg
calcium	162 mg
phosphorus	125 mg
potassium	40 mg
selenium	25 µg
molybdenum	25 µg
chromium	25 µg

Comments:

- This product provides well above 100 percent of the adult RDA for vitamin A, vitamin C, thiamin, riboflavin, B6, B12, and iron.
- Amounts of pantothenic acid and copper are above the recommended intakes for these minerals.
- To prevent iron poisoning, store all supplements out of children's reach.

NATALINS
(multivitamin/mineral prenatal supplement)

Manufacturer: Mead-Johnson Nutritional Div.
Dosage form: Tablets

※

Ingredients:

vitamin A	4,000 IU
vitamin D	400 IU
vitamin E	15 IU
vitamin C	70 mg
folic acid	0.5 mg
thiamin (B_1)	1.5 mg
riboflavin (B_2)	1.6 mg
niacin	17 mg
vitamin B_6	2.6 mg
vitamin B_{12}	2.5 µg
calcium	200 mg
elemental iron	30 mg
zinc	15 mg
copper	1.5 mg

Comments:

- This product provides 100 percent of the RDA for pregnant and breast-feeding women for vitamin D, iron, and zinc.
- This supplement contains more than 100 percent of the RDA for vitamin B_6, vitamin E, and folic acid.
- This product supplies vitamin A, vitamin C, thiamin, riboflavin, and niacin at 100 percent of the RDA for pregnant women but not for breast-feeding women.
- Calcium is supplied at well below the RDAs for both pregnant and breast-feeding women.
- Iron interacts with antacids and oral tetracycline antibiotics, reducing absorption and efficacy of these drugs.

- Accidental iron poisoning is a possibility, especially with young children. Be sure to keep all supplements stored out of their reach.

N'ICE VITAMIN C DROPS
(sugarless vitamin C drops)

Manufacturer: SmithKline Beecham
Dosage form: Capsules
Ingredients:

60 mg of vitamin C (adult flavors: lemon, orange)

45 mg of vitamin C (children's flavor: grape)

Comments:
- This product provides 100 percent of the adult RDA for vitamin C at 60 mg and 100 percent of the RDA for children older than 4 years of age at 45 mg of vitamin C.
- This product contains sorbitol.

OCUVITE
(vitamin/mineral supplement)

Manufacturer: Lederle Laboratories
Dosage form: Tablets
Ingredients:

zinc	40 mg
copper	2 mg
vitamin C	60 mg
vitamin E	30 IU
beta-carotene	5,000 IU
selenium	40 µg

Comments:
- This product provides 200 percent or more of the adult RDA for zinc and vitamin E.
- This supplement provides 100 percent of the RDA for vitamin C and is within the recommended range for copper.
- This product contains half the recommended intake of beta-carotene.
- This product contains lactose.

OCUVITE EXTRA
(antioxidant supplement plus Z and B)

Manufacturer: Lederle Laboratories
Dosage form: Tablets
Ingredients:

beta-carotene	6,000 IU
riboflavin (B2)	3 mg
niacin	40 mg
vitamin C	200 mg
vitamin E	50 IU
zinc	40 mg
copper	2 mg
selenium	40 µg
manganese	5 mg
l-glutathione	5 mg

Comments:
- This product provides 200 percent or greater of the adult RDA for vitamins C and E, niacin, and the mineral zinc.

- It is within the recommended range for copper intake.
- This supplement provides about 50 percent more than the recommended daily amount of beta-carotene.
- The usefulness of added l-glutathione is questionable.
- This product contains lactose.

ONE-A-DAY
ESSENTIAL VITAMINS
(multivitamin supplement)

Manufacturer: Miles Laboratories, Inc.
Dosage form: Tablets
Ingredients:

vitamin A	5,000 IU
vitamin C	60 mg
thiamin (B1)	1.5 mg
riboflavin (B2)	1.7 mg
niacin	20 mg
vitamin D	400 IU
vitamin E	30 IU
vitamin B6	2 mg
folic acid	0.4 mg
vitamin B12	6 µg
pantothenic acid	10 mg

Comments:
- Most of the vitamins in this supplement are supplied in amounts that equal 100 percent of the adult RDA.

- It contains more than 100 percent of the adult RDA for vitamin E, vitamin D, folic acid, and vitamin B12.
- The amount of pantothenic acid is above the range of recommended intake.

ONE-A-DAY MAXIMUM FORMULA (multivitamin/mineral supplement)

Manufacturer: Miles Laboratories, Inc.
Dosage form: Tablets
Ingredients:

vitamin A	5,000 IU
vitamin C	60 mg
thiamin (B1)	1.5 mg
riboflavin (B2)	1.7 mg
niacin	20 mg
vitamin D	400 IU
vitamin E	30 IU
vitamin B6	2 mg
folic acid	0.4 mg
vitamin B12	6 μg
biotin	30 μg
pantothenic acid	10 mg
iron	18 mg
calcium	130 mg
phosphorus	100 mg
iodine	150 μg
magnesium	100 mg

copper	2 mg
zinc	15 mg
chromium	10 µg
selenium	10 µg
molybdenum	10 µg
manganese	2.5 mg
potassium	37.5 mg
chloride	34 mg

Comments:

- This product provides 100 percent of the adult RDA for most nutrients.
- Folic acid and vitamins B6, B12, D, and E are provided in amounts greater than the upper limits of the recommended ranges of intake for these nutrients.
- Iron, iodine, copper, and zinc are the only minerals supplied in amounts high enough to meet the adult RDAs.
- Accidental iron poisoning is a possibility, especially with young children. Be sure to keep all supplements stored out of their reach.

ONE-A-DAY MEN'S
(multivitamin supplement)

Manufacturer: Miles Laboratories, Inc.
Dosage form: Tablets
Ingredients:

vitamin A	5,000 IU
vitamin C	200 mg
thiamin (B1)	2.25 mg
riboflavin (B2)	2.55 mg

niacin	20 mg
vitamin D	400 IU
vitamin E	45 IU
vitamin B6	3 mg
folic acid	0.4 mg
vitamin B12	9 µg
pantothenic acid	10 mg

Comments:

- This product provides more than 100 percent of the adult RDA for men for most of the vitamins it contains.
- This product contains no biotin.
- Antioxidant vitamins are provided in larger amounts than recommended levels; however, this product does not provide the entire spectrum of antioxidants.
- It does not provide iron or any other minerals.

ONE-A-DAY WOMEN'S
(multivitamin supplement with calcium, iron, and zinc)

Manufacturer: Miles Laboratories, Inc.
Dosage form: Tablets
Ingredients:

vitamin A	5,000 IU
vitamin C	60 mg
thiamin (B1)	1.5 mg
riboflavin (B2)	1.7 mg
niacin	20 mg
vitamin D	400 IU

vitamin E	30 IU
vitamin B6	2 mg
folic acid	0.4 mg
vitamin B12	6 µg
pantothenic acid	10 mg
iron	27 mg
calcium	450 mg
zinc	15 mg

Comments:

- This product has 100 percent of the adult RDA for most of the nutrients it contains. Folic acid, iron, and vitamins B6, B12, D, and E are provided in amounts greater than the upper limits of the recommended intake range.
- The only minerals this product provides are calcium, iron, and zinc.
- The amount of calcium provided is higher than in many multivitamins.
- It does not contain biotin.
- Iron interacts with antacids and oral tetracycline antibiotics, reducing the absorption of these drugs.
- To prevent iron poisoning, store all supplements out of children's reach.

ONE-A-DAY 55 PLUS
(multivitamin/mineral supplement)

Manufacturer: Miles Laboratories, Inc.
Dosage form: Tablets

Ingredients:

vitamin A	6,000 IU
vitamin C	120 mg
thiamin (B1)	4.5 mg
riboflavin (B2)	3.4 mg
niacin	20 mg
vitamin D	400 IU
vitamin E	60 IU
vitamin B6	6 mg
folic acid	0.4 mg
vitamin B12	25 µg
biotin	30 µg
pantothenic acid	20 mg
vitamin K	25 µg
calcium	220 mg
iodine	150 µg
magnesium	100 mg
copper	2 mg
zinc	15 mg
chromium	10 µg
selenium	10 µg
molybdenum	10 µg
manganese	2.5 mg
potassium	37.5 mg
chloride	34 mg

Comments:
- This product provides more than 100 percent of the RDA for most vitamins. Iron is not provided.
- It provides 200 percent of the RDA or more for vitamins B1, B2, C, D, E, B6, and B12 and for folic acid.

- Iodine, copper, and zinc are the only minerals supplied in amounts high enough to meet the adult RDAs.

ONE-A-DAY EXTRAS— ANTIOXIDANT
(antioxidant supplement)

Manufacturer: Miles Laboratories, Inc.
Dosage form: Softgels
Ingredients:

beta-carotene	5,000 IU
vitamin C	250 mg
vitamin E	200 IU
zinc	7.5 mg
copper	1 mg
selenium	15 µg
manganese	1.5 mg

Comments:
- This product provides an assortment of antioxidants: Beta-carotene meets the recommended intake for vitamin A; vitamin C is over 400 percent of the adult RDA; vitamin E level is more than ten times the RDA.
- None of the minerals meets the RDAs.

OPTILETS 500
(multivitamin supplement)

Manufacturer: Abbott Laboratories
Dosage form: Tablets

Ingredients:

vitamin C	500 mg
niacin	100 mg
pantothenic acid	20 mg
thiamin (B$_1$)	15 mg
riboflavin (B$_2$)	10 mg
vitamin B$_6$	5 mg
vitamin A	5,000 IU
vitamin B$_{12}$	12 μg
vitamin D	400 IU
vitamin E	30 IU

Comments:

- This product provides more than 500 percent of the RDA for vitamin C, niacin, riboflavin, and vitamin B$_{12}$ and 200 percent or more for vitamin B$_6$, vitamin D, and vitamin E.
- The product also contains well above the upper limit of the recommended range for pantothenic acid.
- Thiamin is provided in a megadose amount (ten or more times the RDA).

OPTILETS-M-500
(multivitamin/mineral supplement)

Manufacturer: Abbott Laboratories
Dosage form: Tablets
Ingredients:

vitamin C	500 mg
niacin	100 mg

pantothenic acid	20 mg
thiamin (B1)	15 mg
riboflavin (B2)	10 mg
vitamin B6	5 mg
vitamin A	5,000 IU
vitamin B12	12 µg
vitamin D	400 IU
vitamin E	30 IU
magnesium	80 mg
iron	20 mg
copper	2 mg
zinc	1.5 mg
manganese	1 mg
iodine	0.15 µg

Comments:

- This product provides more than 500 percent of the adult RDA for vitamin C, niacin, riboflavin, and vitamin B12.
- This supplement provides 200 percent or more of the RDAs for vitamin B6, vitamin D, and vitamin E.
- This product also contains well above the upper limit of the recommended range of intake for pantothenic acid.
- Thiamin is provided by this supplement in a megadose amount (ten or more times the RDA).
- Only copper, iodine, and iron are supplied in amounts that meet the adult RDAs for these minerals.
- Ten percent of the zinc, 50 percent of the manganese, and 25 to 30 percent of the mag-

nesium RDAs are provided by this supplement.

- Accidental iron poisoning is a possibility, especially with young children. Be sure to keep all supplements stored out of their reach.

OS-CAL 500 CHEWABLE TABLETS
(calcium supplement)

Manufacturer: SmithKline Beecham
Dosage form: Chewable tablets
Ingredient:
  elemental calcium   500 mg
Comments:

- This product supplies about 40 percent of the recommended amount of calcium for teenage girls and boys and adult women.
- Taking one tablet twice a day should supplement the diet for teenagers and adult women. Adult men may only need one tablet, depending on their daily intake of dairy products.
- The calcium source is calcium carbonate.

OS-CAL 500 TABLETS
(calcium supplement)

Manufacturer: SmithKline Beecham
Dosage form: Tablets
Ingredient:
  elemental calcium   500 mg

Comment:
- The calcium source is crushed oyster shell powder, which is primarily calcium carbonate.

OS-CAL 500 + D TABLETS
(calcium supplement with vitamin D)

Manufacturer: SmithKline Beecham
Dosage form: Tablets
Ingredients:

elemental calcium	500 mg
vitamin D	125 IU

Comments:
- The calcium source is crushed oyster shell powder, which is primarily calcium carbonate.
- Vitamin D is useful for ensuring the optimum use of calcium.

OS-CAL FORTIFIED TABLETS
(multivitamin/mineral supplement)

Manufacturer: SmithKline Beecham
Dosage form: Tablets
Ingredients:

vitamin D	125 IU
thiamin (B1)	1.7 mg
riboflavin (B2)	1.7 mg
vitamin B6	2 mg

vitamin C	50 mg
vitamin E	0.8 IU
niacin	15 mg
calcium	250 mg
iron	5 mg
magnesium	3.0 mg
manganese	0.5 mg
zinc	0.5 mg

Comments:

- This product contains slightly more than 100 percent of the adult RDAs for thiamin and vitamin C. It also contains about one third of the adult woman's requirement for iron and calcium. Manganese levels do not meet the adult minimum recommended level. Magnesium and zinc levels are way below the adult RDAs.
- The calcium source is crushed oyster shell powder, which is primarily calcium carbonate.
- The calcium is insufficient for teenagers and adult women.

OS-CAL 250 + D TABLETS
(calcium supplement with vitamin D)

Manufacturer: SmithKline Beecham
Dosage form: Tablets
Ingredients:

| elemental calcium | 250 mg |
| vitamin D | 125 IU |

Comments:

- The calcium source is crushed oyster shell powder, which is primarily calcium carbonate.
- The added vitamin D is not necessary if a multivitamin containing it is also being taken.
- Teenagers and adult women may need to take more than three tablets a day if they are taking the product to supplement their diets.

POLY-VI-SOL
(multivitamin children's supplement)

Manufacturer: Mead Johnson Nutritional Division
Dosage form: Liquid
Ingredients:

vitamin A	1,500 IU
vitamin D	400 IU
vitamin E	5 IU
vitamin C	35 mg
thiamin (B1)	0.5 mg
riboflavin (B2)	0.6 mg
niacin	8 mg
vitamin B6	0.4 mg
vitamin B12	2 μg

Comments:

- It provides at least 100 percent of the RDA for infants for most nutrients; it has greater amounts of niacin and vitamins D and B12.
- This product is alcohol free.

POLY-VI-SOL
(multivitamin children's supplement)

Manufacturer: Mead Johnson Nutritional Division

Dosage forms: Chewable tablets

Ingredients:

vitamin A	2,500 IU
vitamin D	400 IU
vitamin E	15 IU
vitamin C	60 mg
folic acid	0.3 mg
thiamin (B_1)	1.05 mg
riboflavin (B_2)	1.2 mg
niacin	13.5 mg
vitamin B_6	1.05 mg
vitamin B_{12}	4.5 µg

Comments:

- For children younger than 4 years of age, this supplement provides at least 100 percent or more of the RDAs for vitamin E, vitamin D, vitamin C, vitamin B_6, and vitamin B_{12}. It also provides 100 percent or more of the following nutrients: folic acid, thiamin, riboflavin, and niacin. For children older than 4 years of age, the RDA is provided for all nutrients except vitamin B_6.
- This product contains sugar.

POLY-VI-SOL WITH IRON
(multivitamin children's supplement with iron)

Manufacturer: Mead Johnson Nutritional Division
Dosage form: Liquid
Ingredients:

vitamin A	1,500 IU
vitamin D	400 IU
vitamin E	5 IU
vitamin C	35 mg
thiamin (B_1)	0.5 mg
riboflavin (B_2)	0.6 mg
niacin	8 mg
vitamin B_6	0.4 mg
iron	10 mg

Comments:

- This supplement provides at least 100 percent of the RDA for infants for most nutrients.
- Niacin, vitamin D, and vitamin B_{12} are provided in amounts greater than the RDA for infants. Only vitamins D and B_{12} would meet the RDAs for older children.
- This product may temporarily darken stools or discolor the gums.
- Accidental iron poisoning is a possibility, especially with young children. Be sure to store all supplements out of their reach.
- This product is alcohol free.

POLY-VI-SOL WITH IRON
(multivitamin children's supplement with iron)

Manufacturer: Mead Johnson Nutritional Division
Dosage form: Chewable tablets
Ingredients:

vitamin A	2,500 IU
vitamin D	400 IU
vitamin E	15 IU
vitamin C	60 mg
folic acid	0.3 mg
thiamin (B_1)	1.05 mg
riboflavin (B_2)	1.2 mg
niacin	13.5 mg
vitamin B_6	1.05 mg
vitamin B_{12}	4.5 µg
iron	12 mg
copper	0.8 mg
zinc	8 mg

Comments:

- This supplement provides 100 percent or more of the RDAs for vitamin E, vitamin D, vitamin C, folic acid, thiamin, riboflavin, niacin, vitamin B_6, and vitamin B_{12} for children younger than 4 years of age. For children older than 4 years of age, the supplement provides the RDA for all nutrients except vitamin B_6.

- This product may temporarily darken stools or discolor the gums.
- Accidental iron poisoning is a possibility, especially with young children. To avoid accidental poisoning, be sure to store all supplements out of their reach.
- This product contains sugar.

POSTURE
(calcium supplement)

Manufacturer: Whitehall Laboratories
Dosage form: Tablets
Ingredient:
  elemental calcium   600 mg
Comment:
- The calcium source is tricalcium phosphate (1,565 mg).

POSTURE-D
(calcium supplement plus vitamin D)

Manufacturer: Whitehall Laboratories
Dosage form: Tablets
Ingredients:
  elemental calcium   600 mg
  vitamin D   125 IU
Comment:
- The calcium source is tricalcium phosphate (1,565 mg).

PROTEGRA
(antioxidant multivitamin/ mineral supplement)

Manufacturer: Lederle Laboratories
Dosage form: Softgels
Ingredients:

vitamin E	200 IU
vitamin C	250 mg
beta-carotene	3 mg
zinc	7.5 mg
copper	1 mg
selenium	15 μg
manganese	1.5 mg

Comments:

- It provides all the antioxidant vitamins.
- This product provides a megadose of vitamin E and more than 400 percent of the RDA for vitamin D. These levels are used in studies examining antioxidant functions of vitamins.
- Beta-carotene and the minerals are provided in amounts less than the recommended RDAs.

SESAME STREET COMPLETE
(multivitamin/mineral children's chewable supplement)

Manufacturer: Johnson & Johnson
Dosage form: Chewable tablets

Ingredients:

vitamin A	2,250 IU
beta-carotene	500 IU
vitamin D	200 IU
thiamin	0.75 mg
riboflavin	0.85 mg
niacin	10 mg
pantothenic acid	5 mg
vitamin B_6	0.7 mg
vitamin B_{12}	3 µg
vitamin C	40 mg
vitamin E	10 IU
folic acid	0.2 mg
biotin	15 µg
iron	10 mg
iodine	75 µg
zinc	8 mg
copper	1 mg
calcium	80 mg
magnesium	20 mg

Comments:

• This product provides much more than 100 percent of the children's RDA for vitamin B_{12} and folic acid.

SLO-NIACIN
(niacin supplement)

Manufacturer: Upsher-Smith Labs
Dosage form: polygel controlled-release capsules

Ingredient:

nicotinic acid   250 mg

Comments:

- This is an effective megadose treatment for extremely high blood cholesterol levels.
- This product may cause flushing and tingling of the skin.
- This slow-release form can cause liver damage and should only be used if liver enzymes are monitored by a physician.

SLOW FE
(iron supplement)

Manufacturer: Ciba Consumer
Dosage form: Wax matrix tablets
Ingredient:

elemental iron   50 mg

Comments:

- Iron is provided as ferrous sulfate (160 mg).
- This product contains more than 300 percent of the RDA for adult women.
- Wax matrix tablets are designed to release iron in the intestines. Slow release of iron makes abdominal discomfort, constipation, and diarrhea less of a problem.
- Iron interacts with antacids and oral tetracycline antibiotics, reducing absorption of these drugs.
- Accidental iron poisoning is a possibility, especially with young children. Be sure to store all supplements out of their reach.

STRESSTABS
(multivitamin supplement)

Manufacturer: Lederle Laboratories
Dosage form: Tablets
Ingredients:

vitamin E	30 IU
vitamin C	500 mg
folic acid	0.4 mg
thiamin (B_1)	10 mg
riboflavin (B_2)	10 mg
niacin	100 mg
vitamin B_6	5 mg
vitamin B_{12}	12 µg
biotin	45 µg
pantothenic acid	20 mg

Comments:
- This product provides more than 100 percent of the adult RDA for riboflavin and vitamin B_6.
- It provides a megadose (ten or more times the RDA) of vitamin C and thiamin.
- This product also provides about five times the adult RDA for niacin and vitamin B_{12}.

STRESSTABS + IRON
(multivitamin supplement with iron)

Manufacturer: Lederle Laboratories
Dosage form: Tablets

Ingredients:

vitamin E	30 IU
vitamin C	500 mg
folic acid	0.4 mg
thiamin (B₁)	10 mg
riboflavin (B₂)	10 mg
niacin	100 mg
vitamin B₆	5 mg
vitamin B₁₂	12 µg
biotin	45 µg
pantothenic acid	20 mg
iron	18 mg

Comments:

- It provides more than 100 percent of the adult RDA for riboflavin and vitamin B₆.
- It provides a megadose (ten or more times the RDA) of vitamin C and thiamin.
- This supplement provides about five times the adult RDA for niacin and vitamin B₁₂.
- To prevent accidental iron poisoning, store all supplements out of the reach of children.

STRESSTABS + ZINC
(multivitamin/mineral supplement)

Manufacturer: Lederle Laboratories
Dosage form: Tablets
Ingredients:

vitamin E	30 IU
vitamin C	500 mg

folic acid	0.4 mg
thiamin (B1)	10 mg
riboflavin (B2)	10 mg
niacin	100 mg
vitamin B6	5 mg
vitamin B12	12 μg
biotin	45 μg
pantothenic acid	20 mg
copper	3 mg
zinc	23.9 mg

Comments:

- This product provides more than 100 percent of the adult RDA for riboflavin, vitamin B6, and zinc.
- This supplement provides more than the recommended range of intake for pantothenic acid.
- This product provides a megadose (ten or more times the RDA) of vitamin C and thiamin.
- It provides about 500 percent, or five times, the adult RDA for niacin and vitamin B12.
- Copper is supplied at the upper limit of the recommended range of intake.

STUART FORMULA, THE
(multivitamin/mineral supplement)

Manufacturer: J & J Merck
Dosage form: Tablets

Ingredients:

vitamin A	5,000 IU
vitamin D	400 IU
vitamin E	10 IU
vitamin C	50 mg
folic acid	0.1 mg
thiamin (B1)	1.5 mg
riboflavin (B2)	1.7 mg
niacin	20 mg
vitamin B6	1 mg
vitamin B12	3 µg
calcium	125 mg
iodine	150 µg
elemental iron	5 mg
copper	1 mg

Comments:

- Most nutrients present are provided at reasonable levels—that is, at or near the recommended daily intake levels.
- The level of vitamin B12 in this supplement exceeds the RDA.
- Calcium is supplied in a relatively insignificant amount.
- Vitamins B6 and C, folic acid, and iron are present in amounts below the RDA.
- The copper level is below the recommended range of intake.
- This supplement does not provide biotin, pantothenic acid, or most minerals, including zinc and selenium.
- This supplement contains sugar.

STUART PRENATAL
(multivitamin/mineral prenatal supplement)

Manufacturer: Wyeth-Ayerst Labs
Dosage form: Tablets
Ingredients:

vitamin A	4,000 IU
vitamin D	400 IU
vitamin E	11 IU
vitamin C	100 mg
folic acid	0.8 mg
thiamin (B_1)	1.84 mg
riboflavin (B_2)	1.7 mg
niacin	18 mg
vitamin B_6	2.6 mg
vitamin B_{12}	4 µg
calcium	200 mg
elemental iron	60 mg
zinc	25 mg

Comments:

- This product provides 100 percent of the RDA for pregnant and breast-feeding women for vitamin D, vitamin E, vitamin C, thiamin, riboflavin, and niacin.
- It provides more than 100 percent of the RDA for vitamin B_6, iron, folic acid, vitamin B_{12}, and zinc.
- This product supplies vitamin A at 100 percent of the RDA for pregnant women, but not for breast-feeding women.

- Calcium is supplied at well below the RDAs for both pregnant and breast-feeding women.
- This supplement contains FD&C Red No. 3. The safety of this food colorant is in question.
- This product can depress zinc absorption.
- Iron interacts with antacids and oral tetracycline antibiotics, reducing the absorption of these drugs.
- Accidental iron poisoning is a possibility, especially with young children. Be sure to store all supplements out of their reach.

SUNKIST MULTIVITAMINS
(children's chewable multivitamin supplement)

Manufacturer: CIBA Consumer Pharmaceuticals

Dosage forms: Chewable tablets

Ingredients:

vitamin A	2,500 IU
folic acid	0.3 mg
thiamin (B_1)	1.05 mg
riboflavin (B_2)	1.2 mg
niacinamide	13.5 mg
vitamin B_6	1.05 mg
vitamin B_{12}	4.5 µg
vitamin C	60 mg
vitamin D	400 IU
vitamin E	15 IU
vitamin K_1	5 µg

Comments:
- Levels are reasonable for most nutrients.
- This product contains phenylalanine and should not be used by those with phenylketonuria.
- This product is sugar free but contains sorbitol and aspartame.

SUNKIST MULTIVITAMINS + EXTRA C

(children's chewable multivitamin supplement with extra C)

Manufacturer: CIBA Consumer Pharmaceuticals
Dosage forms: Chewable tablets
Ingredients:

vitamin A	2,500 IU
folic acid	0.3 mg
thiamin (B_1)	1.05 mg
riboflavin (B_2)	1.2 mg
niacinamide	13.5 mg
vitamin B_6	1.05 mg
vitamin B_{12}	4.5 µg
vitamin C	250 mg
vitamin D	400 IU
vitamin E	15 IU
vitamin K_1	5 µg

Comments:
- Dosage levels are reasonable for most of the nutrients provided.

- Vitamin C is present at 500 percent of the RDA for children.
- This product should not be used by children who have phenylketonuria.
- This product is sugar free but contains sorbitol and aspartame.

SUNKIST MULTIVITAMINS + IRON
(children's chewable multivitamin supplement with iron)

Manufacturer: CIBA Consumer Pharmaceuticals

Dosage forms: Chewable tablets

Ingredients:

vitamin A	2,500 IU
folic acid	0.3 mg
thiamin (B_1)	1.05 mg
riboflavin (B_2)	1.2 mg
niacinamide	13.5 mg
vitamin B_6	1.05 mg
vitamin B_{12}	4.5 µg
vitamin C	60 mg
vitamin D	400 IU
vitamin E	15 IU
vitamin K_1	5 µg
iron	15 mg

Comments:

- Dosage levels are reasonable for most of the nutrients provided.

- This supplement includes vitamin C at a megadose amount: 500 percent of the RDA for children.
- Iron is present at 150 percent of the RDA for children.
- This product contains phenylalanine and should not be used by children who have phenylketonuria.
- Accidental iron poisoning is a possibility, especially with young children. Be sure to store all supplements, especially those designed to be attractive to children, out of their reach.
- This product is sugar free but contains sorbitol and aspartame.

SUNKIST COMPLETE
(children's chewable multivitamin/mineral supplement)

Manufacturer: CIBA Consumer Pharmaceuticals
Dosage forms: Chewable tablets
Ingredients:

vitamin A	5,000 IU
vitamin D	400 IU
vitamin E	30 IU
vitamin C	60 mg
folic acid	0.4 mg
thiamin (B₁)	1.5 mg

riboflavin (B2)	1.7 mg
niacin	20 mg
vitamin B6	2 mg
vitamin B12	6 μg
vitamin K1	10 μg
biotin	40 μg
pantothenic acid	10 mg
iron	18 mg
calcium	100 mg
copper	2 mg
phosphorus	78 mg
iodine	150 μg
magnesium	20 mg
manganese	1 mg
zinc	10 mg

Comments:
- Dosage levels for most of the nutrients are at 100 percent of the adult RDAs, which is more than most of the RDAs for children.
- Calcium and magnesium are well below recommended amounts.
- Iron level is well above recommended level for children.
- This product contains phenylalanine and should not be used by those with phenylketonuria.
- Iron interacts with antacids and oral tetracycline antibiotics, reducing absorption of these drugs.
- Accidental iron poisoning is a possibility, especially with young children. Be sure to

store all supplements, especially those that are designed to be attractive to children, out of their reach.
- This product is sugar free but contains sorbitol and aspartame.

SUNKIST VITAMIN C
(vitamin C supplement)

Manufacturer: CIBA Consumer Pharmaceuticals
Dosage forms: Chewable tablets or caplets
Ingredient:
vitamin C

chewable tablet (sold in rolls)	60 mg
chewable tablet	250 mg
chewable tablet	500 mg
caplet	500 mg

Comments:
- The 60-mg tablet provides 100 percent of the adult RDA.
- The 250-mg tablet provides more than 100 percent of the adult RDA for vitamin C.
- The 500-mg tablet and caplet both provide more than 100 percent of the adult RDA for vitamin C—almost ten times the RDA.
- Long-term use of high-dose chewable vitamin C tablets has been linked to erosion of dental enamel.
- This product contains sugar, sorbitol, and lactose.

SURBEX
(B-complex supplement)

Manufacturer: Abbott Laboratories
Dosage form: Tablets
Ingredients:

niacin	30 mg
pantothenic acid	10 mg
thiamin (B1)	6 mg
riboflavin (B2)	6 mg
vitamin B6	2.5 mg
vitamin B12	5 μg

Comment:
• This supplement provides more than 100 percent of the adult RDA for niacin, thiamin, riboflavin, and vitamin B6.

SURBEX WITH C
(vitamin C and B-complex supplement)

Manufacturer: Abbott Laboratories
Dosage form: Tablets
Ingredients:

niacin	30 mg
pantothenic acid	10 mg
thiamin (B1)	6 mg
riboflavin (B2)	6 mg
vitamin B6	2.5 mg
vitamin B12	5 μg
vitamin C	250 mg

Comment:
- This supplement provides more than 400 percent of the adult RDA for vitamin C and more than 100 percent of the adult RDA for niacin, thiamin, riboflavin, and vitamin B6.

SURBEX-T
(vitamin C and B-complex supplement)

Manufacturer: Abbott Laboratories
Dosage form: Tablets
Ingredients:

vitamin C	500 mg
niacin	100 mg
pantothenic acid	20 mg
thiamin (B1)	15 mg
riboflavin (B2)	10 mg
vitamin B6	5 mg
vitamin B12	10 μg

Comments:
- This product provides more than 500 percent of the RDA for vitamin C.
- This supplement provides more than 100 percent of the RDA for niacin, riboflavin, vitamin B6, and vitamin B12 and more than the recommended safe and sufficient range of intake for pantothenic acid.
- This product provides a megadose (ten or more times the RDA) of the B vitamin thiamin.

SURBEX-750 WITH IRON
(vitamin C, B-complex, and E supplement plus iron)

Manufacturer: Abbott Laboratories
Dosage form: Tablets
Ingredients:

vitamin C	750 mg
niacin	100 mg
vitamin B_6	25 mg
pantothenic acid	20 mg
thiamin (B_1)	15 mg
riboflavin (B_2)	15 mg
vitamin B_{12}	12 µg
folic acid	0.4 mg
vitamin E	30 IU
elemental iron	27 mg

Comments:

- This supplement provides more than 100 percent of the adult RDA for niacin, riboflavin, vitamin B_{12}, and iron. It also provides the recommended range of intake for pantothenic acid.

- This product provides a megadose (ten or more times the RDA) of vitamin C, vitamin B_6, and thiamin.

- Accidental iron poisoning is a possibility, especially with young children. Be sure to store all supplements out of their reach.

SURBEX-750 WITH ZINC
(vitamin C, B-complex, and E supplement plus zinc)

Manufacturer: Abbott Laboratories
Dosage form: Tablets
Ingredients:

vitamin C	750 mg
niacin	100 mg
vitamin B6	20 mg
pantothenic acid	20 mg
thiamin (B1)	15 mg
riboflavin (B2)	15 mg
vitamin B12	12 μg
folic acid	0.4 mg
vitamin E	30 IU
zinc	22.5 mg

Comments:

- This product provides more than 100 percent of the adult RDA for riboflavin, niacin, and vitmain B12 and more than the recommended range of intake for pantothenic acid.
- This product provides a megadose (ten or more times the RDA) of vitamin C, thiamin, and vitamin B6.

THERAGRAN LIQUID
(multivitamin supplement)

Manufacturer: Bristol-Myers Squibb
Dosage form: Liquid

Ingredients:

beta-carotene	5,000 IU
vitamin D	400 IU
vitamin C	200 mg
thiamin (B1)	10 mg
riboflavin (B2)	10 mg
niacin	100 mg
vitamin B6	4.1 mg
vitamin B12	5 μg
pantothenic acid	21.4 mg

Comment:

• This product provides more than the adult RDA for vitamin C, vitamin D, thiamin, riboflavin, niacin, vitamin B6, and vitamin B12 and more than the recommended range of intake for pantothenic acid.

THERAGRAN-M ADVANCED FORMULA (multivitamin/mineral supplement)

Manufacturer: Bristol-Myers Squibb
Dosage form: Tablets
Ingredients:

vitamin A	5,000 IU
vitamin C	90 mg
thiamin (B1)	3 mg
riboflavin (B2)	3.4 mg
niacin	20 mg
vitamin B6	3 mg

vitamin B12	9 µg
vitamin D	400 IU
vitamin E	30 IU
pantothenic acid	10 mg
folic acid	0.4 mg
biotin	30 µg
calcium	40 mg
iodine	150 µg
iron	27 mg
magnesium	100 mg
copper	2 mg
zinc	15 mg
chromium	15 µg
selenium	10 µg
molybdenum	15 µg
phosphorus	31 mg
potassium	7.5 mg
chloride	7.5 mg

Comments:

- This product provides more than 100 percent of the adult RDA for vitamin C, vitamin D, thiamin, riboflavin, niacin, vitamin B6, and iron. The amount of vitamin B12 is more than 400 percent of the adult RDA.
- This product contains insignificant amounts of calcium, potassium, and chloride. The amounts of magnesium, selenium, and chromium are well below recommended intakes.
- Accidental iron poisoning is a possibility, especially with young children. Be sure to store all supplements out of their reach.

THERAGRAN STRESS FORMULA
(multivitamin supplement with iron)

Manufacturer: Bristol-Myers Squibb
Dosage form: Tablets
Ingredients:

vitamin E	30 IU
vitamin C	600 mg
folic acid	0.4 mg
thiamin (B$_1$)	15 mg
riboflavin (B$_2$)	15 mg
niacin	100 mg
vitamin B$_6$	25 mg
vitamin B$_{12}$	12 μg
biotin	45 μg
pantothenic acid	20 mg
iron	27 mg

Comments:

- This product provides more than the adult RDA for vitamins E and B$_{12}$, riboflavin, niacin, folic acid, and for the mineral iron.
- This product provides megadoses (ten or more times the RDA) of vitamin C, thiamin, and vitamin B$_6$.
- Accidental iron poisoning is a possibility, especially with young children. To avoid accidental poisoning, be sure to store all supplements out of their reach.

THERAGRAN ANTIOXIDANT
(antioxidant supplement)

Manufacturer: Bristol-Myers Squibb
Dosage form: Tablets
Ingredients:

beta-carotene	5,000 IU
vitamin C	250 mg
vitamin E	200 IU
copper	1 mg
manganese	1.5 mg
selenium	15 µg
zinc	7.5 mg

Comments:

- In this product, beta-carotene provides 100 percent of the RDA for vitamin A.
- This product provides more than 400 percent of the RDA for vitamin C.
- Vitamin E is present in a megadose.
- The minerals are all present in amounts below the RDAs or recommended intake levels.

TRI-VI-SOL
(multivitamin children's supplement)

Manufacturer: Mead Johnson Nutritional Division
Dosage form: Liquid

Ingredients:

vitamin A	1,500 IU
vitamin D	400 IU
vitamin C	35 mg

Comment:
- This product provides 100 percent of the RDA for each nutrient for infants more than six months of age.

TRI-VI-SOL WITH IRON
(multivitamin children's supplement with iron)

Manufacturer: Mead Johnson Nutritional Division
Dosage form: Liquid
Ingredients:

vitamin A	1,500 IU
vitamin D	400 IU
vitamin C	35 mg
iron	10 mg

Comments:
- This product provides 100 percent of the RDA for each nutrient for infants more than six months of age. The amounts are only slightly higher than the RDA for infants less than six months of age.
- Accidental iron poisoning is a possibility, especially with young children. Be sure to store all supplements out of their reach.

UNICAP
(multivitamin supplement)

Manufacturer: The Upjohn Company
Dosage forms: Tablets, capsules
Ingredients:

vitamin A	5,000 IU
vitamin D	400 IU
vitamin E	30 IU
vitamin C	60 mg
folic acid	0.4 mg
thiamin (B_1)	1.5 mg
riboflavin (B_2)	1.7 mg
niacin	20 mg
vitamin B_6	2 mg
vitamin B_{12}	6 μg

Comments:
- This supplement provides 100 percent of the adult RDA for most nutrients. However, it provides more than 100 percent of the adult RDA for vitamin E, vitamin D, folic acid, and vitamin B_{12}.
- This supplement is sugar and sodium free.

UNICAP JUNIOR
(multivitamin children's supplement)

Manufacturer: The Upjohn Company
Dosage form: Chewable tablets

Ingredients:

vitamin A	5,000 IU
vitamin D	400 IU
vitamin E	30 IU
vitamin C	60 mg
folic acid	0.4 mg
thiamin (B1)	1.5 mg
riboflavin (B2)	1.7 mg
niacin	20 mg
vitamin B6	2 mg
vitamin B12	6 µg
vitamin E	15 IU

Comments:

- This product provides 100 percent or more of the adult RDA for all nutrients. All the nutrients except vitamin D are present at levels greater than 100 percent of the RDAs.
- This supplement contains sugar, mannitol, and lactose.

UNICAP M
(multivitamin/mineral supplement)

Manufacturer: The Upjohn Company
Dosage form: Tablets
Ingredients:

vitamin A	5,000 IU
vitamin D	400 IU
vitamin E	30 IU
vitamin C	60 mg

folic acid	0.4 mg
thiamin (B_1)	1.5 mg
riboflavin (B_2)	1.7 mg
niacin	20 mg
vitamin B_6	2 mg
vitamin B_{12}	6 μg
pantothenic acid	10 mg
iodine	150 μg
iron	18 mg
copper	2 mg
zinc	15 mg
calcium	60 mg
phosphorus	45 mg
manganese	1 mg
potassium	5 mg

Comments:

- This supplemental product provides 100 percent of the adult RDA for all nutrients except vitamin E, folic acid, and vitamin B_{12}, which are provided in larger doses.
- The supplement provides insignificant amounts of the minerals calcium, phosphorus, manganese, and potassium.
- This product is sugar and sodium free.

UNICAP PLUS IRON
(multivitamin supplement with iron)

Manufacturer: The Upjohn Company
Dosage form: Tablets

Ingredients:

vitamin A	5,000 IU
vitamin D	400 IU
vitamin E	30 IU
vitamin C	60 mg
folic acid	0.4 mg
thiamin (B_1)	1.5 mg
riboflavin (B_2)	1.7 mg
niacin	20 mg
vitamin B_6	2 mg
vitamin B_{12}	6 µg
iron	22.5 mg
calcium	100 mg
pantothenic acid	10 mg

Comments:

- This product provides 100 percent of the adult RDA for all nutrients except vitamin E, folic acid, and vitamin B_{12}, which are provided in larger doses.
- Accidental iron poisoning is a possibility, especially with young children. To prevent an accident, be sure to keep all supplements stored out of their reach.
- This supplement contains sugar.

UNICAP SENIOR
(multivitamin/mineral supplement)

Manufacturer: The Upjohn Company
Dosage form: Tablets

Ingredients:

vitamin A	5,000 IU
vitamin D	200 IU
vitamin E	15 IU
vitamin C	60 mg
folic acid	0.4 mg
thiamin (B$_1$)	1.2 mg
riboflavin (B$_2$)	1.4 mg
niacin	16 mg
vitamin B$_6$	2.2 mg
vitamin B$_{12}$	3 μg
pantothenic acid	10 mg
iodine	150 μg
iron	10 mg
copper	2 mg
zinc	15 mg
calcium	100 mg
phosphorus	77 mg
magnesium	30 mg
manganese	1 mg
potassium	5 mg

Comments:

- Amounts of all vitamins included in this product are reasonable.
- This product contains insignificant amounts of magnesium and potassium.
- Calcium is supplied in a small amount.
- Accidental iron poisoning is a possibility, especially with young children. Be sure to store all supplements out of their reach.
- This supplement is sugar and sodium free.

UNICAP T
(multivitamin/mineral supplement)

Manufacturer: The Upjohn Company
Dosage form: Tablets
Ingredients:

vitamin A	5,000 IU
vitamin D	400 IU
vitamin E	30 IU
vitamin C	500 mg
folic acid	0.4 mg
thiamin (B$_1$)	10 mg
riboflavin (B$_2$)	10 mg
niacin	100 mg
vitamin B$_6$	6 mg
vitamin B$_{12}$	18 μg
pantothenic acid	25 mg
iodine	150 μg
iron	18 mg
copper	2 mg
zinc	15 mg
manganese	1 mg
potassium	5 mg
selenium	10 μg

Comments:
- This product provides more than 100 percent of the adult RDA for vitamins C, E, and B$_6$, plus thiamin, riboflavin, niacin, and folic acid.
- This product provides more than the recommended range of intake for pantothenic acid.

- This product contains 900 percent of the adult requirement for vitamin B12.
- The amounts of manganese and potassium are insignificant.
- This supplement is sugar and sodium free.

Z-BEC
(vitamin C, B-complex, and E supplement with zinc)

Manufacturer: A. H. Robins Company
Dosage form: Tablets
Ingredients:

vitamin C	600 mg
thiamin	15 mg
riboflavin	10.2 mg
niacin	100 mg
vitamin B6	10 mg
vitamin B12	6 µg
pantothenic acid	25 mg
vitamin E	45 IU
zinc	22.5 mg

Comments:
- This product provides more than 100 percent of the adult RDA for zinc and vitamin B6 and more than twice the upper limit of the recommended range of intake for pantothenic acid.
- This product provides 500 percent or more of the adult RDA for niacin and riboflavin.
- This product provides a megadose of vitamin C and thiamin.

CHAPTER 13

Recipes for Healthier Living

The recipes that follow provide healthy doses of vitamins and minerals, as well as other nutrients that your body needs. They are designed to fit within the American Heart Association's guidelines for fat intake (which recommend that your daily total fat intake not exceed 30 percent of total calories and your saturated fat intake not exceed 10 percent of total calories). The recipes also tend to be low in sodium and cholesterol.

The nutritional chart that follows each recipe shows the number of calories (kc); grams (g) of protein, carbohydrate, and fat; and milligrams (mg) of cholesterol and sodium in a serving. There is also a listing of the vitamin and mineral content in one serving; units of measure used for these include retinol equivalents (RE) and micrograms (μg), as well as milligrams (mg). You'll notice that different vitamins and minerals are listed under the various recipes. A vitamin or mineral is listed only when the recipe contains a significant amount of it in a serving.

The nutritional information in the chart includes all the ingredients listed in the recipe, except ingredients labeled as "optional" or "for garnish." If a range is given in the yield of a recipe ("Makes 6 to 8 servings," for example), the higher yield was used to calculate the per serving information. If a range is offered for an ingredient (1/4 to 1/8 teaspoon, for example), the first amount given was used to calculate the nutritional information. If an ingredient is presented with an option ("2 tablespoons margarine or oil"), the first ingredient given was used to calculate the nutritional information. Foods offered as "serve with" suggestions at the end of a recipe are not included in the chart unless it is stated in the per serving line. Because numerous variables account for a wide range of values for certain foods, all nutritional information that appears in this book should be considered approximate.

The recipes in this book are NOT intended as a medically therapeutic program, nor as a substitute for medically approved diet plans for people on fat-, cholesterol-, or sodium-restricted diets. Consult your physician before beginning any diet plan.

CREAMY CARROT SOUP

3 cups water
4 cups sliced carrots
½ cup chopped onion
2 tablespoons packed brown sugar
2 teaspoons curry powder
2 garlic cloves, minced
⅛ teaspoon ground ginger
½ cube chicken bouillon
Dash ground cinnamon
½ cup skim milk

In large saucepan, bring water to a boil. Add all remaining ingredients except milk. Reduce heat to low; simmer 40 minutes or until carrots and onion are very tender. Remove from heat; pour mixture in batches into food processor or blender. Process until smooth. Return mixture to saucepan. Over low heat, stir in milk, heating until warm but not boiling. Serve warm. *Makes 6 servings*

NUTRITIONAL INFORMATION PER SERVING

Calories	69.46 kc	Niacin (B3)	0.96 mg
Protein	1.92 g	Pantothenic Acid	0.23 mg
Fat	0.63 g	Phosphorus	67.72 mg
% of Calories		Potassium	338.30 mg
from Fat:	8	Pyridoxine (B6)	0.15 mg
Saturated Fat	0.08 g	Riboflavin (B2)	0.08 mg
Cholesterol	0.33 mg	Thiamin (B1)	0.09 mg
Dietary Fiber	2.80 g	Vitamin A	2,075 RE
Sodium	156.90 mg	Vitamin C	8.24 mg
Beta-carotene	12,377 RE	Copper	0.09 mg
Calcium	56.71 mg	Folate	14.29 µg
Cobalamin (B12)	0.10 µg	Vitamin D	0.22 µg
Iron	0.78 mg	Vitamin E	0.45 mg
Magnesium	17.75 mg	Zinc	0.33 mg

GAZPACHO

- 1 cucumber
- ½ red bell pepper, seeded
- 2 carrots
- 1 medium tomato
- 2 cups spicy tomato juice
- ½ cup water
- ½ cup tomato sauce
- ¼ cup chopped green onions
- 3 tablespoons vinegar
- 2 teaspoons sugar
- 1 garlic clove, minced
- 1 (15-ounce) can navy beans, drained and rinsed

Cut cucumber, bell pepper, carrots, and tomato into large chunks. Place all ingredients except beans in food processor; process until almost puréed but still chunky. Transfer to large bowl. Stir in beans; cover and refrigerate until serving. *Makes 6 servings*

NUTRITIONAL INFORMATION PER SERVING

Calories	129.90 kc	Pantothenic Acid	0.64 mg
Protein	7.04 g	Phosphorus	144.60 mg
Fat	0.59 g	Potassium	674.10 mg
% of Calories		Pyridoxine (B$_6$)	0.29 mg
from Fat:	4	Riboflavin (B$_2$)	0.12 mg
Saturated Fat	0.13 g	Thiamin (B$_1$)	0.21 mg
Dietary Fiber	2.55 g	Vitamin A	774.80 RE
Sodium	737.10 mg	Vitamin C	23.72 mg
Beta-carotene	4220 RE	Copper	.32 mg
Calcium	61.52 mg	Folate	76.96 µg
Iron	2.42 mg	Vitamin E	0.68 mg
Magnesium	58.39 mg	Zinc	0.92 mg
Niacin (B$_3$)	1.65 mg		

FRUITS & VEGETABLES

APRICOT AND RICOTTA STUFFED CELERY

2½ cups (1½-inch) celery pieces
3 tablespoons coarsely chopped dried apricots
½ cup part-skim ricotta cheese
1½ teaspoons sugar
¼ teaspoon grated orange peel
⅛ teaspoon salt

Cut a thin lengthwise slice from the bottom of each celery piece to prevent tipping; set aside. In food processor or blender, process apricots until finely chopped. Set aside 1 tablespoon for garnish. Add ricotta cheese, sugar, orange peel, and salt to food processor or blender; process until cheese is smooth. Fill celery pieces with cheese mixture. Cover and refrigerate up to 3 hours before serving. Just before serving, sprinkle with reserved chopped apricots.

Makes about 25 appetizers

NUTRITIONAL INFORMATION PER SERVING

Calories	10.27 kc	Niacin (B3)	0.07 mg
Protein	0.54 g	Pantothenic Acid	0.03 mg
Fat	0.33 g	Phosphorus	4.14 mg
% of Calories		Potassium	47.88 mg
from Fat:	27	Pyridoxine (B6)	0.01 mg
Saturated Fat	0.01 g	Riboflavin (B2)	0.01 mg
Cholesterol	1.65 mg	Thiamin (B1)	0.01 mg
Dietary Fiber	0.27 g	Vitamin A	10.80 RE
Sodium	25.50 mg	Vitamin C	0.89 mg
Beta-Carotene	51.71 RE	Copper	0.01 mg
Calcium	13.54 mg	Folate	3.47 µg
Iron	0.10 mg	Vitamin E	0.09 mg
Magnesium	1.78 mg	Zinc	0.02 mg

Apple Slices with Citrus-Yogurt Dip

2 to 3 Empire apples, cored and sliced
¼ cup lemon juice
1 cup plain low-fat yogurt
2 tablespoons honey
1 tablespoon frozen orange juice concentrate,
    thawed
1 teaspoon grated orange peel
½ teaspoon grated lemon peel

Dip apple slices in lemon juice to prevent browning;
set aside. Combine remaining ingredients in small
bowl. Cover; refrigerate until chilled. Arrange apple
slices on platter; serve with dip.

Makes 20 (1 tablespoon) servings

NUTRITIONAL INFORMATION PER SERVING

Calories	24.10 kc	Niacin (B3)	0.04 mg
Protein	0.66 g	Pantothenic Acid	0.09 mg
Fat	0.23 g	Phosphorus	18.11 mg
% of Calories		Potassium	53.62 mg
from Fat:	8	Pyridoxine (B6)	0.01 mg
Saturated Fat	0.12 g	Riboflavin (B2)	0.03 mg
Cholesterol	0.70 mg	Thiamin (B1)	0.01 mg
Dietary Fiber	0.33 g	Vitamin A	3.35 RE
Sodium	8.21 mg	Vitamin C	3.83 mg
Beta-Carotene	5.09 RE	Copper	0.01 mg
Calcium	22.58 mg	Folate	3.44 µg
Cobalamin (B12)	0.06 µg	Vitamin E	0.10 mg
Iron	0.05 mg	Zinc	0.11 mg
Magnesium	3.17 mg		

ZUCCHINI WITH PIMIENTO

- 2 cups thin zucchini slices (about 2 medium zucchini)
- 1 small onion, chopped
- 1 jar (2 ounces) pimiento, drained and diced
- ½ teaspoon salt (optional)
- ½ teaspoon dried oregano leaves, crushed
- ⅛ teaspoon garlic powder
- ⅛ teaspoon ground red pepper

In 2-quart microwavable casserole, combine all ingredients; cover. Microwave at HIGH (100% power) 6 to 7 minutes or until fork-tender, stirring halfway through cooking time.   *Makes 4 servings*

NUTRITIONAL INFORMATION PER SERVING

Calories	21.68 kc	Pantothenic Acid	0.08 mg
Protein	1.16 g	Phosphorus	30.69 mg
Fat	0.23 g	Potassium	236.60 mg
% of Calories		Pyridoxine (B6)	0.11 mg
from Fat:	8	Riboflavin (B2)	0.03 mg
Saturated Fat	0.04 g	Thiamin (B1)	0.06 mg
Dietary Fiber	1.65 g	Vitamin A	58.36 RE
Sodium	273.50 mg	Vitamin C	20.59 mg
Beta-Carotene	180.50 RE	Copper	0.07 mg
Calcium	19.66 mg	Folate	19.89 µg
Iron	0.62 mg	Vitamin E	0.31 mg
Magnesium	17.65 mg	Zinc	0.21 mg
Niacin (B3)	0.37 mg		

Ratatouille

- ½ pound eggplant, cut into ½-inch cubes
- 1 small onion, sliced and separated into rings
- 1 small zucchini, thinly sliced
- ½ medium green bell pepper, chopped
- 1 medium tomato, cut into wedges
- 1 stalk celery, chopped
- 1 tablespoon grated Parmesan cheese
- ¼ teaspoon salt (optional)
- ¼ teaspoon dried chervil, crushed
- ¼ teaspoon dried oregano, crushed
- ⅛ teaspoon instant minced garlic
- ⅛ teaspoon dried thyme, crushed
- Dash black pepper

Combine all ingredients in 2-quart microwavable casserole; cover. Microwave at HIGH (100% power) 7 to 10 minutes or until eggplant is translucent, stirring every 3 minutes. *Makes 6 servings*

NUTRITIONAL INFORMATION PER SERVING

Calories	28.98 kc	Niacin (B3)	0.48 mg
Protein	1.40 g	Pantothenic Acid	0.13 mg
Fat	0.53 g	Phosphorus	34.79 mg
% of Calories		Potassium	230.20 mg
from Fat:	15	Pyridoxine (B6)	0.10 mg
Saturated Fat	0.24 g	Riboflavin (B2)	0.03 mg
Cholesterol	0.82 mg	Thiamin (B1)	0.06 mg
Dietary Fiber	1.97 g	Vitamin A	29.41 RE
Sodium	29.20 mg	Vitamin C	13.09 mg
Beta-Carotene	81.71 RE	Copper	0.08 mg
Calcium	28.25 mg	Folate	18.11 µg
Cobalamin (B12)	0.02 µg	Vitamin E	0.30 mg
Iron	0.46 mg	Zinc	0.19 mg
Magnesium	14.52 mg		

ORANGE-SPIKED ZUCCHINI AND CARROTS

- 1 pound zucchini, cut into ¼-inch slices
- 1 (10-ounce) package frozen sliced carrots, thawed
- 1 cup unsweetened orange juice
- 1 stalk celery, finely chopped
- 2 tablespoons chopped onion
  Salt and pepper to taste (optional)

Combine all ingredients in large nonstick saucepan. Simmer, covered, 10 to 12 minutes or until zucchini is tender. Uncover and continue to simmer, stirring occasionally, until most of the liquid has evaporated.

Makes 7 servings

NUTRITIONAL INFORMATION PER SERVING

Calories	40.84 kc	Pantothenic Acid	0.21 mg
Protein	1.14 g	Phosphorus	39.89 mg
Fat	0.16 g	Potassium	288.60 mg
% of Calories		Pyridoxine (B6)	0.12 mg
from Fat:	3	Riboflavin (B2)	0.05 mg
Saturated Fat	0.03 g	Thiamin (B1)	0.07 mg
Dietary Fiber	2.70 g	Vitamin A	737.20 RE
Sodium	30.80 mg	Vitamin C	21.84 mg
Beta-Carotene	4,368 RE	Copper	0.09 mg
Calcium	24.88 mg	Folate	34.76 µg
Iron	0.48 mg	Vitamin E	0.40 mg
Magnesium	20.35 mg	Zinc	0.22 mg
Niacin (B3)	0.57 mg		

FRUIT SOUP

- **5 fresh California nectarines, diced**
- **1 cup plain low-fat yogurt**
- **½ cup low-fat milk**
- **1 tablespoon sugar**
- **1 teaspoon almond extract**
- **¼ teaspoon curry powder**
- **½ cup strawberries, diced**
- **Mint leaves (optional)**

Reserve ½ cup nectarines. Place remaining nectarines, yogurt, milk, sugar, almond extract, and curry powder in blender; cover. Blend until smooth. Pour into bowl. Stir in reserved nectarines and strawberries. Chill; garnish with mint leaves.

Makes 6 servings

NUTRITIONAL INFORMATION PER SERVING

Calories	103.40 kc	Niacin (B3)	1.22 mg
Protein	3.81 g	Pantothenic Acid	0.51 mg
Fat	1.56 g	Phosphorus	94.48 mg
% of Calories		Potassium	381.80 mg
from Fat:	13	Pyridoxine (B6)	0.06 mg
Saturated Fat	0.68 g	Riboflavin (B2)	0.17 mg
Cholesterol	3.83 mg	Thiamin (B1)	0.05 mg
Dietary Fiber	2.17 g	Vitamin A	103.80 RE
Sodium	36.85 mg	Vitamin C	13.66 mg
Beta-Carotene	86.72 RE	Copper	0.10 mg
Calcium	101.70 mg	Folate	11.56 µg
Cobalamin (B12)	0.29 µg	Vitamin D	0.21 µg
Iron	0.28 mg	Vitamin E	1.26 mg
Magnesium	19.95 mg	Zinc	0.54 mg

CELERY AND CHICKPEA CURRY WITH APPLE

- 1 tablespoon vegetable oil
- 2 cups diagonally sliced celery
- 1 cup tart apple slices
- ½ cup chopped onion
- 2 teaspoons curry powder
- 1 teaspoon minced garlic
- 1 can (10½ ounces) chickpeas, rinsed and drained
- 1 can (8 ounces) stewed tomatoes, broken up
- 3 cups cooked brown rice

Heat oil in large skillet until hot. Add celery, apple, onion, curry powder, and garlic; cook and stir until vegetables are crisp-tender, 8 minutes. Stir in chickpeas and tomatoes. Bring to a boil; reduce heat and simmer, uncovered, until flavors are blended, about 5 minutes. Serve over cooked rice.   *Makes 4 servings*

NUTRITIONAL INFORMATION PER SERVING

Calories	318.40 kc	Pantothenic Acid	0.63 mg
Protein	8.72 g	Phosphorus	241.10 mg
Fat	6.50 g	Potassium	599.40 mg
% of Calories		Pyridoxine (B6)	0.31 mg
from Fat:	18	Riboflavin (B2)	0.12 mg
Saturated Fat	0.94 g	Thiamin (B1)	0.22 mg
Dietary Fiber	8.98 g	Vitamin A	42.89 RE
Sodium	500.20 mg	Vitamin C	18.42 mg
Beta-Carotene	143.10 RE	Copper	0.42 mg
Calcium	98.29 mg	Folate	30.44 µg
Iron	3.54 mg	Vitamin E	9.28 mg
Magnesium	106.50 mg	Zinc	1.89 mg
Niacin (B3)	3.15 mg		

FRUITS & VEGETABLES

DELICIOUS APPLE COMPOTE

- 2 Red or Golden Delicious apples
- 2 cups seeded watermelon cubes
- 1 cup seedless grapes
- 1 orange, peeled, sliced, and seeded
- 1 banana, peeled and sliced
- 2 cups chilled ginger ale
- 2 tablespoons lime juice

Core apples; cut into bite-sized pieces. Toss with watermelon, grapes, orange, and banana. Combine ginger ale and lime juice. Pour over fruit. Serve immediately.
Makes 6 servings

NUTRITIONAL INFORMATION PER SERVING

Calories	120.00 kc	Pantothenic Acid	0.26 mg
Protein	1.02 g	Phosphorus	18.68 mg
Fat	0.67 g	Potassium	285.40 mg
% of Calories		Pyridoxine (B6)	0.25 mg
from Fat:	5	Riboflavin (B2)	0.06 mg
Saturated Fat	0.12 g	Thiamin (B1)	0.10 mg
Dietary Fiber	2.37 g	Vitamin A	29.90 RE
Sodium	7.86 mg	Vitamin C	25.45 mg
Beta-Carotene	179.30 RE	Copper	0.11 mg
Calcium	23.33 mg	Folate	14.18 µg
Iron	0.46 mg	Vitamin E	0.65 mg
Magnesium	18.27 mg	Zinc	0.17 mg
Niacin (B3)	0.39 mg		

SPICED PEAR-CRANBERRY SOUP

2 fresh California Bartlett pears, peeled and
    chopped
2 thin slices fresh ginger (optional)
¼ teaspoon ground cinnamon
⅛ teaspoon ground cloves
1½ cups low-calorie cranberry juice cocktail
    Plain low-fat yogurt (optional)

Combine pears, ginger, cinnamon, and cloves in food
processor or blender; cover. Process until smooth.
With machine running, slowly add cranberry juice
until mixture is well blended. Garnish each serving
with a dollop of yogurt, if desired. Soup may be
served warm or cold. *Makes 4 servings*

NUTRITIONAL INFORMATION PER SERVING

Calories	75.23 kc	Pantothenic Acid	0.13 mg
Protein	0.33 g	Phosphorus	9.74 mg
Fat	0.35 g	Potassium	112.00 mg
% of Calories		Pyridoxine (B$_6$)	0.02 mg
from Fat:	4	Riboflavin (B$_2$)	0.04 mg
Saturated Fat	0.02 g	Thiamin (B$_1$)	0.02 mg
Dietary Fiber	2.16 g	Vitamin A	2.19 RE
Sodium	1.60 mg	Vitamin C	13.09 mg
Beta-Carotene	10.33 RE	Copper	0.10 mg
Calcium	13.68 mg	Folate	6.05 µg
Iron	0.31 mg	Vitamin E	0.55 mg
Magnesium	6.17 mg	Zinc	0.12 mg
Niacin (B$_3$)	0.09 mg		

DILLED GREEN BEANS

1 (10-ounce) package frozen cut green beans
½ cup plus 2 tablespoons water
2 green onions, finely chopped
2 teaspoons cornstarch
1 teaspoon instant chicken bouillon granules
1 teaspoon cider vinegar
¼ teaspoon grated lime peel
¼ teaspoon dill weed
  Dash pepper

Place beans and 2 tablespoons water in 1-quart microwavable casserole; cover. Microwave at HIGH (100% power) 4 to 7 minutes or until beans are tender, stirring after 3 minutes. Drain. Cover; set aside. In small microwavable bowl, blend remaining ingredients. Microwave at HIGH (100% power) 1½ to 2 minutes or until clear and thickened. Pour over beans. Toss to coat.   *Makes 4 servings*

Tip: For low-salt diets, substitute low-salt bouillon.

NUTRITIONAL INFORMATION PER SERVING

Calories	75.23 kc	Pantothenic Acid	0.13 mg
Protein	0.33 g	Phosphorus	9.74 mg
Fat	0.35 g	Potassium	112.00 mg
% of Calories		Pyridoxine (B6)	0.02 mg
from Fat:	4	Riboflavin (B2)	0.04 mg
Saturated Fat	0.02 g	Thiamin (B1)	0.02 mg
Dietary Fiber	2.16 g	Vitamin A	2.19 RE
Sodium	1.60 mg	Vitamin C	13.09 mg
Beta-Carotene	10.33 RE	Copper	0.10 mg
Calcium	13.68 mg	Folate	6.05 µg
Iron	0.31 mg	Vitamin E	0.55 mg
Magnesium	6.17 mg	Zinc	0.12 mg
Niacin (B3)	0.09 mg		

TODAY'S SLIM TUNA STUFFED TOMATOES

- 6 medium tomatoes
- 1 cup dry curd cottage cheese
- ½ cup plain low-fat yogurt
- ¼ cup chopped cucumber
- ¼ cup chopped green bell pepper
- ¼ cup thinly sliced radishes
- ¼ cup chopped green onion
- ½ teaspoon dried basil, crushed
- ⅛ teaspoon garlic powder
- 1 (6½-ounce) can tuna, packed in water, drained and flaked
- Lettuce leaves

Cut each tomato into 6 wedges, cutting to, but not through, each base. Refrigerate. Just before serving, in medium bowl, combine cottage cheese and yogurt; mix well. Stir in remaining ingredients except lettuce leaves. Place tomatoes on lettuce-lined plates; spread wedges apart. Spoon cottage cheese mixture into center of each tomato.   *Makes 6 servings*

NUTRITIONAL INFORMATION PER SERVING

Calories	98.48 kc	Niacin (B$_3$)	4.72 mg
Protein	14.00 g	Pantothenic Acid	0.51 mg
Fat	1.39 g	Phosphorus	131.80 mg
% of Calories		Potassium	414.40 mg
from Fat:	12	Pyridoxine (B$_6$)	0.19 mg
Saturated Fat	0.39 g	Riboflavin (B$_2$)	0.18 mg
Cholesterol	8.36 mg	Thiamin (B$_1$)	0.11 mg
Dietary Fiber	1.97 g	Vitamin A	113.30 RE
Sodium	47.66 mg	Vitamin C	34.53 mg
Beta-Carotene	250.70 RE	Copper	0.12 mg
Calcium	58.71 mg	Folate	29.47 µg
Cobalamin (B$_{12}$)	1.12 µg	Vitamin D	0.01 µg
Iron	1.19 mg	Vitamin E	1.11 mg
Magnesium	29.61 mg	Zinc	0.58 mg

GLAZED FRUIT KABOBS

- 2 fresh California nectarines, each cut into 6 wedges
- 3 fresh California plums, quartered
- ½ fresh pineapple, peeled and cut into 2-inch cubes
- ¼ cup firmly packed brown sugar
- 2 tablespoons water
- 1½ teaspoons cornstarch
- ¾ teaspoon rum extract

Alternately thread fruit onto skewers. Combine sugar, water, cornstarch, and rum extract in small saucepan. Bring to a boil, stirring constantly, until thickened and clear. Place fruit kabobs in shallow pan. Brush with glaze mixture.*

Grill kabobs about 4 to 5 inches from heat, 6 to 8 minutes or until hot, turning once, brushing occasionally with glaze mixture.   *Makes 4 servings*

*Kabobs may be prepared early and refrigerated until grilling time.

NUTRITIONAL INFORMATION PER SERVING

Calories	163.00 kc	Pantothenic Acid	0.33 mg
Protein	1.10 g	Phosphorus	25.58 mg
Fat	0.81 g	Potassium	358.60 mg
% of Calories		Pyridoxine (B6)	0.14 mg
from Fat:	4	Riboflavin (B2)	0.08 mg
Saturated Fat	0.07 g	Thiamin (B1)	0.13 mg
Dietary Fiber	2.94 g	Vitamin A	58.63 RE
Sodium	5.37 mg	Vitamin C	22.34 mg
Beta-Carotene	102.30 RE	Copper	0.23 mg
Calcium	25.53 mg	Folate	15.28 µg
Iron	1.08 mg	Vitamin E	1.04 mg
Magnesium	25.97 mg	Zinc	0.21 mg
Niacin (B3)	1.26 mg		

FETA POCKETS

- 2 cups bean sprouts
- 1 small cucumber, chopped
- ½ cup (2 ounces) crumbled Wisconsin Feta cheese
- ¼ cup plain yogurt
- 1 tablespoon sesame seed, toasted
- ¼ teaspoon black pepper
- 2 pita bread rounds, halved
- 1 medium tomato, cut into 4 slices

In medium bowl, stir together sprouts, cucumber, cheese, yogurt, sesame seed, and pepper. Spoon mixture into pita bread halves. Place tomato slice on filling in each bread half.   *Makes 4 servings*

NUTRITIONAL INFORMATION PER SERVING

Calories	145.10 kc	Niacin (B3)	1.77 mg
Protein	7.46 g	Pantothenic Acid	0.69 mg
Fat	5.04 g	Phosphorus	151.50 mg
% of Calories		Potassium	334.50 mg
from Fat:	30	Pyridoxine (B6)	0.22 mg
Saturated Fat	2.58 g	Riboflavin (B2)	0.29 mg
Cholesterol	13.90 mg	Thiamin (B1)	0.22 mg
Dietary Fiber	2.61 g	Vitamin A	45.53 RE
Sodium	288.70 mg	Vitamin C	16.56 mg
Beta-Carotene	41.52 RE	Copper	0.27 mg
Calcium	154.90 mg	Folate	66.02 µg
Cobalamin (B12)	0.33 µg	Vitamin E	2.01 mg
Iron	1.75 mg	Zinc	1.27 mg
Magnesium	40.00 mg		

CRUNCHY APPLE STIR-FRY

- 1 cup thinly sliced carrots (2 medium carrots)
- ½ cup onion slices
- 1 teaspoon dried basil, crushed
- 1½ teaspoons vegetable oil
- 1 cup fresh or thawed frozen snow peas
- 1 tablespoon water
- 1 medium Washington Golden Delicious or Criterion apple, cored and thinly sliced

Stir-fry carrots, onion, and basil in oil in nonstick skillet until carrots are tender. Stir in snow peas and water; stir-fry 2 minutes. Remove from heat; stir in apple slices. Serve hot.   *Makes 4 servings*

NUTRITIONAL INFORMATION PER SERVING

Calories	70.95 kc	Pantothenic Acid	0.37 mg
Protein	1.65 g	Phosphorus	42.18 mg
Fat	2.00 g	Potassium	244.40 mg
% of Calories		Pyridoxine (B6)	0.14 mg
from Fat:	24	Riboflavin (B2)	0.06 mg
Saturated Fat	0.26 g	Thiamin (B1)	0.10 mg
Dietary Fiber	2.90 g	Vitamin A	783.70 RE
Sodium	12.04 mg	Vitamin C	27.74 mg
Beta-Carotene	4,693 RE	Copper	0.07 mg
Calcium	37.03 mg	Folate	23.75 µg
Iron	1.15 mg	Vitamin E	2.84 mg
Magnesium	17.82 mg	Zinc	0.22 mg
Niacin (B3)	0.56 mg		

APPLE AND CARROT CASSEROLE

- **6 large carrots, sliced**
- **4 large apples, peeled and sliced**
- **5 tablespoons all-purpose flour**
- **1 tablespoon firmly packed brown sugar**
- **½ teaspoon ground nutmeg**
- **1 tablespoon margarine**
- **½ cup orange juice**

Preheat oven to 350°F. Cook carrots in large saucepan in boiling water for 5 minutes; drain. Layer carrots and apples in large casserole. In small bowl, mix flour, sugar, and nutmeg; sprinkle over carrots and apples. Dot with margarine; pour orange juice over flour mixture. Bake 30 minutes or until carrots are tender. *Makes 6 servings*

NUTRITIONAL INFORMATION PER SERVING

Calories	144.30 kc	Pantothenic Acid	0.27 mg
Protein	1.77 g	Phosphorus	50.59 mg
Fat	2.52 g	Potassium	396.90 mg
% of Calories		Pyridoxine (B6)	0.16 mg
from Fat:	15	Riboflavin (B2)	0.10 mg
Saturated Fat	0.51 g	Thiamin (B1)	0.16 mg
Dietary Fiber	4.67 g	Vitamin A	2,057 RE
Sodium	48.65 mg	Vitamin C	22.24 mg
Beta-Carotene	12,206 RE	Copper	0.10 mg
Calcium	31.83 mg	Folate	25.78 µg
Iron	0.96 mg	Vitamin D	0.19 µg
Magnesium	19.51 mg	Vitamin E	2.38 mg
Niacin (B3)	1.21 mg	Zinc	0.24 mg

FRUITS & VEGETABLES

MINT-GLAZED CARROTS AND SNOW PEAS

    1 tablespoon margarine
    3 medium carrots, thinly sliced diagonally
    ½ pound fresh snow peas, trimmed
    2 tablespoons sugar
    1 tablespoon fresh lemon juice
    1 tablespoon chopped fresh mint leaves or
    1 teaspoon dried mint, crushed

In large nonstick skillet, melt margarine over medium heat. Cook and stir carrots 3 to 4 minutes. Add snow peas, sugar, lemon juice, and mint. Cook and stir an additional 1 to 2 minutes until vegetables are glazed and crisp-tender.   *Makes 4 servings*

NUTRITIONAL INFORMATION PER SERVING

Calories	94.39 kc	Pantothenic Acid	0.47 mg
Protein	2.34 g	Phosphorus	54.39 mg
Fat	3.05 g	Potassium	309.20 mg
% of Calories		Pyridoxine (B6)	0.16 mg
from Fat:	28	Riboflavin (B2)	0.07 mg
Saturated Fat	0.59 g	Thiamin (B1)	0.12 mg
Dietary Fiber	3.24 g	Vitamin A	1,561 RE
Sodium	54.01 mg	Vitamin C	32.52 mg
Beta-Carotene	9,132 RE	Copper	0.07 mg
Calcium	38.38 mg	Folate	23.59 µg
Iron	1.33 mg	Vitamin D	0.28 µg
Magnesium	22.43 mg	Vitamin E	2.95 mg
Niacin (B3)	0.80 mg	Zinc	0.31 mg

COUNTRY BEAN SOUP

½ pound (1¼ cups) dried navy beans or lima
   beans
2½ cups water
   4 ounces salt pork or fully cooked ham, chopped
   ¼ cup chopped onion
   ½ teaspoon dried oregano, crushed
   ¼ teaspoon salt
   ¼ teaspoon ground ginger
   ¼ teaspoon dried sage, crushed
   ¼ teaspoon black pepper
   2 cups skim milk
   2 tablespoons butter

Rinse navy beans. Place beans in large saucepan; add
enough water to cover. Bring to a boil; reduce heat
and simmer 2 minutes. Remove from heat; cover and
let stand for 1 hour.*

Drain; return beans to saucepan. Stir in 2½ cups
water, salt pork, chopped onion, oregano, salt,
ground ginger, sage, and pepper. Bring to a boil;
reduce heat. Cover and simmer for 2 to 2½ hours or
until beans are tender. (If necessary, add more water
during cooking time.)

Add milk and butter, stirring until mixture is heated through and butter is melted. Season to taste with additional salt and pepper.   *Makes 6 servings*

*Or, cover beans with water and let soak 8 hours or overnight.

NUTRITIONAL INFORMATION PER SERVING

Calories	229.70 kc	Pantothenic Acid	0.59 mg
Protein	15.12 g	Phosphorus	259.90 mg
Fat	6.93 g	Potassium	519.80 mg
% of Calories		Pyridoxine (B6)	0.27 mg
from Fat:	27	Riboflavin (B2)	0.24 mg
Saturated Fat	3.82 g	Selenium	0.01 mg
Cholesterol	26.63 mg	Thiamin (B1)	0.34 mg
Dietary Fiber	0.13 g	Vitamin A	86.07 RE
Sodium	420.10 mg	Vitamin C	2.16 mg
Beta-Carotene	10.21 RE	Copper	0.29 mg
Calcium	166.80 mg	Folate	127.20 mc
Cobalamin (B12)	0.43 µg	Vitamin D	0.89 µg
Iron	2.49 mg	Vitamin E	0.29 mg
Magnesium	67.71 mg	Zinc	1.75 mg
Niacin (B3)	1.51 mg		

CRISPY VEGETABLES WITH ORANGE FLAVOR

      1 tablespoon vegetable oil
      2 cups diagonally sliced celery
      1 cup broccoli florets
    ¾ cup red bell pepper chunks
    ½ cup sliced green onions
      4 strips (2×½-inch) orange peel
   1½ teaspoons ground ginger
   1½ cups (about 8 ounces) firm tofu, cut into
            1-inch pieces
      1 tablespoon soy sauce
      1 packet low-sodium vegetable bouillon dissolved
            in 1½ cups water or 1½ cups no-salt-added
            tomato juice
      2 tablespoons cornstarch
      6 ounces thin spaghetti, cooked
         Orange slices (optional)

Heat oil in large nonstick skillet or wok until hot.
Add celery, broccoli, red pepper, green onions,
orange peel, and ginger; cook and stir until vegetables are crisp-tender, 4 to 5 minutes.

Meanwhile, in small bowl, toss tofu with soy sauce
until well coated; set aside. In measuring cup, combine bouillon and cornstarch. When vegetables are
cooked, add cornstarch mixture to skillet; bring to a
boil, stirring constantly until mixture is slightly
thickened, about 1 minute. Gently stir in tofu mixture; cook until heated through, about 1 minute.
Serve over cooked spaghetti. Garnish with orange
slices, if desired.   *Makes 4 servings*

Tip: Tofu, or soybean curd, is sometimes fortified with calcium. It is very perishable and should be used within one week of purchasing. Store tofu covered with water in the refrigerator. For maximum freshness, change the water every day, making sure to recover tofu each time.

NUTRITIONAL INFORMATION PER SERVING

Calories	341.10 kc	Pantothenic Acid	0.56 mg
Protein	17.20 g	Phosphorus	219.30 mg
Fat	9.65 g	Potassium	533.20 mg
% of Calories		Pyridoxine (B6)	0.31 mg
from Fat:	25	Riboflavin (B2)	0.28 mg
Saturated Fat	1.32 g	Thiamin (B1)	0.42 mg
Dietary Fiber	3.74 g	Vitamin A	106.40 RE
Sodium	342.10 mg	Vitamin C	73.14 mg
Beta-Carotene	484.30 RE	Copper	0.41 mg
Calcium	181.50 mg	Folate	69.93 µg
Iron	8.72 mg	Vitamin E	3.87 mg
Magnesium	95.95 mg	Zinc	1.83 mg
Niacin (B3)	3.58 mg		

Broccoli & Cauliflower with Mustard Sauce

> 2 cups fresh broccoli flowerets
> 2 cups fresh cauliflowerets
> 1/3 to 1/2 cup skim milk
> 1 tablespoon all-purpose flour
> 1 1/2 teaspoons prepared mustard
> 1/4 teaspoon salt (optional)
>   Dash garlic powder
>   Dash white pepper

To Microwave: Combine broccoli and cauliflower in medium microwavable baking dish. Cover. Microwave at HIGH (100% power) 8 to 11 minutes or until tender, stirring after half the cooking time. Drain; set aside.

In medium microwavable bowl, whisk together remaining ingredients. Microwave at HIGH (100% power) 2 to 3 minutes, or until thickened, stirring every minute. Pour over vegetables. Toss to coat.

Makes 4 servings

NUTRITIONAL INFORMATION PER SERVING

Calories	39.34 kc	Iron	0.70 mg
Protein	3.19 g	Magnesium	18.71 mg
Carbohydrate	6.95 g	Manganese	0.19 mg
Fat	0.41 g	Molybdenum	0.49 µg
% of Calories		Niacin (B3)	0.64 mg
from Fat:	8	Pantothenic Acid	0.36 mg
Saturated Fat	0.09 g	Phosphorus	67.30 mg
Cholesterol	0.33 mg	Potassium	315.40 mg
Dietary Fiber	2.50 g	Pyridoxine (B6)	0.17 mg
Sodium	49.84 mg	Riboflavin (B2)	0.11 mg
Beta-Carotene	68.74 RE	Thiamin (B1)	0.08 mg
Biotin	0.44 µg	Vitamin A	74.10 RE
Calcium	60.51 mg	Vitamin C	58.40 mg
Cobalamin (B12)	0.08 µg	Vitamin D	0.22 µg
Copper	0.07 mg	Vitamin E	0.39 mg
Fluoride	6.73 mg	Vitamin K	0.82 µg
Folate	47.25 µg	Zinc	0.38 mg

FRENCH CARROT MEDLEY

2 cups fresh or thawed frozen carrot slices
¾ cup unsweetened orange juice
1 (4-ounce) can sliced mushrooms, undrained
4 stalks celery, sliced
2 tablespoons chopped onion
½ teaspoon dillweed
   Salt and pepper to taste (optional)
2 teaspoons cornstarch or arrowroot
¼ cup cold water

Combine all ingredients except cornstarch and water in medium saucepan. Simmer, covered, 12 to 15 minutes or until carrots are tender. Combine cornstarch and water in small bowl. Stir into vegetable mixture; cook and stir until mixture thickens and bubbles. *Makes 6 servings*

NUTRITIONAL INFORMATION PER SERVING

Calories	42.49 kc	Pantothenic Acid	0.33 mg
Protein	1.17 g	Phosphorus	41.43 mg
Fat	0.22 g	Potassium	281.90 mg
% of Calories		Pyridoxine (B$_6$)	0.12 mg
from Fat:	4	Riboflavin (B$_2$)	0.05 mg
Saturated Fat	0.04 g	Thiamin (B$_1$)	0.08 mg
Dietary Fiber	2.22 g	Vitamin A	1,040 RE
Sodium	117.60 mg	Vitamin C	16.48 mg
Beta-Carotene	6,240 RE	Copper	0.09 mg
Calcium	27.46 mg	Folate	32.56 µg
Iron	0.63 mg	Vitamin E	0.48 mg
Magnesium	15.42 mg	Zinc	0.28 mg
Niacin (B$_3$)	0.83 mg		

PLUM RATATOUILLE

2½ cups diced eggplant
2 cups sliced zucchini
1 onion, cut into wedges
1 tablespoon vegetable oil
2 cups diced tomatoes
4 fresh California plums, cut into wedges (2 cups)
2 teaspoons minced garlic
1½ teaspoons dried basil, crumbled
1 teaspoon dried oregano, crumbled
¼ teaspoon black pepper
Fresh lemon juice

In large nonstick skillet, cook and stir eggplant, zucchini, and onion in vegetable oil 15 minutes or until tender. Add remaining ingredients except lemon wedges. Reduce heat and cover. Cook, stirring occasionally, until plums are tender, about 4 minutes. Drizzle with fresh lemon juice just before serving.

Makes 6 servings

NUTRITIONAL INFORMATION PER SERVING

Calories	69.17 kc	Iron	0.81 mg
Protein	1.43 g	Magnesium	23.86 mg
Carbohydrate	12.13 g	Manganese	0.22 mg
Fat	2.56 g	Niacin (B3)	0.69 mg
% of Calories		Pantothenic Acid	0.15 mg
from Fat:	30	Phosphorus	42.25 mg
Saturated Fat	0.34 g	Potassium	351.10 mg
Dietary Fiber	3.41 g	Pyridoxine (B6)	0.14 mg
Sodium	4.17 mg	Riboflavin (B2)	0.04 mg
Beta-Carotene	155.70 RE	Thiamin (B1)	0.10 mg
Biotin	0.30 µg	Vitamin A	28.76 RE
Calcium	29.82 mg	Vitamin C	7.47 mg
Chromium	0.01 mg	Vitamin E	2.23 mg
Copper	0.12 mg	Vitamin K	1.50 µg
Fluoride	19.92 µg	Zinc	0.28 mg
Folate	23.88 µg		

Applesauce Berry Salad

1 (3-ounce) package sugar-free strawberry gelatin
1 cup boiling water
1 (10-ounce) package frozen strawberries, thawed
1 cup applesauce
1 cup plain low-fat yogurt or low-fat sour cream

Dissolve gelatin in boiling water. Stir in strawberries and applesauce; pour into 10×6-inch dish. Chill until set. Spread yogurt on top of gelatin mixture. Cover and chill 2 hours. Cut into squares.

Makes 6 to 8 servings

NUTRITIONAL INFORMATION PER SERVING

Calories	77.56 kc	Niacin (B3)	0.25 mg
Protein	7.54 g	Pantothenic Acid	0.24 mg
Fat	0.49 g	Phosphorus	184.60 mg
% of Calories		Potassium	142.90 mg
from Fat:	6	Pyridoxine (B6)	0.03 mg
Saturated Fat	0.29 g	Riboflavin (B2)	0.08 mg
Cholesterol	1.75 mg	Thiamin (B1)	0.02 mg
Dietary Fiber	1.39 g	Vitamin A	8.07 RE
Sodium	250.80 mg	Vitamin C	15.20 mg
Beta-Carotene	6.67 RE	Copper	0.03 mg
Calcium	58.45 mg	Folate	9.25 µg
Cobalamin (B12)	0.16 µg	Vitamin E	0.18 mg
Iron	0.33 mg	Zinc	0.31 mg
Magnesium	9.82 mg		

ARTICHOKE WILD RICE SALAD

SALAD:

2 cups cooked wild rice
1 cup frozen peas, thawed
1 (8-ounce) can sliced water chestnuts, drained
1 (6-ounce) jar marinated artichoke hearts
4 ounces shredded mozzarella cheese (optional)
1 (2-ounce) jar diced pimiento, drained

DRESSING:

2 tablespoons canola oil
2 tablespoons reserved liquid from artichokes
1 tablespoon balsamic vinegar
½ teaspoon dried tarragon leaves, crumbled
½ teaspoon Dijon mustard
2 to 3 drops hot pepper sauce (or to taste)

Drain artichokes, reserving liquid. In large bowl, combine salad ingredients. In small bowl, mix dressing ingredients; pour over salad and toss. Chill 4 hours or overnight to allow flavors to blend.

Makes 6 to 8 servings

NUTRITIONAL INFORMATION PER SERVING

Calories	129.00 kc	Pantothenic Acid	0.23 mg
Protein	3.80 g	Phosphorus	80.65 mg
Fat	3.83 g	Potassium	201.90 mg
% of Calories		Pyridoxine (B6)	0.16 mg
from Fat:	22	Riboflavin (B2)	0.08 mg
Saturated Fat	0.30 g	Thiamin (B1)	0.10 mg
Dietary Fiber	2.85 g	Vitamin A	36.89 RE
Sodium	48.17 mg	Vitamin C	11.12 mg
Beta-Carotene	132.30 RE	Copper	0.13 mg
Calcium	20.75 mg	Folate	36.90 µg
Iron	1.34 mg	Vitamin E	0.28 mg
Magnesium	34.86 mg	Zinc	0.97 mg
Niacin (B3)	1.20 mg		

CALIFORNIA APRICOT FRUIT SALAD

- **2** cups sliced fresh California apricots (about 1 pound)
- **1½** cups sliced fresh strawberries
- **1½** cups peeled and sliced kiwifruit
- **¼** cup California apricot nectar
- **¼** cup flake coconut, lightly toasted
- **1** tablespoon finely chopped fresh mint

In medium bowl, combine all ingredients. Refrigerate until chilled. Serve as salad or arrange on wooden skewers for fresh fruit kabobs.

Makes 5 servings

NUTRITIONAL INFORMATION PER SERVING

Calories	114.70 kc	Pantothenic Acid	0.42 mg
Protein	2.18 g	Phosphorus	50.02 mg
Fat	2.38 g	Potassium	523.80 mg
% of Calories		Pyridoxine (B6)	0.13 mg
from Fat:	17	Riboflavin (B2)	0.09 mg
Saturated Fat	1.50 g	Thiamin (B1)	0.05 mg
Dietary Fiber	4.71 g	Vitamin A	266.70 RE
Sodium	16.48 mg	Vitamin C	83.18 mg
Calcium	33.23 mg	Copper	0.20 mg
Iron	1.03 mg	Folate	34.73 µg
Magnesium	28.46 mg	Vitamin E	1.76 mg
Niacin (B3)	0.94 mg	Zinc	0.47 mg

HEARTY HEALTHY CHICKEN SALAD

- 1 broiler-fryer chicken, cooked, skinned, boned, and cut into chunks
- 1 cup small macaroni, cooked
- 3 tomatoes, cubed
- 1 cup sliced celery
- ½ cup chopped red bell pepper
- 3 tablespoons chopped green onion
- 1 teaspoon salt
- ½ teaspoon ground black pepper
- ¼ teaspoon oregano
- 1 cup chicken broth
- 1 clove garlic, split
- ¼ cup wine vinegar

In large bowl, mix warm chicken, macaroni, tomatoes, celery, bell pepper, and onion. Sprinkle with salt, black pepper, and oregano. Place broth and garlic in small saucepan; bring to a boil over high heat and boil 10 minutes or until broth is reduced to ½ cup. Add vinegar; pour over salad, mixing well. Chill until cold. *Makes 6 servings*

NUTRITIONAL INFORMATION PER SERVING

Calories	249.10 kc	Niacin	10.13 mg
Protein	30.07 g	Pantothenic Acid	1.31 mg
Fat	8.18 g	Phosphorus	236.70 mg
% of Calories		Potassium	512.80 mg
from Fat:	30	Pyridoxine (B6)	0.58 mg
Saturated Fat	2.08 g	Riboflavin (B2)	0.29 mg
Cholesterol	85.34 mg	Thiamin (B1)	0.18 mg
Dietary Fiber	1.96 g	Vitamin A	80.95 RE
Sodium	698.50 mg	Vitamin C	31.49 mg
Beta-Carotene	172.80 RE	Copper	0.18 mg
Calcium	35.86 mg	Folate	27.52 µg
Cobalamin (B12)	0.35 µg	Vitamin E	1.22 mg
Iron	2.19 mg	Zinc	2.30 mg
Magnesium	40.47 mg		

SPICY BEEF AND RICE SALAD

- **1 pound boneless beef top sirloin steak, 1 inch thick**
- **2 teaspoons Spicy Seasoning Mix (recipe follows), divided**
  Salt to taste
- **2 cups Spicy Cooked Rice (recipe follows)**
- **1 medium red apple, cut into small chunks**
- **2 to 3 green onions, thinly sliced**
- **¼ cup coarsely chopped walnuts, toasted***
  Leaf lettuce (optional)
  Additional apple chunks (optional)

Prepare Spicy Seasoning Mix; set aside. Heat large nonstick skillet over medium heat 5 minutes. Meanwhile, rub 1 teaspoon Spicy Seasoning into sides of steak. Place steak in skillet and cook 12 to 14 minutes for rare (140°F) to medium (160°F), turning once. Season with salt, if desired.

Meanwhile, combine Spicy Cooked Rice, apple, onions, and walnuts. Cut steak into thin slices; arrange over rice mixture. Garnish with leaf lettuce and apple, if desired.   *Makes 4 servings*

*To toast walnuts, spread walnuts in single layer on baking sheet. Bake at 350°F, 5 to 8 minutes, stirring occasionally, until lightly browned. Cool.

SPICY SEASONING MIX

  3 tablespoons chili powder
  2 teaspoons ground cumin
1½ teaspoons garlic powder
  ¾ teaspoon dried oregano leaves
  ½ teaspoon ground red pepper

Combine chili powder, cumin, garlic powder, oregano, and red pepper. Store, covered, in airtight container. Shake before using to blend.

Makes about ⅓ cup.

Spicy Cooked Rice: Cook ⅔ cup rice according to package directions, adding 1 teaspoon Spicy Seasoning Mix to water before cooking.

NUTRITIONAL INFORMATION PER SERVING

Calories	378.50 kc	Niacin (B3)	5.82 mg
Protein	34.85 g	Pantothenic Acid	0.88 mg
Fat	10.39 g	Phosphorus	328.80 mg
% of Calories		Potassium	525.40 mg
from Fat:	25	Pyridoxine (B6)	0.60 mg
Saturated Fat	2.54 g	Riboflavin (B2)	0.32 mg
Cholesterol	71.62 mg	Thiamin (B1)	0.32 mg
Dietary Fiber	2.39 g	Vitamin A	16.66 RE
Sodium	67.81 mg	Vitamin C	3.33 mg
Beta-Carotene	87.04 RE	Copper	0.30 mg
Calcium	30.90 mg	Folate	19.82 µg
Cobalamin (B12)	2.82 µg	Vitamin E	2.34 mg
Iron	4.81 mg	Zinc	7.23 mg
Magnesium	62.44 mg		

SALADS

FRUIT AND GREEN SALAD

- 2 tablespoons plain yogurt
- 1 teaspoon lemon juice
- 1 teaspoon sugar
- 1½ cups torn lettuce
- 1 orange, cubed
- 1 apple, cubed
- 1 teaspoon walnuts

In small bowl, mix yogurt, lemon juice, and sugar. In salad bowl, toss lettuce, orange, and apple. Pour dressing over salad and top with nuts.

Makes 2 servings

NUTRITIONAL INFORMATION PER SERVING

Calories	101.70 kc	Niacin (B3)	0.34 mg
Protein	2.24 g	Pantothenic Acid	0.32 mg
Fat	1.36 g	Phosphorus	48.97 mg
% of Calories		Potassium	306.30 mg
from Fat:	11	Pyridoxine (B6)	0.10 mg
Saturated Fat	0.25 g	Riboflavin (B2)	0.08 mg
Cholesterol	0.88 mg	Thiamin (B1)	0.10 mg
Dietary Fiber	3.59 g	Vitamin A	34.05 RE
Sodium	14.22 mg	Vitamin C	41.68 mg
Beta-Carotene	116.70 RE	Copper	0.09 mg
Calcium	65.94 mg	Folate	47.64 µg
Cobalamin (B12)	0.08 µg	Vitamin E	1.21 mg
Iron	0.45 mg	Zinc	0.33 mg
Magnesium	18.54 mg		

FRUITED SLAW

- 1 (8¼-ounce) can pineapple chunks in syrup
- 1 (8-ounce) carton orange-flavored yogurt
- 1 tablespoon lemon juice
- 3 cups finely shredded cabbage
- 1 (11-ounce) can mandarin orange sections, drained
- 1 cup thin celery slices
- ½ cup chopped walnuts
- ¼ cup raisins
- 1 medium banana, sliced

Drain pineapple, reserving 2 tablespoons syrup. In small bowl, combine reserved syrup, yogurt, and lemon juice. In large bowl, combine pineapple, cabbage, oranges, celery, nuts, and raisins; fold in yogurt mixture. Gently fold in banana. Cover; chill.

Makes 8 servings

NUTRITIONAL INFORMATION PER SERVING

Calories	140.60 kc	Niacin (B3)	0.51 mg
Protein	4.52 g	Pantothenic Acid	0.33 mg
Fat	5.04 g	Phosphorus	96.71 mg
% of Calories		Potassium	383.60 mg
from Fat:	30	Pyridoxine (B6)	0.24 mg
Saturated Fat	0.54 g	Riboflavin (B2)	0.13 mg
Cholesterol	1.25 mg	Thiamin (B1)	0.12 mg
Dietary Fiber	2.49 g	Vitamin A	27.10 RE
Sodium	37.97 mg	Vitamin C	32.96 mg
Beta-Carotene	103.00 RE	Copper	0.19 mg
Calcium	84.12 mg	Folate	43.54 µg
Cobalamin (B12)	0.13 µg	Vitamin E	2.55 mg
Iron	0.84 mg	Zinc	0.72 mg
Magnesium	42.26 mg		

PASTA AND WALNUT FRUIT SALAD

8 ounces medium pasta shells, uncooked
1 (8-ounce) container nonfat plain yogurt
¼ cup frozen orange juice concentrate, thawed
1 (15-ounce) can juice-packed mandarin oranges, drained
1 cup seedless red grapes, halved
1 cup seedless green grapes, halved
1 apple, cored and chopped
½ cup sliced celery
½ cup walnut halves

Cook shells according to package directions; drain. In small bowl, blend yogurt and orange juice concentrate. In large bowl, combine shells and remaining ingredients. Add yogurt mixture; toss to coat. Cover and chill thoroughly.   *Makes 6 to 8 servings*

NUTRITIONAL INFORMATION PER SERVING

Calories	231.00 kc	Niacin (B3)	1.13 mg
Protein	8.44 g	Pantothenic Acid	0.45 mg
Fat	5.66 g	Phosphorus	148.40 mg
% of Calories		Potassium	334.50 mg
from Fat:	21	Pyridoxine (B6)	0.18 mg
Saturated Fat	0.51 g	Riboflavin (B2)	0.25 mg
Cholesterol	24.98 mg	Thiamin (B1)	0.29 mg
Dietary Fiber	2.93 g	Vitamin A	31.88 RE
Sodium	35.47 mg	Vitamin C	33.07 mg
Beta-Carotene	137.90 RE	Copper	0.22 mg
Calcium	85.95 mg	Folate	42.25 µg
Cobalamin (B12)	0.28 µg	Vitamin E	2.27 mg
Iron	1.39 mg	Zinc	1.13 mg
Magnesium	47.29 mg		

FRUITED LAMB SALAD

- **3 cups cooked American lamb cubes or slices**
- **3 cups cooked brown and wild rice, chilled**
- **1½ cups sliced strawberries**
- **1½ cups orange cubes**
- **¾ cup green grapes**
- **½ cup banana slices**
- **¼ cup walnuts**
- **2 tablespoons honey**
- **2 tablespoons lemon juice**
- **12 large Romaine lettuce leaves**

In large bowl, combine lamb, rice, fruit, and nuts. In small bowl, mix together honey and lemon juice; toss with lamb mixture. Chill. Serve on lettuce leaves.

Makes 12 servings

NUTRITIONAL INFORMATION PER SERVING

Calories	167.40 kc	Niacin (B3)	2.99 mg
Protein	12.90 g	Pantothenic Acid	0.47 mg
Fat	5.15 g	Phosphorus	133.40 mg
% of Calories		Potassium	311.30 mg
from Fat:	27	Pyridoxine (B6)	0.20 mg
Saturated Fat	1.35 g	Riboflavin (B2)	0.18 mg
Cholesterol	32.52 mg	Thiamin (B1)	0.10 mg
Dietary Fiber	2.19 g	Vitamin A	12.65 RE
Sodium	30.70 mg	Vitamin C	25.08 mg
Beta-Carotene	20.38 RE	Copper	0.16 mg
Calcium	24.29 mg	Folate	43.29 µg
Cobalamin (B12)	0.93 µg	Vitamin E	1.01 mg
Iron	1.30 mg	Zinc	2.60 mg
Magnesium	35.41 mg		

TURKEY, MANDARIN, AND POPPY SEED SALAD

- 5 cups red leaf lettuce, torn
- 2 cups spinach leaves, torn
- ½ pound honey roasted turkey, cut into ½-inch julienne strips
- 1 can (10½ ounces) mandarin oranges, drained
- ¼ cup orange juice
- 1½ tablespoons red wine vinegar
- 1½ teaspoons poppy seed
- 1½ teaspoons olive oil
- 1 teaspoon Dijon-style mustard
- ⅛ teaspoon pepper

In large bowl, combine lettuce, spinach, turkey, and oranges. In small bowl, combine orange juice, vinegar, poppy seed, oil, mustard, and pepper. Pour dressing over turkey mixture. Serve immediately.

Makes 4 servings

NUTRITIONAL INFORMATION PER SERVING

Calories	142.80 kc	Niacin (B3)	4.26 mg
Protein	14.87 g	Pantothenic Acid	0.19 mg
Fat	3.20 g	Phosphorus	174.80 mg
% of Calories		Potassium	600.30 mg
from Fat:	20	Pyridoxine (B6)	0.42 mg
Saturated Fat	1.69 g	Riboflavin (B2)	0.24 mg
Cholesterol	42.92 mg	Thiamin (B1)	0.17 mg
Dietary Fiber	2.28 g	Vitamin A	347.00 RE
Sodium	726.50 mg	Vitamin C	48.94 mg
Beta-Carotene	1,318 RE	Copper	0.15 mg
Calcium	119.10 mg	Folate	115.40 µg
Cobalamin (B12)	0.20 µg	Vitamin E	2.04 mg
Iron	2.88 mg	Zinc	1.80 mg
Magnesium	58.68 mg		

CONFETTI APPLESLAW

- 2 tablespoons orange or apple juice concentrate, thawed
- 1 unpeeled red apple, cored and diced
- 4 cups shredded cabbage
- 2 small red onions, finely shredded
- 1 red or green bell pepper, thinly sliced
- 3 tablespoons raisins
- 1 tablespoon reduced-calorie mayonnaise
- ½ cup plain low-fat yogurt
- ½ teaspoon dry mustard
  - Paprika to taste
  - Freshly ground black pepper to taste

In large bowl, combine juice concentrate and diced apple. Add cabbage, onions, bell pepper, and raisins. In small bowl, stir together mayonnaise, yogurt, mustard, paprika, and black pepper. Add to vegetable mixture. Cover tightly, and refrigerate until ready to serve. *Makes 7 servings*

NUTRITIONAL INFORMATION PER SERVING

Calories	69.78 kc	Niacin (B3)	0.34 mg
Protein	2.11 g	Pantothenic Acid	0.24 mg
Fat	1.08 g	Phosphorus	52.28 mg
% of Calories		Potassium	298.40 mg
from Fat:	13	Pyridoxine (B6)	0.14 mg
Saturated Fat	0.27 g	Riboflavin (B2)	0.07 mg
Cholesterol	1.71 mg	Thiamin (B1)	0.07 mg
Dietary Fiber	2.24 g	Vitamin A	18.71 RE
Sodium	24.46 mg	Vitamin C	42.21 mg
Beta-Carotene	26.57 RE	Copper	0.06 mg
Calcium	64.11 mg	Folate	44.62 µg
Cobalamin (B12)	0.09 µg	Vitamin D	0.02 µg
Iron	0.53 mg	Vitamin E	2.52 mg
Magnesium	17.44 mg	Zinc	0.32 mg

GOLDEN FRUIT SALAD

1 **Golden Delicious or Crispin apple, cored and sliced**

1 **Red Delicious or Empire apple, cored and sliced**

1 **banana, peeled and sliced**

½ **cup red or green grapes**

Lettuce

Orange Yogurt Dressing (recipe follows)

Combine fruit; mix well. Serve on lettuce-lined salad plates with Orange Yogurt Dressing.

Makes 3 servings

Orange Yogurt Dressing: Combine ½ cup plain low-fat yogurt, 2 to 3 tablespoons orange juice, and dash nutmeg; mix well.

NUTRITIONAL INFORMATION PER SERVING

Calories	136.60 kc	Niacin (B3)	0.44 mg
Protein	2.81 g	Pantothenic Acid	0.40 mg
Fat	1.27 g	Phosphorus	73.55 mg
% of Calories		Potassium	414.80 mg
from Fat:	8	Pyridoxine (B6)	0.32 mg
Saturated Fat	0.56 g	Riboflavin (B2)	0.15 mg
Cholesterol	2.33 mg	Thiamin (B1)	0.08 mg
Dietary Fiber	3.04 g	Vitamin A	19.43 RE
Sodium	28.12 mg	Vitamin C	16.99 mg
Beta-Carotene	71.62 RE	Copper	0.11 mg
Calcium	82.23 mg	Folate	20.74 µg
Cobalamin (B12)	0.21 µg	Vitamin E	0.97 mg
Iron	0.40 mg	Zinc	0.45 mg
Magnesium	24.39 mg		

CURRY RICE SALAD WITH APPLES

- ⅓ cup plain or vanilla yogurt
- 1½ tablespoons dry sherry or cider vinegar
- 1 to 2 teaspoons curry powder
- ⅛ teaspoon ground cloves
  Salt and pepper to taste
- ¾ cup finely diced celery
- ¼ to ½ cup currants or raisins
- 2 Empire, McIntosh, or Cortland apples,
  unpeeled and cubed*
- 4 cups cooked brown rice

In large bowl, combine yogurt, sherry, curry powder, cloves, salt, and pepper. Mix well. Add celery, currants, and apples. Mix well. Add rice; mix well. Salad keeps well for a few days in the refrigerator.

Makes 6 servings

*Mix apples with a small amount of lemon juice to prevent browning.

NUTRITIONAL INFORMATION PER SERVING

Calories	226.10 kc	Niacin (B3)	2.15 mg
Protein	4.99 g	Pantothenic Acid	0.70 mg
Fat	0.93 g	Phosphorus	101.30 mg
% of Calories		Potassium	214.70 mg
from Fat:	4	Pyridoxine (B6)	0.18 mg
Saturated Fat	0.33 g	Riboflavin (B2)	0.08 mg
Cholesterol	1.17 mg	Thiamin (B1)	0.25 mg
Dietary Fiber	2.99 g	Vitamin A	9.07 RE
Sodium	29.69 mg	Vitamin C	5.79 mg
Beta-Carotene	29.20 RE	Copper	0.12 mg
Calcium	63.05 mg	Folate	12.66 µg
Cobalamin (B12)	0.11 µg	Vitamin E	0.95 mg
Iron	1.82 mg	Zinc	0.86 mg
Magnesium	26.21 mg		

WILD RICE SEAFOOD SALAD

- ⅓ cup low-fat mayonnaise
- ⅓ cup nonfat sour cream
- ¼ cup low-sodium chili sauce
- 1 tablespoon lemon juice
- 1 teaspoon Dijon-style mustard
- 3 cups cooked wild rice
- ½ cup thin green onion slices
- 1 large tomato, peeled, seeded, and diced
- 1 cup thin slices celery
- ½ pound imitation crabmeat
  Salt and pepper (optional)
  Lettuce cups (optional)
  Chopped parsley (optional)

For dressing, in medium bowl, blend mayonnaise, sour cream, chili sauce, lemon juice, and mustard. Refrigerate. Combine wild rice, onions, tomato, celery, and crabmeat. Season with salt and pepper to taste, if desired. Place salad in individual lettuce cups and garnish with parsley, if desired. Serve with dressing. *Makes 6 servings*

NUTRITIONAL INFORMATION PER SERVING

Calories	186.40 kc	Niacin (B₃)	1.32 mg
Protein	9.20 g	Pantothenic Acid	0.30 mg
Fat	4.49 g	Phosphorus	187.10 mg
% of Calories		Potassium	242.40 mg
from Fat:	21	Pyridoxine (B₆)	0.16 mg
Saturated Fat	0.58 g	Riboflavin (B₂)	0.11 mg
Cholesterol	12.00 mg	Thiamin (B₁)	0.08 mg
Dietary Fiber	2.08 g	Vitamin A	57.26 RE
Sodium	372.00 mg	Vitamin C	9.48 mg
Beta-Carotene	245.00 RE	Copper	0.14 mg
Calcium	21.70 mg	Folate	32.31 µg
Cobalamin (B₁₂)	0.61 µg	Vitamin D	0.12 µg
Iron	0.96 mg	Vitamin E	7.78 mg
Magnesium	48.87 mg	Zinc	1.32 mg

SPINACH CHICKPEA SALAD

2 tablespoons red wine vinegar
2 tablespoons water
1 teaspoon sesame oil
1 teaspoon lite soy sauce
1 teaspoon sugar
3 cups spinach
2 carrots, sliced
1 cup canned chickpeas, drained and rinsed
1½ tablespoons sesame seeds

In small bowl, mix vinegar, water, oil, soy sauce, and sugar to make dressing. In salad bowl, toss dressing with spinach, carrots, and chickpeas. Sprinkle with sesame seeds. *Makes 4 servings*

NUTRITIONAL INFORMATION PER SERVING

Calories	114.20 kc	Pantothenic Acid	0.10 mg
Protein	4.83 g	Phosphorus	119.90 mg
Fat	4.05 g	Potassium	479.00 mg
% of Calories		Pyridoxine (B6)	0.16 mg
from Fat	30	Riboflavin (B2)	0.13 mg
Saturated Fat	0.57 g	Thiamin (B1)	0.10 mg
Dietary Fiber	5.55 g	Vitamin A	1,295 RE
Sodium	323.60 mg	Vitamin C	17.96 mg
Beta-Carotene	7,773 RE	Copper	0.33 mg
Calcium	107.20 mg	Folate	89.49 µg
Iron	3.30 mg	Vitamin E	4.26 mg
Magnesium	69.60 mg	Zinc	1.09 mg
Niacin (B3)	0.96 mg		

JAPANESE PETAL SALAD

    Romaine lettuce leaves
 1 pound medium shrimp, cooked, or 2 cups
      chicken, cooked, shredded
 2 fresh California nectarines, thinly sliced
 2 cups cucumber, sliced
 2 celery stalks, cut into 3-inch matchstick pieces
 ⅓ cup red radishes, shredded
    Sesame Dressing (recipe follows) or low-calorie
      dressing
 2 teaspoons sesame seeds (optional)

Center shrimp on 4 lettuce-lined salad plates. Fan
nectarines to right side of shrimp; overlap cucumber
slices to left side. Place celery pieces at top of plate;
mound radishes at bottom of plate. Prepare dressing;
pour 3 tablespoons over each salad. Sprinkle with
sesame seeds, if desired.   *Makes 4 servings*

SESAME DRESSING

½ cup rice wine vinegar (not seasoned-type)
2 tablespoons low-sodium soy sauce
2 teaspoons sugar
2 teaspoons dark sesame oil

In small bowl, combine all ingredients. Stir to dissolve sugar. Makes about ⅔ cup.

NUTRITIONAL INFORMATION PER SERVING

Calories	192.00 kc	Iodine	40.82 µg
Protein	25.31 g	Iron	4.21 mg
Carbohydrate	14.67 g	Magnesium	55.31 mg
Fat	3.93 g	Manganese	0.11 mg
% of Calories		Molybdenum	0.84 µg
from Fat:	18	Niacin (B3)	4.15 mg
Saturated Fat	0.71 g	Pantothenic Acid	0.69 mg
Cholesterol	221.50 mg	Phosphorus	193.00 mg
Dietary Fiber	2.03 g	Potassium	516.70 mg
Sodium	573.30 mg	Pyridoxine (B6)	0.22 mg
Beta-Carotene	66.37 RE	Riboflavin (B2)	0.10 mg
Biotin	0.54 µg	Thiamin (B1)	0.08 mg
Calcium	67.24 mg	Vitamin A	130.10 RE
Chromium	0.01 mg	Vitamin C	11.04 mg
Cobalamin (B12)	1.68 µg	Vitamin E	6.81 mg
Copper	0.32 mg	Vitamin K	2.87 µg
Fluoride	16.80 µg	Zinc	2.03 mg
Folate	21.96 µg		

INDONESIAN CHICKEN AND PEAR SALAD

Curry Dressing (recipe follows)
1½ cups cold cooked chicken, cubed
3 fresh California Bartlett pears, halved, cored, divided
½ cup macadamia nuts or peanuts, coarsely chopped (optional)
½ cup cucumber, sliced
3 tablespoons crystallized ginger, slivered (optional)
2 tablespoons green onion, thinly sliced
Lemon juice
Iceberg lettuce cups
Toasted shredded coconut (optional)

Prepare Curry Dressing; set aside. Place chicken in large bowl. Cube 2 pear halves; add to chicken along with nuts, cucumber, ginger and onion. Add Curry Dressing; mix gently.

Dip remaining 4 pear halves in lemon juice and arrange in lettuce cup on salad plate. Spoon salad over pear halves. Sprinkle with toasted coconut, if desired.   *Makes 4 servings*

Curry Dressing: Combine ½ cup plain low fat yogurt, ½ teaspoon curry powder, and ¼ teaspoon each dry mustard, ground allspice, and garlic powder; mix well. Prepare dressing about 20 minutes before using to allow flavors to blend. Makes about ⅔ cup.

Tip: Chicken is an excellent source of high-quality protein and B vitamins, yet is low in saturated fat. As a rule, one broiler-fryer chicken (about 3 pounds) yields about 2½ cups of chopped, cooked chicken.

NUTRITIONAL INFORMATION PER SERVING

Calories	179.80 kc	Niacin (B_3)	5.62 mg
Protein	14.86 g	Pantothenic Acid	0.71 mg
Fat	4.37 g	Phosphorus	150.60 mg
% of Calories		Potassium	360.10 mg
from Fat:	21	Pyridoxine (B_6)	0.28 mg
Saturated Fat	1.25 g	Riboflavin (B_2)	0.17 mg
Cholesterol	37.77 mg	Selenium	0.01 mg
Dietary Fiber	3.52 g	Thiamin (B_1)	0.07 mg
Sodium	50.45 mg	Vitamin A	33.48 RE
Beta-Carotene	92.00 RE	Vitamin C	7.03 mg
Calcium	77.69 mg	Copper	0.18 mg
Cobalamin (B_{12})	0.30 µg	Folate	15.66 µg
Iron	0.97 mg	Vitamin E	1.02 mg
Magnesium	27.05 mg		

SUN COUNTRY CHICKEN SALAD

- 1 large cantaloupe
- 2 cups cooked chicken chunks
- 1 cup cucumber chunks
- 1 cup green grapes
- ½ cup chopped green onions
- 2 tablespoons chopped parsley
- 1 cup plain nonfat yogurt
- 3 tablespoons prepared chutney
- ¼ teaspoon grated lemon peel
- 1 tablespoon lemon juice
- ¼ cup whole blanched California almonds, toasted*
- 1 large bunch watercress

Cut cantaloupe into 12 wedges, removing seeds and peel. In large bowl, combine chicken, cucumber, grapes, onions, and parsley. In small bowl, blend together yogurt, chutney, lemon peel, and juice. Toss lightly with chicken mixture. Fold in almonds.

Arrange watercress on 4 salad plates. Place 3 wedges of cantaloupe on each plate. Spoon chicken salad mixture over cantaloupe.   *Makes 4 servings*

*To toast almonds, spread almonds in single layer on baking sheet. Bake at 350°F, 5 to 8 minutes, stirring occasionally, until lightly browned. Cool.

Tip: Cantaloupe is a very good source of potassium and vitamins A and C. Look for well-shaped melons with a smoothly rounded, depressed area at stem end. A fragrant aroma is a good sign of ripeness.

NUTRITIONAL INFORMATION PER SERVING

Calories	355.50 kc	Niacin (B3)	10.37 mg
Protein	25.23 g	Pantothenic Acid	1.55 mg
Fat	9.42 g	Phosphorus	325.00 mg
% of Calories		Potassium	1,259 mg
from Fat:	23	Pyridoxine (B6)	0.75 mg
Saturated Fat	1.80 g	Riboflavin (B2)	0.32 mg
Cholesterol	49.02 mg	Selenium	0.02 mg
Dietary Fiber	5.78 g	Thiamin (B1)	0.23 mg
Sodium	153.70 mg	Vitamin A	1,283 RE
Beta-Carotene	517.40 RE	Vitamin C	131.90 mg
Calcium	206.10 mg	Copper	0.31 mg
Cobalamin (B12)	0.53 µg	Folate	25.49 µg
Iron	2.16 mg	Vitamin E	2.93 mg
Magnesium	99.80 mg	Zinc	2.09 mg

BLUEBERRY-PEACH SALAD

    1 (6-ounce) package orange-flavored gelatin
    ⅓ cup sugar
    1 teaspoon finely shredded orange peel
    2¼ cups orange juice, divided
    2 cups buttermilk
    1 (8-ounce) can crushed pineapple, drained
    2 medium peaches, peeled and chopped (1 cup)
    1 cup fresh or frozen unsweetened blueberries,
        thawed
    1 (8-ounce) carton dairy sour cream

In medium saucepan, combine gelatin and sugar; stir
in orange peel and 2 cups orange juice. Cook and stir
until gelatin is dissolved; cool. Stir in buttermilk.
Chill until partially set. Fold in fruit; spoon into 10
individual molds. Chill for 6 hours or until firm.
Combine sour cream and remaining orange juice;
chill. Unmold salad; serve with sour cream mixture.

Makes 10 servings

NUTRITIONAL INFORMATION PER SERVING

Calories	204.00 kc	Iodine	18.20 µg
Protein	4.65 g	Iron	0.30 mg
Carbohydrate	36.34 g	Magnesium	20.80 mg
Fat	5.46 g	Manganese	0.31 mg
% of Calories		Niacin (B3)	0.56 mg
from Fat:	23	Pantothenic Acid	0.39 mg
Saturated Fat	3.29 g	Phosphorus	104.70 mg
Cholesterol	12.00 mg	Potassium	295.70 mg
Dietary Fiber	1.27 g	Pyridoxine (B6)	0.07 mg
Sodium	113.70 mg	Riboflavin (B2)	0.15 mg
Beta-Carotene	132.10 RE	Thiamin (B1)	0.11 mg
Biotin	1.53 µg	Vitamin A	81.92 RE
Calcium	95.34 mg	Vitamin C	33.63 mg
Cobalamin (B12)	0.18 µg	Vitamin D	0.05 µg
Copper	0.09 mg	Vitamin E	0.36 mg
Fluoride	18.36 µg	Vitamin K	1.99 µg
Folate	38.23 µg	Zinc	0.38 mg

CALIFORNIA BROWN RICE SALAD

1 (16-ounce) can California fruit cocktail in juice
   or extra light syrup
1 cup brown rice
1 medium tomato, diced
1 cup celery slices
½ cup green onion slices
2 tablespoons red wine vinegar
1 tablespoon vegetable oil
1 tablespoon Dijon-style mustard
½ teaspoon dried tarragon, crumbled
⅛ teaspoon garlic powder

Drain fruit cocktail, reserving ¼ cup liquid; save
remainder for other uses. Cook rice according to
package directions; chill thoroughly. In large bowl,
toss rice with fruit cocktail, tomato, celery, and green
onions. In small bowl, combine reserved fruit cocktail liquid, vinegar, oil, mustard, tarragon, and garlic
powder. Stir into rice mixture; chill to allow flavors
to blend. *Makes 6 servings*

NUTRITIONAL INFORMATION PER SERVING

Calories	181.70 kc	Pantothenic Acid	0.65 mg
Protein	3.43 g	Phosphorus	133.50 mg
Fat	3.46 g	Potassium	269.40 mg
% of Calories		Pyridoxine (B$_6$)	0.23 mg
from Fat:	17	Riboflavin (B$_2$)	0.07 mg
Saturated Fat	0.51 g	Thiamin (B$_1$)	0.16 mg
Dietary Fiber	3.01 g	Vitamin A	72.28 RE
Sodium	58.28 mg	Vitamin C	10.36 mg
Beta-Carotene	265.60 RE	Copper	0.16 mg
Calcium	31.18 mg	Folate	17.60 µg
Iron	1.03 mg	Vitamin E	2.71 mg
Magnesium	56.26 mg	Zinc	0.78 mg
Niacin (B$_3$)	2.08 mg		

TODAY'S SLIM NOODLES ROMANOV

    8 ounces uncooked noodles
    1 cup low-fat yogurt
    1 cup low-fat (1%) cottage cheese
    ¼ cup finely chopped onion
    ¼ cup chopped fresh parsley
    2 tablespoons Worcestershire sauce
    ½ teaspoon salt
    3 drops hot pepper sauce
    2 tablespoons grated Wisconsin Parmesan cheese

Cook and drain noodles. Preheat oven to 350°F. In large bowl, combine all remaining ingredients except Parmesan cheese. Fold in cooked noodles. Spoon into 1½-quart buttered casserole; sprinkle with Parmesan cheese. Bake 30 minutes or until hot.

Makes 6 to 8 servings

NUTRITIONAL INFORMATION PER SERVING

Calories	149.90 kc	Niacin (B3)	1.21 mg
Protein	9.34 g	Pantothenic Acid	0.36 mg
Fat	2.31 g	Phosphorus	147.00 mg
% of Calories		Potassium	161.50 mg
from Fat:	14	Pyridoxine (B6)	0.07 mg
Saturated Fat	1.00 g	Riboflavin (B2)	0.19 mg
Cholesterol	28.71 mg	Thiamin (B1)	0.16 mg
Dietary Fiber	0.17 g	Vitamin A	28.22 RE
Sodium	340.00 mg	Vitamin C	9.12 mg
Beta-Carotene	63.06 RE	Copper	0.09 mg
Calcium	107.80 mg	Folate	16.56 µg
Cobalamin (B12)	0.43 µg	Vitamin D	0.02 µg
Iron	1.62 mg	Vitamin E	0.30 mg
Magnesium	23.28 mg	Zinc	0.90 mg

NOT FRIED ASIAN RICE

- 2 teaspoons sesame oil
- ¾ cup chopped green onions
- ½ cup chopped red bell pepper
- 2 cloves garlic, minced
- 2 cups water
- 1 cup uncooked converted rice
- 2 egg whites
- 1 tablespoon lite soy sauce
- 2 teaspoons sugar

In large nonstick skillet, heat oil over medium-high heat. Add onions, bell pepper, and garlic; cook and stir 1 minute. Add water; bring to a boil. Reduce heat to low; stir in rice and egg whites. Simmer, stirring frequently, 20 minutes or until rice is tender. Stir in soy sauce and sugar. Cook and stir for 3 to 5 minutes or until sugar caramelizes. *Makes 6 servings*

NUTRITIONAL INFORMATION PER SERVING

Calories	147.40 kc	Pantothenic Acid	0.47 mg
Protein	3.78 g	Phosphorus	54.35 mg
Fat	1.79 g	Potassium	120.30 mg
% of Calories		Pyridoxine (B6)	0.18 mg
from Fat:	11	Riboflavin (B2)	0.09 mg
Saturated Fat	0.27 g	Thiamin (B1)	0.21 mg
Dietary Fiber	1.17 g	Vitamin A	61.92 RE
Sodium	124.60 mg	Vitamin C	21.65 mg
Beta-Carotene	310.00 RE	Copper	0.08 mg
Calcium	30.14 mg	Folate	11.42 µg
Cobalamin (B12)	0.02 µg	Vitamin E	0.75 mg
Iron	1.45 mg	Zinc	0.38 mg
Magnesium	15.77 mg		
Niacin (B3)	1.24 mg		

BRYANI

- 1 onion, chopped
- 1 clove garlic, minced
  Curry Rice (recipe follows)
- 2 large fresh California peaches, coarsely
  chopped (2½ cups)
- ½ cup roasted cashews, chopped (optional)
- 1 (9-ounce) package frozen cut green beans,
  thawed

In large bowl, combine onion, garlic, and Curry
Rice. Spoon half of Curry Rice mixture into 1½
quart casserole. Top with peaches, cashews, and
green beans. Spoon remaining Curry Rice mixture
over top. Microwave until heated through or cover
with foil and bake in 375°F oven 50 minutes. Serve
with plain low-fat yogurt, additional sliced peaches,
and raisins, if desired.

CURRY RICE

- **2 cups water**
- **2 teaspoons curry powder**
- **½ teaspoon ground turmeric**
- **¼ teaspoon ground cinnamon**
- **1 cup long grain white rice**

Combine water, curry powder, ground turmeric, and ground cinnamon in large saucepan. Cover; bring to boil. Add long grain white rice. Cover; return to a boil. Reduce heat; simmer 20 minutes or until liquid is absorbed.

Makes 6 servings

NUTRITIONAL INFORMATION PER SERVING

Calories	149.80 kc	Iron	2.09 mg
Protein	3.43 g	Magnesium	23.53 mg
Carbohydrate	33.54 g	Manganese	0.61 mg
Fat	0.45 g	Molybdenum	28.07 µg
% of Calories		Niacin (B$_3$)	1.83 mg
from fat:	3	Pantothenic Acid	0.42 mg
Saturated Fat	0.08 g	Phosphorus	61.61 mg
Dietary Fiber	2.11 g	Potassium	199.40 mg
Sodium	8.41 mg	Pyridoxine (B$_6$)	0.12 mg
Beta-Carotene	112.00 RE	Riboflavin (B$_2$)	0.07 mg
Biotin	2.23 µg	Thiamin (B$_1$)	0.22 mg
Calcium	40.37 mg	Vitamin A	38.75 RE
Chromium	0.02 mg	Vitamin C	7.42 mg
Copper	0.14 mg	Vitamin E	0.36 mg
Fluoride	37.00 µg	Vitamin K	13.75 µg
Folate	12.23 µg	Zinc	0.74 mg

Pinwheel Appetizers

   1 (8-ounce) package nonfat pasteurized process
      cream cheese product
   ⅓ cup grated Parmesan cheese
   1 teaspoon dried parsley flakes
   ½ teaspoon garlic powder
   ½ teaspoon Dijon-style mustard
   2 to 3 drops hot pepper sauce (optional)
   3 cups cooked wild rice
   3 (12-inch) soft flour tortillas
   2½ ounces wafer-thin corned beef
   9 fresh spinach leaves

In large bowl, combine cream cheese, Parmesan
cheese, parsley, garlic, mustard, and hot sauce; mix
well. Stir in rice. Spread mixture evenly over tortillas, leaving ½-inch border on one half of each
tortilla bare. Place single layer of corned beef over
rice and cheese mixture. Top with layer of spinach
leaves. Roll up each tortilla tightly toward border.

Moisten border of tortilla with water. Press to seal
roll. Wrap tightly in plastic wrap; refrigerate several
hours or overnight. Cut into 1-inch slices.

Makes 36 appetizers

NUTRITIONAL INFORMATION PER SERVING

Calories	42.03 kc	Iron	16.25 mg
Protein	2.69 g	Magnesium	6.97 mg
Carbohydrate	6.19 g	Manganese	0.05 mg
Fat	0.66 g	Molybdenum	0.19 µg
% of Calories		Niacin (B3)	0.41 mg
from Fat:	14	Pantothenic Acid	0.03 mg
Saturated Fat	0.40 g	Phosphorus	25.93 mg
Cholesterol	3.78 mg	Potassium	27.79 mg
Dietary Fiber	0.37 g	Pyridoxine (B6)	0.03 mg
Sodium	98.58 mg	Riboflavin (B2)	0.03 mg
Beta-Carotene	31.37 RE	Thiamin (B1)	0.01 mg
Biotin	0.08 µg	Vitamin A	7.40 RE
Calcium	21.97 mg	Vitamin C	0.54 mg
Cobalamin (B12)	0.05 µg	Vitamin E	0.17 mg
Copper	0.03 mg	Vitamin K	2.07 µg
Fluoride	1.58 µg	Zinc	0.35 mg
Folate	5.99 µg		

GRAINS & PASTA

LINGUINE AND FRESH FRUIT COOLER

- **1 cup fresh berries**
- **1 cup (1-inch) honeydew or cantaloupe chunks**
- **1 cup kiwifruit or plum slices**
- **¼ cup lemon juice**
- **1 teaspoon finely grated orange peel**
- **2 tablespoons cornstarch**
- **1½ cups apricot nectar**
- **1 stick cinnamon**
- **4 whole cloves**
- **4 whole allspice berries**
- **¼ cup dry white wine**
- **½ pound linguine, vermicelli, or angel hair pasta, cooked and drained**
- **½ cup fresh mint leaves**

In large bowl, combine berries, honeydew chunks, kiwifruit slices, lemon juice, and orange peel; set aside. Place cornstarch in 2-quart saucepan. Slowly add apricot nectar, over high heat, stirring until well blended. Add cinnamon stick, cloves, and allspice berries. Bring to a boil, stirring frequently. Reduce heat; simmer, uncovered, 15 minutes or until thick.

Remove cinnamon stick, cloves, and allspice berries. Stir apricot mixture into fruit mixture. Add wine and linguine; garnish with mint leaves.

Makes 4 lunch or 8 dessert servings

Tip: The tangy-sweet flavor of kiwifruit has been described as a combination of pineapple, melon, and strawberry. It's high in vitamin C, and the little black seeds inside make it a good source of fiber.

NUTRITIONAL INFORMATION PER SERVING

Calories	346.40 kc	Niacin (B3)	3.17 mg
Protein	8.97 g	Pantothenic Acid	0.54 mg
Fat	2.82 g	Phosphorus	149.30 mg
% of Calories		Potassium	575.00 mg
from Fat:	7	Pyridoxine (B6)	0.18 mg
Saturated Fat	0.47 g	Riboflavin (B2)	0.21 mg
Cholesterol	48.96 mg	Thiamin (B1)	0.37 mg
Dietary Fiber	4.09 g	Vitamin A	226.40 RE
Sodium	23.49 mg	Vitamin C	144.30 mg
Beta-Carotene	1,255 RE	Copper	0.33 mg
Calcium	81.03 mg	Folate	42.04 µg
Cobalamin (B12)	0.13 µg	Vitamin E	1.10 mg
Iron	3.69 mg	Zinc	1.17 mg
Magnesium	59.28 mg		

Radiatore Salad with Salmon and Papaya

- 1 pound uncooked radiatore or other medium-size pasta
- 2 tablespoons vegetable oil
  Freshly ground black pepper to taste
- 1 pound skinless, boneless, fresh or frozen salmon fillets, cooked and chopped *or* 2 (7½-ounce) cans salmon, drained and flaked
- 1 papaya, peeled, seeded, and chopped *or* 1 mango or 2 peaches or 2 nectarines, peeled, seeded, and chopped *or* 1 (15-ounce) can papaya or other fruit in light syrup, drained and chopped
- 1 cup cherry tomatoes
- 1 bunch green onions, thinly sliced
- 1 yellow bell pepper, seeded and chopped
- 1 medium cucumber, quartered lengthwise and sliced
- 1 small jalapeño, seeded and finely minced
- 2 tablespoons chopped fresh cilantro
- 3 tablespoons rice wine vinegar
- 3 tablespoons white wine vinegar
- 3 drops hot pepper sauce

Prepare pasta according to package directions; transfer to medium bowl. Toss warm pasta with oil; season with black pepper. Set aside until cool. Add salmon, papaya, tomatoes, green onions, yellow bell pepper, and cucumber; toss until well mixed.

In small bowl, combine jalapeño, cilantro, vinegars, and hot pepper sauce. Pour over pasta mixture; toss until well coated. Cover; refrigerate until chilled.

Makes 6 to 8 servings

Tip: One serving or more of seafood each week is linked to a lower risk of heart disease. All seafood is low in saturated fat and most is low in cholesterol.

NUTRITIONAL INFORMATION PER SERVING

Calories	343.30 kc	Niacin (B₃)	5.66 mg
Protein	21.08 g	Pantothenic Acid	0.92 mg
Fat	8.59 g	Phosphorus	251.80 mg
% of Calories		Potassium	544.60 mg
from Fat:	23	Pyridoxine (B₆)	0.34 mg
Saturated Fat	1.32 g	Riboflavin (B₂)	0.40 mg
Cholesterol	71.37 mg	Selenium	0.02 mg
Dietary Fiber	3.54 g	Thiamin (B₁)	0.46 mg
Sodium	92.51 mg	Vitamin A	215.30 RE
Beta-Carotene	1,098 RE	Vitamin C	41.35 mg
Calcium	54.90 mg	Copper	0.23 mg
Cobalamin (B₁₂)	1.84 µg	Folate	27.90 µg
Iron	2.98 mg	Vitamin E	4.24 mg
Magnesium	54.96 mg	Zinc	1.25 mg

Pasta Primavera

- ⅓ cup broccoli flowerets
- ⅓ cup cauliflower flowerets
- 1 baby carrot, peeled and cut into julienne strips
- 1 tablespoon premium olive oil
- ⅓ cup each red and yellow bell peppers, peeled and cut into julienne strips
- ⅓ cup snow peas
- ¼ cup shiitake, morel, or chanterelle mushrooms
- 1 clove garlic, minced
- 1 (16-ounce) package linguine or other long pasta, cooked and drained
- 4 leaves minced fresh basil or 2 teaspoons minced fresh chervil

Steam broccoli, cauliflower, and carrot until crisp-tender, about 3 minutes. Heat olive oil in large skillet over medium heat. Add steamed vegetables, peppers, snow peas, mushrooms, and garlic. Cook and stir for 3 minutes. Toss with hot linguine. Sprinkle with basil; serve immediately.   *Makes 4 servings*

NUTRITIONAL INFORMATION PER SERVING

Calories	438.70 kc	Niacin (B3)	3.36 mg
Protein	16.15 g	Pantothenic Acid	0.64 mg
Fat	6.62 g	Phosphorus	207.50 mg
% of Calories		Potassium	204.50 mg
from Fat:	14	Pyridoxine (B6)	0.21 mg
Saturated Fat	0.94 g	Riboflavin (B2)	0.48 mg
Cholesterol	97.91 mg	Thiamin (B1)	0.66 mg
Dietary Fiber	5.59 g	Vitamin A	287.90 RE
Sodium	24.05 mg	Vitamin C	28.26 mg
Beta-Carotene	1,563 RE	Copper	0.35 mg
Calcium	32.82 mg	Folate	36.31 µg
Cobalamin (B12)	0.42 µg	Vitamin E	1.32 mg
Iron	3.82 mg	Zinc	1.85 mg
Magnesium	61.41 mg		

TOMATO ZUCCHINI PESTO

6 ounces uncooked pasta
1 cup fresh basil leaves, chopped
1 teaspoon sugar
1 teaspoon vegetable oil
2 cloves garlic, minced
1 tablespoon grated Parmesan cheese
¼ cup part-skim ricotta cheese
1 medium zucchini, sliced
2 teaspoons water
1 cup quartered cherry tomatoes
½ teaspoon salt (optional)

Prepare pasta according to package directions. Rinse and drain; cover. In food processor or blender container, process basil, sugar, oil, and garlic until blended. Add Parmesan and ricotta cheeses; process until blended. Set aside. Place zucchini in large casserole dish; add water. Cover; microwave on HIGH (100% power) 4 minutes. Drain. Stir in pasta and cheese mixture. Garnish with tomatoes. Sprinkle with salt, if desired. *Makes 4 servings*

NUTRITIONAL INFORMATION PER SERVING

Calories	211.70 kc	Niacin (B3)	1.82 mg
Protein	9.43 g	Pantothenic Acid	0.47 mg
Fat	4.35 g	Phosphorus	143.30 mg
% of Calories		Potassium	342.20 mg
from Fat:	18	Pyridoxine (B6)	0.15 mg
Saturated Fat	1.42 g	Riboflavin (B2)	0.26 mg
Cholesterol	42.70 mg	Thiamin (B1)	0.31 mg
Dietary Fiber	3.56 g	Vitamin A	158.40 RE
Sodium	67.41 mg	Vitamin C	28.34 mg
Beta-Carotene	631.00 RE	Copper	0.19 mg
Calcium	101.10 mg	Folate	54.71 µg
Cobalamin (B12)	0.22 µg	Vitamin E	1.95 mg
Iron	2.75 mg	Zinc	1.13 mg
Magnesium	43.73 mg		

FISH STEAKS WITH PEAR JARDINIÈRE

- 2 teaspoons vegetable oil
- 1 cup thin onion slices
- 1 cup julienne carrot strips
- ½ teaspoon dry mustard
- ¼ teaspoon each dried basil leaves, crushed, and dill weed
- 2 fresh California Bartlett pears, cored and quartered
- 1½ pounds firm fish fillets, such as sea bass, haddock, or salmon
- 2 tomatoes, sliced
- 1 lemon, thinly sliced

Heat oil in large nonstick skillet. Add onion and carrots; stir to mix well. Cover and cook over medium heat 5 to 10 minutes. Mix mustard, basil, and dill weed in large bowl. Add pears; toss lightly. Add fish, tomatoes, lemon slices, and pear mixture to skillet. Cover; simmer 10 minutes or until fish flakes easily with fork.   *Makes 4 servings*

NUTRITIONAL INFORMATION PER SERVING

Calories	278.00 kc	Niacin (B₃)	3.91 mg
Protein	33.27 g	Pantothenic Acid	0.33 mg
Fat	6.38 g	Phosphorus	382.50 mg
% of Calories		Potassium	849.80 mg
from Fat:	20	Pyridoxine (B₆)	0.90 mg
Saturated Fat	1.23 g	Riboflavin (B₂)	0.33 mg
Cholesterol	70.55 mg	Thiamin (B₁)	0.31 mg
Dietary Fiber	4.63 g	Vitamin A	898.90 RE
Sodium	132.60 mg	Vitamin C	31.52 mg
Beta-Carotene	4,728 RE	Copper	0.21 mg
Calcium	48.70 mg	Folate	38.60 μg
Cobalamin (B₁₂)	0.60 μg	Vitamin D	0.03 μg
Iron	1.30 mg	Vitamin E	5.34 mg
Magnesium	91.56 mg	Zinc	0.98 mg

BAKED SOLE PACIFICA

1 can (16 ounces) California cling peach slices in
    juice or extra light syrup
4 sole fillets (about 1 pound)
$1/2$ teaspoon dill weed
1 tablespoon olive oil
2 onions, cut into wedges
4 cups julienne zucchini strips
2 cups red pepper strips
$1/2$ teaspoon herb pepper seasoning

Preheat broiler. Drain peaches, reserving liquid.
Place fish on broiler pan. Brush both sides of fillets
with peach liquid; sprinkle with dill. Broil about 4
inches from heat 10 minutes, or until fish flakes
easily with fork, turning halfway through cooking.
Heat oil over medium-high heat in large skillet. Add
onions; cook and stir until crisp-tender. Stir in
zucchini; cook and stir 2 minutes. Add red peppers
and peach slices. Cook until heated through. Stir in
seasoning. Place peach mixture on serving plate; top
with fish.   *Makes 4 servings*

NUTRITIONAL INFORMATION PER SERVING

Calories	240.50 kc	Niacin (B3)	3.80 mg
Protein	22.55 g	Pantothenic Acid	0.77 mg
Fat	5.18 g	Phosphorus	321.40 mg
% of Calories		Potassium	969.70 mg
from Fat:	18	Pyridoxine (B6)	0.68 mg
Saturated Fat	0.86 g	Riboflavin (B2)	0.20 mg
Cholesterol	53.20 mg	Thiamin (B1)	0.28 mg
Dietary Fiber	6.19 g	Vitamin A	155.10 RE
Sodium	95.65 mg	Vitamin C	119.90 mg
Beta-Carotene	364.70 RE	Copper	0.26 mg
Calcium	61.28 mg	Folate	75.96 µg
Cobalamin (B12)	1.96 µg	Vitamin E	2.98 mg
Iron	1.82 mg	Zinc	1.11 mg
Magnesium	96.87 mg		

FRUITFUL SOLE AND NECTARINES REMOULADE

Remoulade Sauce (recipe follows)
4 **sole fillets (1 pound)**
 Pepper
 Dill weed
2 **tablespoons water**
2 **fresh California nectarines or peaches, sliced (2 cups)**

Microwave directions: Prepare Remoulade Sauce. Roll up sole fillets and fasten with wooden picks. (If fillets are large, cut in half lengthwise before rolling.) Stand on end, turban-fashion, in microwave-safe dish. Season with pepper and dill weed to taste. Add water to dish. Cover and microwave on HIGH (100%) 3 to 4 minutes or until fish flakes easily when tested with fork. Add nectarine slices to dish and microwave, covered, 1 minute more or until hot. Transfer fish and fruit to warm serving platter and remove picks. Serve with Remoulade Sauce.

Makes 4 servings

REMOULADE SAUCE

- 1 cup plain low-fat yogurt
- 1/4 cup chopped dill pickle or capers
- 2 tablespoons chopped green onion
- 2 teaspoons Dijon-style mustard
- 1 teaspoon tarragon leaves, crushed.

Combine all ingredients. Mix well. Makes about 1 1/4 cups.

NUTRITIONAL INFORMATION PER SERVING

Calories	164.70 kc	Iodine	26.00 µg
Protein	22.69 g	Iron	0.60 mg
Carbohydrate	12.52 g	Magnesium	62.44 mg
Fat	2.55 g	Manganese	0.05 mg
% of Calories		Niacin (B3)	2.44 mg
from Fat:	14	Pantothenic Acid	0.92 mg
Saturated Fat	0.92 g	Phosphorus	324.20 mg
Cholesterol	56.70 mg	Potassium	569.70 mg
Dietary Fiber	1.28 g	Pyridoxine (B6)	0.24 mg
Sodium	207.90 mg	Riboflavin (B2)	0.24 mg
Beta-Carotene	125.50 RE	Thiamin (B1)	0.10 mg
Biotin	0.78 µg	Vitamin A	82.34 RE
Calcium	125.90 mg	Vitamin C	5.25 mg
Cobalamin (B12)	2.28 µg	Vitamin E	0.87 mg
Copper	0.09 mg	Vitamin K	0.01 mg
Fluoride	1.50 µg	Zinc	1.09 mg
Folate	16.55 µg		

SNAPPER FILLETS WITH ORANGE-SHALLOT SAUCE

    2 Florida oranges
    6 red snapper* fillets (about 2¼ pounds)
    1 tablespoon olive oil
    1 cup finely chopped shallots
    2 cloves garlic, minced
    3 tablespoons all-purpose flour
    1 cup chicken broth
    1 cup Florida orange juice
    1 tablespoon grated orange peel
    2 tablespoons cooking sherry
1½ teaspoons dried oregano leaves, crushed
     Salt and pepper to taste
    2 tablespoons chopped parsley for garnish

Preheat broiler. Thinly slice oranges; set aside. Place fillets, skin side down, on nonstick jelly-roll pan. Broil about 4 inches from heat source 5 to 8 minutes until fish flakes easily with fork. Remove from broiler; set aside.

Meanwhile, in large nonstick skillet, heat oil over medium-high heat until hot. Add shallots and garlic; cook and stir 3 to 4 minutes until shallots begin to brown. Add flour; cook and stir about 30 seconds or until well blended. Stir in broth, orange juice, orange peel, sherry, oregano, salt, and pepper. Bring to a boil, stirring constantly, until slightly thickened. Add orange slices and fish fillets, skin side up. Cook 1 to 2 minutes until fish is heated through and orange slices are slightly softened. Garnish with parsley, if desired. Serve immediately. *Makes 6 servings*

*You may substitute any lightly textured fish, such as tuna, flounder, grouper, swordfish, or scrod, for red snapper.

Tip: While fish broils, prepare the sauce, then assemble. Total preparation and cooking time is 15 minutes.

NUTRITIONAL INFORMATION PER SERVING

Calories	282.00 kc	Niacin (B$_3$)	1.53 mg
Protein	37.09 g	Pantothenic Acid	0.29 mg
Fat	5.48 g	Phosphorus	313.70 mg
% of Calories		Potassium	990.90 mg
from Fat:	18	Pyridoxine (B$_6$)	0.15 mg
Saturated Fat	0.91 g	Riboflavin (B$_2$)	0.07 mg
Cholesterol	62.42 mg	Thiamin (B$_1$)	0.20 mg
Dietary Fiber	1.54 g	Vitamin A	353.40 RE
Sodium	316.00 mg	Vitamin C	44.14 mg
Beta-Carotene	2,074 RE	Copper	0.16 mg
Calcium	96.75 mg	Folate	41.51 µg
Cobalamin (B$_{12}$)	0.04 µg	Vitamin E	0.58 mg
Iron	1.15 mg	Zinc	0.84 mg
Magnesium	66.07 mg		

FLORIDA GRAPEFRUIT MARINATED SHRIMP

- 1 cup frozen Florida grapefruit juice concentrate, thawed
- 2 cloves garlic, minced
- 3 tablespoons chopped cilantro or parsley
- 1 tablespoon honey
- 2 teaspoons ketchup
- 1/2 teaspoon salt
- 1/4 teaspoon red pepper flakes
- 1 pound medium shrimp, shelled and deveined
- 2 teaspoons cornstarch
- 1 cup uncooked long-grain white rice
- 1 tablespoon olive oil
- 1 large red bell pepper, cut into strips
- 2 ribs celery, sliced diagonally into 1/4-inch-thick slices
- 2 Florida grapefruit, peeled and sectioned

Combine grapefruit juice concentrate, garlic, cilantro, honey, ketchup, salt, and red pepper flakes in medium bowl. Stir in shrimp. Marinate 20 minutes, turning shrimp once. Drain shrimp, reserving marinade; set shrimp aside. Combine reserved marinade and cornstarch. Meanwhile, prepare rice according to package directions.

Heat oil over medium-high heat in large nonstick skillet; add shrimp. Cook and stir 2 to 3 minutes until shrimp turn orange and just begin to caramelize. Add red bell pepper, celery, and reserved marinade. Bring to a boil over high heat until shrimp turn opaque and marinade thickens slightly, stirring constantly. Add grapefruit and heat 30 seconds. Garnish with fresh sprigs of cilantro. Serve over rice.

Makes 4 servings

NUTRITIONAL INFORMATION PER SERVING

Calories	441.60 kc	Niacin (B3)	5.20 mg
Protein	24.29 g	Pantothenic Acid	1.28 mg
Fat	5.14 g	Phosphorus	226.90 mg
% of Calories		Potassium	772.40 mg
from Fat:	10	Pyridoxine (B6)	0.42 mg
Saturated Fat	0.90 g	Riboflavin (B2)	0.14 mg
Cholesterol	174.20 mg	Selenium	0.07 mg
Dietary Fiber	3.02 g	Thiamin (B1)	0.46 mg
Sodium	518.90 mg	Vitamin A	138.50 RE
Beta-Carotene	322.50 RE	Vitamin C	137.10 mg
Calcium	99.68 mg	Copper	0.43 mg
Cobalamin (B12)	1.33 µg	Folate	41.37 µg
Iron	5.61 mg	Vitamin E	6.51 mg
Magnesium	79.79 mg	Zinc	2.19 mg

ORIENTAL BAKED SEAFOOD

¼ cup chopped California almonds
2 cups water
½ teaspoon salt
1 cup uncooked long-grain white rice
1 tablespoon sesame oil
1 tablespoon grated ginger root
1 teaspoon grated lemon peel
1 pound halibut
½ pound large scallops
¼ pound medium shrimp, shelled and deveined
1 clove garlic, minced
1 tablespoon light soy sauce
½ cup slivered green onions

Preheat oven to 350°F. Spread almonds in shallow baking pan. Toast in oven 5 to 8 minutes until lightly browned, stirring occasionally; cool. Bring water and salt to a boil in medium saucepan. Stir in rice, sesame oil, ginger root, and lemon peel. Bring to a boil; cover and reduce heat to low. Simmer 20 to 25 minutes until water is absorbed. Meanwhile, preheat oven to 400°F or preheat broiler or grill. Remove skin and bones from halibut; cut into large pieces. Cut 4 (12-inch) squares of foil. Divide halibut, scallops, and shrimp among foil squares. Sprinkle seafood with garlic and soy sauce; seal squares tightly. Bake 12 minutes or broil or grill 4 inches from heat 15 minutes, turning once. Stir almonds into rice. Pour seafood mixture and juices over rice. Sprinkle with green onions.   *Makes 4 servings*

Microwave Directions: Spread almonds in shallow pan. Microwave on HIGH (100%) power 2 minutes, stirring often; cool. Combine water, salt, rice, sesame oil, ginger root, and lemon peel in 3-quart microwave-safe dish. Cover with plastic wrap. Microwave on HIGH 12 minutes, stirring halfway through. Let stand 10 minutes. Prepare fish packets as directed on parchment paper instead of foil. Bring edges up and seal with rubber band. Place packets in microwave-safe baking dish halfway through. Microwave on HIGH 5 minutes, rotating dish, halfway through. Serve as directed.

NUTRITIONAL INFORMATION PER SERVING

Calories	417.20 kc	Niacin (B3)	9.77 mg
Protein	43.13 g	Pantothenic Acid	0.69 mg
Fat	7.84 g	Phosphorus	510.30 mg
% of Calories		Potassium	887.40 mg
from Fat:	17	Pyridoxine (B6)	0.57 mg
Saturated Fat	0.97 g	Riboflavin (B2)	0.23 mg
Cholesterol	98.69 mg	Selenium	0.12 mg
Dietary Fiber	1.49 g	Thiamin (B1)	0.37 mg
Sodium	628.80 mg	Vitamin A	124.20 RE
Beta-Carotene	300.10 RE	Vitamin C	7.76 mg
Calcium	121.90 mg	Copper	0.30 mg
Cobalamin (B12)	2.41 µg	Folate	20.71 µg
Iron	4.37 mg	Vitamin E	3.49 mg
Magnesium	173.60 mg	Zinc	2.17 mg

CALIFORNIA BLACKENED SNAPPER

1 can (16 ounces) California cling peach halves in juice or extra light syrup
1 tablespoon sweet paprika
1 teaspoon onion powder
1 teaspoon garlic powder
¾ teaspoon white pepper
¾ teaspoon black pepper
½ teaspoon ground red pepper (cayenne)
½ teaspoon dried thyme leaves, crushed
½ teaspoon dried oregano leaves, crushed
6 red snapper fillets (about 1½ pounds)
2 tablespoons soft tub margarine

Drain peaches, reserving liquid; set aside. Combine paprika, onion powder, garlic powder, white pepper, black pepper, red pepper, thyme, and oregano; mix well. Dip fish fillet in reserved peach liquid. Sprinkle both sides of each fish fillet with paprika mixture.

Heat 10-inch skillet on high heat for 5 minutes. Carefully place half the fish fillets in skillet. Cut margarine into small pieces; add half to skillet. (Skillet will smoke as margarine pieces are added.) Cook about 1½ to 2 minutes on each side or until fish flakes easily with fork. Repeat with remaining fish fillets and margarine. Fan peach halves over fish fillets to serve.   *Makes 6 servings*

Tip: There are more than 250 species of snapper. The fish used in this recipe, red snapper, is by far the most popular. Red snapper's firm-textured flesh contains very little fat and is suitable for virtually any type of cooking.

NUTRITIONAL INFORMATION PER SERVING

Calories	187.30 kc	Pantothenic Acid	0.04 mg
Protein	24.02 g	Phosphorus	196.10 mg
Fat	5.63 g	Potassium	567.90 mg
% of Calories		Pyridoxine (B6)	0.02 mg
from Fat:	27	Riboflavin (B2)	0.05 mg
Saturated Fat	1.11 g	Thiamin (B1)	0.08 mg
Cholesterol	41.61 mg	Vitamin A	156.60 RE
Dietary Fiber	0.77 g	Vitamin C	3.53 mg
Sodium	98.54 mg	Copper	0.09 mg
Beta-Carotene	422.90 RE	Folate	2.67 µg
Calcium	49.28 mg	Vitamin D	0.37 µg
Iron	0.96 mg	Vitamin E	3.50 mg
Magnesium	40.46 mg	Zinc	0.54 mg
Niacin (B3)	1.15 mg		

LOBSTER WILD RICE BISQUE

- 2 tablespoons light margarine
- 1 cup chopped onion
- 1 can (4 ounces) sliced mushrooms, drained
- 1 tablespoon all-purpose flour
- 2 teaspoons rosemary leaves, crushed
- ½ teaspoon salt
- ½ teaspoon pepper
- 4 cups low-sodium chicken broth
- 1 cup skim milk
- ¼ cup cooking sherry
- 2 cups cooked wild rice
- 1 cup chopped canned tomatoes
- 6 ounces imitation lobster, in 1-inch chunks
- 1 cup shredded low-fat Cheddar cheese

Heat margarine in large skillet until melted. Add onion and mushrooms; cook and stir until tender. Stir in flour, rosemary, salt, and pepper. Cook until bubbly. Gradually stir in broth; bring to a boil, stirring often. Stir in milk and sherry. Add rice, tomatoes, and lobster. Cook until heated through. Fold in cheese.   *Makes 10 servings*

NUTRITIONAL INFORMATION PER SERVING

Calories	134.50 kc	Niacin (B3)	1.83 mg
Protein	9.07 g	Pantothenic Acid	0.28 mg
Fat	3.97 g	Phosphorus	125.20 mg
% of Calories		Potassium	199.10 mg
from Fat:	26	Pyridoxine (B6)	0.11 mg
Saturated Fat	1.46 g	Riboflavin (B2)	0.12 mg
Cholesterol	14.59 mg	Thiamin (B1)	0.08 mg
Dietary Fiber	1.20 g	Vitamin A	62.43 RE
Sodium	436.00 mg	Vitamin C	4.89 mg
Beta-Carotene	86.86 RE	Copper	0.12 mg
Calcium	132.30 mg	Folate	18.52 µg
Cobalamin (B12)	0.19 µg	Vitamin D	0.56 µg
Iron	0.94 mg	Vitamin E	0.55 mg
Magnesium	23.38 mg	Zinc	1.05 mg

DILLED TUNA SANDWICHES

1 can (12½ ounces) chunk light tuna in water,
   drained
¼ cup thinly sliced green onion with tops
¼ cup chopped seeded cucumber
3 tablespoons reduced-calorie mayonnaise
1½ teaspoons drained capers
1 teaspoon Dijon-style mustard
½ to 1 teaspoon lemon juice
¾ teaspoon dried dill weed
   White pepper
4 slices multigrain bread, toasted
8 slices cucumber
2 slices tomato, cut into halves

Break tuna into chunks in small bowl; add green
onion and cucumber. Stir in mayonnaise, capers,
mustard, lemon juice, and dill weed; season with
pepper to taste. Spread tuna mixture on toasted
bread slices (open-faced); garnish with cucumber and
tomato slices.   *Makes 4 servings*

NUTRITIONAL INFORMATION PER SERVING

Calories	200.00 kc	Niacin (B₃)	12.07 mg
Protein	24.58 g	Pantothenic Acid	0.22 mg
Fat	5.57 g	Phosphorus	187.40 mg
% of Calories		Potassium	213.70 mg
from Fat:	24	Pyridoxine (B₆)	0.13 mg
Saturated Fat	0.58 g	Riboflavin (B₂)	0.21 mg
Cholesterol	19.69 mg	Thiamin (B₁)	0.12 mg
Dietary Fiber	1.07 g	Vitamin A	46.49 RE
Sodium	179.90 mg	Vitamin C	2.85 mg
Beta-Carotene	155.10 RE	Copper	0.09 mg
Calcium	41.98 mg	Folate	22.57 µg
Cobalamin (B₁₂)	2.35 µg	Vitamin D	0.11 mg
Iron	2.08 mg	Vitamin E	7.02 mg
Magnesium	39.99 mg	Zinc	0.75 mg

CHINESE STEAMED FISH

12 ounces firm white fish fillets, such as swordfish
   Pepper
2 teaspoons cornstarch
2 teaspoons low-sodium soy sauce
2 teaspoons dry sherry
1 tablespoon finely chopped green onion
¼ teaspoon minced ginger root
1 garlic clove, minced
1½ fresh California peaches, sliced (1½ cups)

Cut fish lengthwise into 2-inch-wide strips. Sprinkle
with pepper to taste. Combine cornstarch, soy sauce,
and sherry in small bowl. Add fish to cornstarch
mixture; turn fish to coat. Arrange fish strips in
spirals in small, shallow baking dish, and sprinkle
with onion, ginger, garlic, and peaches. Place low
rack in large skillet. Pour hot water into bottom of
skillet, under rack; bring to a boil. Place baking dish
on rack. Cover. Steam 10 to 15 minutes or just until
fish flakes easily with fork. Transfer fish and peaches
to serving dish using wide spatula. Spoon sauce over
fish, if desired.   *Makes 4 servings*

NUTRITIONAL INFORMATION PER SERVING

Calories	128.60 kc	Niacin (B3)	8.25 mg
Protein	17.29 g	Pantothenic Acid	0.08 mg
Fat	3.45 g	Phosphorus	233.20 mg
% of Calories		Potassium	323.10 mg
from Fat:	25	Pyridoxine (B6)	0.28 mg
Saturated Fat	0.94 g	Riboflavin (B2)	0.10 mg
Cholesterol	33.52 mg	Thiamin (B1)	0.04 mg
Dietary Fiber	0.58 g	Vitamin A	51.08 RE
Sodium	176.70 mg	Vitamin C	3.66 mg
Beta-Carotene	145.50 RE	Copper	0.14 mg
Calcium	8.38 mg	Folate	4.21 µg
Cobalamin (B12)	1.34 µg	Vitamin E	1.23 mg
Iron	0.84 mg	Zinc	1.05 mg
Magnesium	26.68 mg		

TURKEY WILD RICE CHILI

- 1 tablespoon canola oil
- 1 medium onion, chopped
- 1 garlic clove, minced
- 1¼ pounds turkey breast slices, cut into ½-inch pieces
- 2 cups cooked wild rice
- 1 can (15 ounces) great northern white beans, drained
- 1 can (11 ounces) white corn (optional)
- 2 cans (4 ounces) diced green chilies
- 1 can (14½ ounces) low-sodium chicken broth
- 1 teaspoon ground cumin
  Hot pepper sauce (optional)
- 4 ounces low-fat Monterey Jack cheese, shredded

Heat oil in large pan over medium heat; add onion and garlic. Cook until tender. Add turkey, wild rice, beans, corn, chilies, broth, and cumin. Cover and simmer over low heat 30 minutes or until turkey is tender. Stir hot pepper sauce into chili to taste. Serve with shredded cheese.   *Makes 8 servings*

NUTRITIONAL INFORMATION PER SERVING

Calories	272.00 kc	Niacin (B3)	4.95 mg
Protein	26.00 g	Pantothenic Acid	0.79 mg
Fat	5.75 g	Phosphorus	315.30 mg
% of Calories		Potassium	529.70 mg
from Fat:	19	Pyridoxine (B6)	0.40 mg
Saturated Fat	1.36 g	Riboflavin (B2)	0.25 mg
Cholesterol	35.96 mg	Thiamin (B1)	0.16 mg
Dietary Fiber	1.88 g	Vitamin A	40.64 RE
Sodium	199.10 mg	Vitamin C	27.51 mg
Beta-Carotene	64.92 RE	Copper	0.19 mg
Calcium	202.10 mg	Folate	80.88 µg
Cobalamin (B12)	0.28 µg	Vitamin E	0.47 mg
Iron	2.58 mg	Zinc	2.44 mg
Magnesium	67.11 mg		

POULTRY

CRUNCHY APPLE SALSA WITH GRILLED CHICKEN

2 cups Washington Gala apples, halved, cored, and chopped
¾ cup (1 large) Anaheim chile pepper, seeded and chopped
½ cup chopped onion
¼ cup lime juice
   Salt and pepper to taste
   Grilled Chicken (recipe follows)

Combine all ingredients except chicken and mix well; allow flavors to blend about ½ hour. Serve salsa over or alongside Grilled Chicken.

Makes 4 servings (3 cups salsa)

Grilled Chicken: Marinate 2 whole boneless, skinless chicken breasts in a mixture of ¼ cup dry white wine, ¼ cup apple juice, ½ teaspoon grated lime peel, ½ teaspoon salt, and dash pepper for 20 to 30 minutes. Drain and grill over medium-hot coals, turning once, until center is no longer pink.

NUTRITIONAL INFORMATION PER SERVING

Calories	272.00 kc	Niacin (B3)	4.95 mg
Protein	26.00 g	Pantothenic Acid	0.79 mg
Fat	5.75 g	Phosphorus	315.30 mg
% of Calories		Potassium	529.70 mg
from Fat:	19	Pyridoxine (B6)	0.40 mg
Saturated Fat	1.36 g	Riboflavin (B2)	0.25 mg
Cholesterol	35.96 mg	Thiamin (B1)	0.16 mg
Dietary Fiber	1.88 g	Vitamin A	40.64 RE
Sodium	199.10 mg	Vitamin C	27.51 mg
Beta-Carotene	64.92 RE	Copper	0.19 mg
Calcium	202.10 mg	Folate	80.88 µg
Cobalamin (B12)	0.28 µg	Vitamin E	0.47 mg
Iron	2.58 mg	Zinc	2.44 mg
Magnesium	67.11 mg		

TURKEY-POTATO CASSEROLE

- ½ cup chopped green bell pepper
- ½ cup sliced green onions
- 3 tablespoons margarine
- 1 can (15 ounces) cream-style corn
- 2 cups skim milk
- ½ teaspoon salt
- ⅛ teaspoon ground black pepper
- 2 cups cooked turkey, cut into ½-inch cubes
- 2 cups instant potato flakes
- ¼ cup grated Parmesan cheese
- 2 tablespoons sliced green onion tops

Preheat oven to 375°F. In large saucepan, over medium-high heat, cook and stir bell pepper and sliced onions in margarine until tender. Add corn, milk, salt, and pepper. Reduce heat and cook until mixture bubbles; remove from heat. Fold in turkey and potato flakes. Pour turkey mixture into greased 9-inch square casserole. Sprinkle with cheese and onion tops. Bake 25 minutes or until lightly browned.   *Makes 6 servings*

NUTRITIONAL INFORMATION PER SERVING

Calories	300.70 kc	Niacin (B₃)	3.70 mg
Protein	18.83 g	Pantothenic Acid	0.78 mg
Fat	7.67 g	Phosphorus	244.90 mg
% of Calories		Potassium	776.50 mg
from Fat:	23	Pyridoxine (B₆)	0.35 mg
Saturated Fat	2.14 g	Riboflavin (B₂)	0.24 mg
Cholesterol	36.13 mg	Thiamin (B₁)	0.09 mg
Dietary Fiber	1.48 g	Vitamin A	189.00 RE
Sodium	619.10 mg	Vitamin C	24.72 mg
Beta-Carotene	308.90 RE	Copper	0.13 mg
Calcium	175.00 mg	Folate	44.23 µg
Cobalamin (B₁₂)	0.52 µg	Vitamin D	1.42 µg
Iron	1.18 mg	Vitamin E	4.44 mg
Magnesium	38.31 mg	Zinc	1.55 mg

TURKEY PISTACHIO SANDWICH

- ½ cup plain yogurt
- ¼ cup salted pistachio nuts, chopped
- 1 teaspoon dried dill weed
- 4 lettuce leaves
- 8 slices whole-wheat bread
- 8 ounces cooked turkey breast, sliced

In small bowl, combine yogurt, pistachio nuts, and dill weed. Cover and refrigerate at least 1 hour or overnight to allow flavors to blend.

To serve, place 1 lettuce leaf on bread slice; top with ¼ of turkey. Spoon 2 tablespoons yogurt mixture over turkey; top with bread slice. If desired, repeat with remaining ingredients. Turkey mixture will keep up to four days in refrigerator. *Makes 4 servings*

NUTRITIONAL INFORMATION PER SERVING

Calories	283.90 kc	Niacin (B3)	6.03 mg
Protein	25.93 g	Pantothenic Acid	1.10 mg
Fat	6.83 g	Phosphorus	340.00 mg
% of Calories		Potassium	503.70 mg
from Fat:	21	Pyridoxine (B6)	0.47 mg
Saturated Fat	1.29 g	Riboflavin (B2)	0.23 mg
Cholesterol	50.70 mg	Thiamin (B1)	0.23 mg
Dietary Fiber	4.34 g	Vitamin A	14.15 RE
Sodium	349.60 mg	Vitamin C	1.59 mg
Beta-Carotene	18.10 RE	Copper	0.24 mg
Calcium	129.00 mg	Folate	53.32 µg
Cobalamin (B12)	0.38 µg	Vitamin E	1.30 mg
Iron	3.06 mg	Zinc	2.36 mg
Magnesium	68.27 mg		

TURKEY, CORN, AND SWEET POTATO SOUP

½ cup chopped onion
1 small jalapeño pepper, minced
1 teaspoon margarine
5 cups turkey broth or reduced-sodium chicken
   bouillon
1½ pounds sweet potatoes, peeled and cut into
   1-inch cubes
2 cups cooked turkey, cut into ½-inch cubes
½ teaspoon salt
1½ cups frozen corn
   Cilantro (optional)

In 5-quart saucepan, over medium-high heat, cook and stir onion and pepper in margarine 5 minutes or until onion is soft. Add broth, potatoes, turkey, and salt; bring to a boil. Reduce heat to low; cover and simmer 20 to 25 minutes or until potatoes are tender. Stir in corn. Increase heat to medium and cook 5 to 6 minutes. Spoon 1 cup soup. Garnish with cilantro, if desired. *Makes 8 servings*

NUTRITIONAL INFORMATION PER SERVING

Calories	154.70 kc	Niacin (B3)	4.36 mg
Protein	12.14 g	Pantothenic Acid	0.71 mg
Fat	1.27 g	Phosphorus	119.70 mg
% of Calories		Potassium	376.70 mg
from Fat:	7	Pyridoxine (B6)	0.37 mg
Saturated Fat	0.18 g	Riboflavin (B2)	0.20 mg
Cholesterol	23.63 mg	Thiamin (B1)	0.10 mg
Dietary Fiber	3.30 g	Vitamin A	1,462 RE
Sodium	254.20 mg	Vitamin C	18.22 mg
Beta-Carotene	1,863 RE	Copper	0.18 mg
Calcium	36.24 mg	Folate	25.74 µg
Cobalamin (B12)	0.11 µg	Vitamin D	0.05 µg
Iron	1.32 mg	Vitamin E	5.62 mg
Magnesium	29.02 mg	Zinc	0.82 mg

SWEET 'N' SOUR WITH RICE

4 (3-ounce) boneless skinless chicken breasts
1½ cups water
¼ cup vinegar
1 cup uncooked converted rice
2 tablespoons brown sugar
8 ounces canned chunk pineapple, drained,
   reserving 2 tablespoons juice

Broil chicken for 10 to 15 minutes or until cooked
through, turning once. Meanwhile, in medium
saucepan, bring water and vinegar to a boil. Add rice
and brown sugar. Cover; cook 20 minutes or until
water is absorbed and rice is fluffy. Stir in pineapple
and reserved juice. Serve chicken over rice.

Makes 4 servings

NUTRITIONAL INFORMATION PER SERVING

Calories	283.80 kc	Niacin (B3)	7.41 mg
Protein	15.94 g	Pantothenic Acid	0.97 mg
Fat	1.75 g	Phosphorus	160.00 mg
% of Calories		Potassium	256.70 mg
from Fat:	6	Pyridoxine (B6)	0.45 mg
Saturated Fat	0.48 g	Riboflavin (B2)	0.10 mg
Cholesterol	34.30 mg	Thiamin (B1)	0.36 mg
Dietary Fiber	1.29 g	Vitamin A	3.39 RE
Sodium	34.61 mg	Vitamin C	4.36 mg
Beta-Carotene	1.13 RE	Copper	0.20 mg
Calcium	49.36 mg	Folate	11.88 µg
Cobalamin (B12)	0.14 µg	Vitamin E	0.47 mg
Iron	2.62 mg	Zinc	0.93 mg
Magnesium	37.58 mg		

PERUVIAN CHICKEN WITH PLUMS

- 1 chicken (3½ pounds), skinned, cut up
- 1 teaspoon vegetable oil
- 1 cup chopped onion
- 1 cup diced green bell pepper
- 2 teaspoons minced garlic
- 1 tomato, chopped
- 1 fresh jalapeño pepper, seeded, diced
- ¼ teaspoon powdered saffron (optional)
- 3½ cups low-sodium chicken broth
- 1 bay leaf
- 4 fresh California plums, quartered
- 4 cups cooked brown rice

Cook chicken in oil in large nonstick skillet, turning often until golden brown on all sides, about 12 minutes. Add onion, bell pepper, and garlic; cook and stir 2 minutes longer. Add tomato, chili, saffron, broth, and bay leaf. Bring to a boil; cover and simmer 10 minutes. Add plums and rice; heat through. Discard bay leaf.   *Makes 8 servings*

NUTRITIONAL INFORMATION PER SERVING

Calories	344.20 kc	Niacin (B3)	12.04 mg
Protein	33.23 g	Pantothenic Acid	1.50 mg
Fat	9.36 g	Phosphorus	296.80 mg
% of Calories		Potassium	432.10 mg
from Fat:	25	Pyridoxine (B6)	0.75 mg
Saturated Fat	2.32 g	Riboflavin (B2)	0.26 mg
Cholesterol	89.61 mg	Thiamin (B1)	0.22 mg
Dietary Fiber	3.06 g	Vitamin A	50.96 RE
Sodium	173.90 mg	Vitamin C	30.61 mg
Beta-Carotene	96.78 RE	Copper	0.22 mg
Calcium	42.72 mg	Folate	23.51 µg
Cobalamin (B12)	0.33 µg	Vitamin E	3.62 mg
Iron	2.33 mg	Zinc	2.84 mg
Magnesium	75.22 mg		

TURKEY SPLIT PEA SOUP

- 1 pound dried split peas, washed and drained
- 7 cups Turkey Broth (recipe follows) or low sodium chicken bouillon
- 2 cups chopped onions
- 1 cup chopped carrots
- ½ cup chopped celery
- 1 clove garlic, minced
- 3 tablespoons dried parsley
- 1 bay leaf
- 1 pound turkey ham, cut into ½-inch cubes

In 5-quart saucepan, over high heat, combine peas, Turkey Broth, onions, carrots, celery, garlic, parsley, and bay leaf; bring to a boil. Reduce heat to simmer; cover and cook 1 hour. Remove saucepan from heat; discard bay leaf.

With wire whisk, gently whisk soup to blend peas. If desired, soup may be puréed in blender for smoother texture.

Return soup to medium-high heat, add turkey ham and bring to a boil. Reduce heat to simmer, and cook, uncovered, 10 to 15 minutes.   *Makes 8 servings*

TURKEY BROTH

    4 cups water
      Turkey giblets
    1 stalk celery, sliced
    1 carrot, sliced
    1 onion, sliced
    1 bay leaf
    3 sprigs parsley
    4 peppercorns

In large saucepan, over high heat, bring water, giblets, celery, carrot, onion, bay leaf, parsley, and peppercorns to a boil. Reduce heat to low, cover and simmer 1 hour.

Strain broth and refrigerate until needed. Store giblets in refrigerator until ready to make gravy or dressing.

NUTRITIONAL INFORMATION PER SERVING

Calories	242.50 kc	Niacin (B3)	5.26 mg
Protein	23.42 g	Pantothenic Acid	0.09 mg
Fat	4.15 g	Phosphorus	232.10 mg
% of Calories		Potassium	662.80 mg
from Fat:	15	Pyridoxine (B6)	0.27 mg
Saturated Fat	1.05 g	Riboflavin (B2)	0.37 mg
Cholesterol	33.94 mg	Thiamin (B1)	0.26 mg
Dietary Fiber	7.18 g	Vitamin A	400.60 RE
Sodium	754.10 mg	Vitamin C	5.37 mg
Beta-carotene	2,331 RE	Copper	0.38 mg
Calcium	51.94 mg	Folate	88.58 µg
Cobalamin (B12)	0.14 µg	Vitamin E	3.29 mg
Iron	4.53 mg	Zinc	2.99 mg
Magnesium	57.89 mg		

CHICKEN AND
VEGETABLE COUSCOUS

- 1 tablespoon vegetable oil
- 3 (3-ounce) boneless chicken breasts, cut into 3-inch cubes
- 3 garlic cloves, minced
- ½ cup chopped green onions
- 1¼ cups tomato sauce
- 1½ cups water, divided
- 1¼ cups chopped carrots
- 1 large potato, cut into cubes
- 1 yellow squash, chopped
- 1 medium tomato, chopped
- 1 cup canned small white beans, rinsed and drained
- ¼ cup chopped red bell pepper
- ¼ cup raisins
- 2 tablespoons brown sugar
- 2 teaspoons ground cumin
- ¾ teaspoon ground cinnamon
- 3 to 4 drops hot sauce
- 1 cup dry couscous

Place oil in medium skillet. Add chicken breasts and brown over medium heat. Add garlic and green onions; cook and stir for 1 minute. Stir in tomato sauce and ¼ cup water. Add carrots, potato, squash, tomato, beans, red bell pepper, raisins, brown sugar, cumin, cinnamon, and hot sauce. Bring to a simmer and cook 15 minutes.

Meanwhile, bring remaining 1¼ cups water to a boil. Add couscous; cover and remove from heat. Let stand 5 minutes. Serve chicken and vegetables over couscous.

Makes 6 servings

Tip: Couscous is a granular pasta that is a staple in North African cuisine. It is readily available in large supermarkets, usually shelved with rice and other grains.

NUTRITIONAL INFORMATION PER SERVING

Calories	322.40 kc	Niacin (B₃)	6.25 mg
Protein	16.93 g	Pantothenic Acid	1.19 mg
Fat	4.12 g	Phosphorus	229.40 mg
% of Calories		Potassium	833.00 mg
from Fat:	11	Pyridoxine (B₆)	0.50 mg
Saturated Fat	0.71 g	Riboflavin (B₂)	0.17 mg
Cholesterol	21.72 mg	Selenium	0.01 mg
Dietary Fiber	9.25 g	Thiamin (B₁)	0.27 mg
Sodium	347.70 mg	Vitamin A	757.80 RE
Beta-carotene	4,109 RE	Vitamin C	26.13 mg
Calcium	80.07 mg	Copper	0.39 mg
Soluble Fiber	1.60 g	Folate	70.55 µg
Cobalamin (B₁₂)	0.09 µg	Vitamin E	2.51 mg
Iron	3.32 mg	Zinc	1.34 mg
Magnesium	77.37 mg		

LEMON TURKEY
STIR-FRY AND PASTA

  1 pound linguine or other long pasta
1½ pounds turkey cutlets, cut into ½-inch strips
  1 tablespoon soy sauce
  1 tablespoon white wine vinegar
  2 teaspoons cornstarch
  1 teaspoon lemon pepper
  2 tablespoons olive oil
  6 medium green onions, sliced
  1 medium fresh lemon, cut into 10 thin slices and
      slivered
  1 clove garlic, finely minced
  1 (10-ounce) bag fresh spinach, washed, drained,
      and chopped
    Parsley (optional)
    Lemon slices (optional)

In resealable plastic food storage bag, combine
turkey cutlets, soy sauce, white wine vinegar, cornstarch, and lemon pepper. Shake bag to coat turkey
cutlets thoroughly. Refrigerate 30 minutes to allow
flavors to blend. Cook linguine according to package
directions; drain.

In large skillet, over medium heat, cook and stir turkey cutlets and marinade in olive oil 2 to 3 minutes or until turkey is no longer pink. Add sliced green onions, lemon slivers, and garlic; continue to cook until onions are soft. Stir in chopped spinach and cook until spinach is just wilted. Spoon mixture over hot linguine and garnish with parsley and lemon slices, if desired.

Makes 6 servings

NUTRITIONAL INFORMATION PER SERVING

Calories	433.00 kc	Niacin (B3)	7.34 mg
Protein	33.48 g	Pantothenic Acid	0.97 mg
Fat	9.12 g	Phosphorus	314.10 mg
% of Calories		Potassium	579.40 mg
from Fat:	19	Pyridoxine (B6)	0.58 mg
Saturated Fat	1.71 g	Riboflavin (B2)	0.50 mg
Cholesterol	114.80 mg	Thiamin (B1)	0.51 mg
Dietary Fiber	4.57 g	Vitamin A	354.70 RE
Sodium	267.20 mg	Vitamin C	29.97 mg
Beta-carotene	2,058 RE	Copper	0.34 mg
Calcium	89.48 mg	Folate	112.20 µg
Cobalamin (B12)	0.54 µg	Vitamin E	2.43 mg
Iron	4.92 mg	Zinc	2.88 mg
Magnesium	97.85 mg		

CHICKEN WILD RICE SOUP

- ⅓ cup instant nonfat dry milk
- 2 tablespoons cornstarch
- 2 teaspoons low-sodium instant chicken bouillon
- ¼ teaspoon dried onion flakes
- ¼ teaspoon dried basil
- ¼ teaspoon dried thyme leaves
- ⅛ teaspoon ground black pepper
- 4 cups low-sodium chicken broth
- ½ cup sliced celery
- ½ cup sliced carrots
- ½ cup chopped onion
- 2 cups cooked wild rice
- 1 cup cooked cubed chicken breasts

In small bowl, combine dry milk, cornstarch, bouillon, onion flakes, basil, thyme, and pepper. Stir in small amount of chicken broth; set aside. In large saucepan, combine remaining broth, celery, carrots, and onion. Cook until vegetables are crisp-tender. Gradually add dry milk mixture. Stir in wild rice and chicken. Simmer 5 to 10 minutes.   *Makes 8 servings*

NUTRITIONAL INFORMATION PER SERVING

Calories	102.90 kc	Niacin (B3)	3.78 mg
Protein	8.48 g	Pantothenic Acid	0.33 mg
Fat	1.11 g	Phosphorus	102.70 mg
% of Calories		Potassium	188.60 mg
from Fat:	10	Pyridoxine (B6)	0.18 mg
Saturated Fat	0.19 g	Riboflavin (B2)	0.15 mg
Cholesterol	12.53 mg	Thiamin (B1)	0.07 mg
Dietary Fiber	1.19 g	Vitamin A	216.00 RE
Sodium	70.21 mg	Vitamin C	2.07 mg
Beta-carotene	1,169 RE	Copper	0.07 mg
Calcium	54.97 mg	Folate	17.71 µg
Cobalamin (B12)	0.16 µg	Vitamin E	0.30 mg
Iron	0.87 mg	Zinc	0.87 mg
Magnesium	24.00 mg		

PERSIAN CHICKEN

2 cups low-sodium chicken broth
1 cup cracked wheat
½ teaspoon dried basil leaves, crushed
½ teaspoon grated lemon peel
¼ teaspoon mint flakes
¼ cup whole natural California almonds, chopped
1 tablespoon almond or olive oil
½ cup sliced green onions
⅓ cup raisins
2 tablespoons chopped parsley
1 tablespoon lemon juice
1 cup diced cooked chicken or turkey

Combine broth, wheat, basil, lemon peel, and mint flakes in large saucepan; heat to boiling. Cover; reduce heat to low and cook 15 minutes. Meanwhile, lightly brown almonds in oil in small skillet, stirring constantly, over medium heat. When wheat is cooked, add almonds, onions, raisins, parsley, and lemon juice; toss lightly to mix. Add chicken; heat 1 minute before serving. *Makes 3 servings*

NUTRITIONAL INFORMATION PER SERVING

Calories	370.30 kc	Niacin (B3)	6.84 mg
Protein	21.70 g	Pantothenic Acid	0.42 mg
Fat	11.29 g	Phosphorus	330.10 mg
% of Calories		Potassium	410.40 mg
from Fat:	27	Pyridoxine (B6)	0.28 mg
Saturated Fat	0.88 g	Riboflavin (B2)	0.31 mg
Cholesterol	31.50 mg	Thiamin (B1)	0.25 mg
Dietary Fiber	3.18 g	Vitamin A	84.27 RE
Sodium	70.45 mg	Vitamin C	12.03 mg
Beta-carotene	501.20 RE	Copper	0.26 mg
Calcium	96.00 mg	Folate	10.32 µg
Cobalamin (B12)	0.15 µg	Vitamin E	5.12 mg
Iron	3.93 mg	Zinc	1.27 mg
Magnesium	60.65 mg		

TURKEY WALDORF SANDWICH

- **6 ounces cooked turkey breast, cubed**
- **½ cup diced celery**
- **1 small Red Delicious apple, cored and cut into small cubes**
- **2 tablespoons walnuts, chopped**
- **1 tablespoon reduced-calorie mayonnaise**
- **1 tablespoon nonfat yogurt**
- **⅛ teaspoon nutmeg**
- **⅛ teaspoon cinnamon**
- **4 lettuce leaves**
- **8 slices reduced-calorie raisin bread**

In medium bowl, combine turkey, celery, apple, walnuts, mayonnaise, yogurt, nutmeg, and cinnamon. Cover and refrigerate at least 1 hour to allow flavors to blend. To serve, arrange 1 lettuce leaf on each bread slice. Spoon ¾ cup turkey mixture over lettuce, and top with 1 bread slice. Turkey mixture will keep up to four days in refrigerator.

Makes 4 servings

NUTRITIONAL INFORMATION PER SERVING

Calories	187.80 kc	Niacin (B₃)	4.36 mg
Protein	16.37 g	Pantothenic Acid	0.53 mg
Fat	4.72 g	Phosphorus	151.30 mg
% of Calories		Potassium	335.80 mg
from Fat:	22	Pyridoxine (B₆)	0.31 mg
Saturated Fat	0.61 g	Riboflavin (B₂)	0.24 mg
Cholesterol	36.75 mg	Thiamin (B₁)	0.13 mg
Dietary Fiber	1.95 g	Vitamin A	19.94 RE
Sodium	136.80 mg	Vitamin C	4.38 mg
Beta-carotene	30.05 RE	Copper	0.13 mg
Calcium	54.39 mg	Folate	30.63 µg
Cobalamin (B₁₂)	0.19 µg	Vitamin D	0.04 µg
Iron	1.75 mg	Vitamin E	3.29 mg
Magnesium	32.42 mg	Zinc	1.13 mg

WASHINGTON APPLE TURKEY GYROS

- 1 cup onion slices
- 1 cup each thinly sliced red and green bell peppers
- 2 tablespoons lemon juice
- 1 tablespoon vegetable oil
- ½ pound cooked turkey breast, cut into thin strips
- 1 medium Washington Golden Delicious or Winesap apple, cored and thinly sliced
- 6 pita rounds, lightly toasted
- ½ cup plain low-fat yogurt

Cook and stir onion, peppers, and lemon juice in oil in nonstick skillet until crisp-tender. Stir in turkey; cook until turkey is thoroughly heated. Remove from heat; stir in apple. Fill each pita with apple mixture; drizzle with yogurt. Serve warm.   *Makes 6 servings*

NUTRITIONAL INFORMATION PER SERVING

Calories	219.5 kc	Niacin (B3)	4.45 mg
Protein	16.83 g	Pantothenic Acid	0.45 mg
Fat	3.60 g	Phosphorus	165.33 mg
% of Calories		Potassium	316.67 mg
from Fat:	15	Pyridoxine (B6)	0.32 mg
Saturated Fat	0.60 g	Riboflavin (B2)	0.18 mg
Cholesterol	32.50 mg	Thiamin (B1)	0.23 mg
Dietary Fiber	1.95 g	Vitamin A	20.66 RE
Sodium	250.5 mg	Vitamin C	26.50 mg
Beta-carotene	48.01 RE	Copper	.072 mg
Calcium	79.67 mg	Folate	16.01 µg
Iron	1.73 mg	Zinc	.91 mg
Magnesium	20.83 mg		

Apple-icious Lamb Kebabs

1½ pounds fresh American lamb (leg or shoulder),
    cut into 1¼-inch cubes
1 cup apple juice or cider
2 tablespoons Worcestershire sauce
½ teaspoon lemon pepper
2 cloves garlic, peeled and sliced
1 large apple, cut into 12 wedges
    Assorted vegetables, such as 1 large green or
    red bell pepper, 1 large onion, 1 small
    summer squash, cut into wedges
    Apple Barbecue Sauce (recipe follows)

Mix apple juice, Worcestershire sauce, lemon pepper, and garlic in plastic bag or nonmetal container. Add lamb cubes and coat well. To marinate, place in refrigerator for at least 2 hours or up to 24 hours.

Preheat grill or broiler. Remove meat from marinade and thread onto skewers, alternating meat, apple, and vegetables.

To grill, place kebabs 4 inches from medium coals. Cook about 10 to 12 minutes for medium-rare, turning occasionally and brushing with Apple Barbecue Sauce. (To broil, place kebabs on broiler pan that has been lightly oiled or sprayed with nonstick cooking spray. Broil lamb 4 inches from heat source. Cook about 10 to 12 minutes for medium-rare, turning occasionally and brushing with Apple Barbecue Sauce.) *Makes 6 servings*

Apple Barbecue Sauce

- ½ cup apple juice or cider
- ½ cup finely chopped onion
- 1 cup chili sauce
- ½ cup unsweetened applesauce
- 2 tablespoons packed brown sugar
- 1 tablespoon Worcestershire sauce
- 1 teaspoon dry mustard
- 5 drops hot pepper sauce

Combine apple juice and onion in 1-quart saucepan; bring to a boil. Reduce heat and simmer for 2 minutes. Stir in chili sauce, applesauce, brown sugar, Worcestershire sauce, dry mustard, and hot pepper sauce. Simmer 10 minutes, stirring occasionally. Remove from heat.

NUTRITIONAL INFORMATION PER SERVING
(includes about 1½ tablespoons sauce)

Calories	224.38 kc	Niacin (B3)	5.81 mg
Protein	25.20 g	Pantothenic Acid	0.56 mg
Fat	6.85 g	Phosphorus	159.30 mg
% of Calories		Potassium	513.97 mg
from Fat:	29	Pyridoxine (B6)	0.21 mg
Saturated Fat	2.36 g	Riboflavin (B2)	0.29 mg
Cholesterol	75.65 mg	Thiamin (B1)	0.15 mg
Dietary Fiber	2.11 g	Vitamin A	14.97 RE
Sodium	242.60 mg	Vitamin C	12.90 mg
Beta-carotene	22.77 RE	Copper	0.15 mg
Calcium	25.72 mg	Folate	29.28 µg
Cobalamin (B12)	1.70 µg	Vitamin E	0.44 mg
Iron	2.30 mg	Zinc	3.38 mg
Magnesium	29.73 mg		

Beef Chili

    2 teaspoons vegetable oil
    1 pound lean beef cubed steaks
 4½ teaspoons Spicy Seasoning Mix (recipe fol-
        lows), divided
    1 medium onion, chopped
    1 can (28 ounces) plum tomatoes, undrained
    2 cups frozen whole kernel corn

Heat oil in deep large skillet or wok, over medium
heat 5 minutes. Meanwhile, cut each beef steak
lengthwise into 1-inch-wide strips; cut crosswise into
1-inch pieces. Sprinkle beef with 2 teaspoons Spicy
Seasoning Mix. Stir-fry beef and onion in hot oil 2
to 3 minutes. Season with salt, if desired. Add
tomatoes (breaking up with back of spoon), corn,
and remaining 2½ teaspoons Spicy Seasoning Mix.
Bring to a boil; reduce heat to medium-low and
simmer, uncovered, 18 to 20 minutes until beef is
tender.   *Makes 4 servings*

SPICY SEASONING MIX

   3 tablespoons chili powder
   2 teaspoons ground cumin
1½ teaspoons garlic powder
   ¾ teaspoon dried oregano leaves, crushed
   ½ teaspoon ground red pepper (cayenne)

Combine all ingredients. Cover; store in airtight container. Shake before using.   *Makes about ⅓ cup.*

Tip: Serve with tortilla chips and melon wedges.

NUTRITIONAL INFORMATION PER SERVING

Calories	301.20 kc	Folate	43.22 µg
Protein	26.52 g	Iron	4.73 mg
Carbohydrate	29.30 g	Magnesium	68.87 mg
Fat	10.29 g	Manganese	0.51 mg
% of Calories		Niacin (B3)	5.70 mg
from Fat:	29	Pantothenic Acid	0.83 mg
Saturated Fat	3.15 g	Phosphorus	276.10 mg
Cholesterol	63.94 mg	Potassium	961.60 mg
Dietary Fiber	4.38 g	Pyridoxine (B6)	0.63 mg
Sodium	393.20 mg	Riboflavin (B2)	0.37 mg
Beta-carotene	1,187 RE	Thiamin (B1)	0.27 mg
Biotin	8.28 µg	Vitamin A	200.50 RE
Calcium	73.84 mg	Vitamin C	35.16 mg
Chromium	0.04 mg	Vitamin E	3.32 mg
Cobalamin (B12)	1.96 µg	Vitamin K	52.97 µg
Copper	0.41 mg	Zinc	4.97 mg
Fluoride	49.35 µg		

Beef and Pineapple Kabobs

1 pound boneless beef top sirloin steak, cut
   1-inch-thick*
1 small onion, finely chopped
½ cup bottled teriyaki sauce
16 pieces (1×1-inch) fresh pineapple
1 can (8 ounces) water chestnuts, drained

Prepare grill for medium coals. Cut beef steak into
¼-inch-thick strips. For marinade, combine onion
and teriyaki sauce. Place beef strips in small bowl;
add marinade, stirring to coat. Alternately thread
beef strips (weaving back and forth), pineapple
cubes, and water chestnuts on bamboo** or thin
metal skewers. Place kabobs on grid over medium
coals. Grill 4 minutes, turning once.

Makes 4 servings

Tip: Serve with hot cooked rice and stir-fried broccoli, mushrooms, and red bell peppers.

*You may substitute beef top round steak, cut 1-inch
thick, for the sirloin steak.

**Soak bamboo skewers in cold water 20 minutes
before grilling to prevent scorching.

NUTRITIONAL INFORMATION PER SERVING

Calories	308.30 kc	Folate	33.16 µg
Protein	37.60 g	Iron	5.25 mg
Carbohydrate	24.11 g	Magnesium	73.30 mg
Fat	6.75 g	Manganese	1.42 mg
% of Calories		Niacin (B3)	5.87 mg
from Fat:	20	Pantothenic Acid	0.78 mg
Saturated Fat	2.50 g	Phosphorus	355.00 mg
Cholesterol	101.40 mg	Potassium	723.90 mg
Dietary Fiber	1.27 g	Pyridoxine (B6)	0.72 mg
Sodium	1460 mg	Riboflavin (B2)	0.41 mg
Beta-carotene	11.96 RE	Thiamin (B1)	0.24 mg
Biotin	0.22 µg	Vitamin A	1.99 RE
Calcium	32.89 mg	Vitamin C	13.95 mg
Cobalamin (B12)	3.23 µg	Vitamin E	0.54 mg
Copper	0.36 mg	Vitamin K	0.10 µg
Fluoride	22.85 µg	Zinc	7.75 mg

THAI BEEF WITH NOODLES

1 pound boneless beef top sirloin, 1 inch thick
$1/4$ cup dry sherry
$1\frac{1}{2}$ tablespoons reduced-sodium soy sauce
1 teaspoon each grated fresh ginger, minced
    garlic, and Oriental dark roasted sesame oil
$1/4$ to $1/2$ teaspoon crushed red pepper
2 teaspoons cornstarch
$1/4$ cup water
2 cups cooked ramen noodles or linguine
$1/4$ cup chopped green onion tops

Combine sherry, soy sauce, ginger, garlic, sesame oil, and pepper. Place beef in plastic bag; add marinade. Close bag securely and marinate 15 minutes. Pour off marinade; reserve. Heat nonstick skillet over medium heat 5 minutes. Add steak; cook 12 to 15 minutes for rare (140°F) to medium (160°F), turning once. Remove beef; keep warm. Dissolve cornstarch in reserved marinade and water; add to skillet. Bring to a boil, stirring constantly. Stir in noodles. Cut beef into thin slices and serve over noodles. Sprinkle with onions. *Makes 4 servings*

NUTRITIONAL INFORMATION PER SERVING

Calories	310.3 kc	Niacin (B3)	4.86 mg
Protein	31.32 g	Pantothenic Acid	0.40 mg
Fat	10.55 g	Phosphorus	270.40 mg
% of Calories		Potassium	452.30 mg
from Fat:	30	Pyridoxine (B6)	0.46 mg
Saturated Fat	2.33 g	Riboflavin (B2)	0.33 mg
Cholesterol	98.86 mg	Thiamin (B1)	0.21 mg
Dietary Fiber	1.15 g	Vitamin A	135.60 RE
Sodium	673.40 mg	Vitamin C	2.34 mg
Beta-carotene	248.90 RE	Copper	0.21 mg
Calcium	24.62 mg	Folate	14.34 µg
Cobalamin (B12)	2.59 µg	Vitamin E	0.63 mg
Iron	4.30 mg	Zinc	6.31 mg
Magnesium	43.14 mg		

MEAT

LAMB TORTELLINI MINESTRONE

- **2 cups cooked cubed lean American lamb (leg or shoulder) or 1 pound ground lamb, cooked and drained**
- **2 cans (14 ounces each) reduced-sodium beef broth**
- **1 can (8 ounces) tomato sauce**
- **1 clove garlic, minced or ¼ teaspoon garlic powder**
- **1 package (8 ounces) dry cheese tortellini or 16 ounces fresh cheese tortellini**
- **1 bag (16 ounces) frozen cauliflower, zucchini, carrot, and red pepper combination**
- **1 can (15 ounces) white northern beans or kidney beans, drained**
- **1½ teaspoon dried Italian seasonings**

Bring broth and tomato sauce to a boil in large saucepan over high heat. Add all other ingredients and reduce heat to medium-low. Simmer 10 to 15 minutes until tortellini and vegetables are tender, stirring occasionally. *Makes 8 servings*

NUTRITIONAL INFORMATION PER SERVING

Calories	218.70 kc	Magnesium	40.81 mg
Manganesium	0.31 mg	Niacin (B3)	3.29 mg
Protein	16.74 g	Pantothenic Acid	0.44 mg
Fat	4.27 g	Phosphorus	140.50 mg
% of Calories		Potassium	504.50 mg
from Fat:	18	Pyridoxine (B6)	0.15 mg
Saturated Fat	1.86 g	Riboflavin (B2)	0.18 mg
Cholesterol	30.23 mg	Selenium	0.01 mg
Dietary Fiber	1.68 g	Thiamin (B1)	0.16 mg
Sodium	277.10 mg	Vitamin A	29.72 RE
Beta-carotene	11.70 RE	Vitamin C	4.50 mg
Soluble Fiber	0.16 g	Copper	0.18 mg
Calcium	62.90 mg	Folate	52.40 µg
Cobalamin (B12)	0.75 µg	Vitamin E	0.02 mg
Iron	1.91 mg	Zinc	1.83 mg

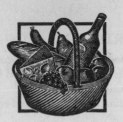

Vitamin and Mineral Counter

The Vitamin and Mineral Counter will give you a good idea of your vitamin intake (pages 459–503) and your mineral intake (pages 504–547), using the following abbreviations.

VIT A = vitamin A
BETA-C = beta-carotene
VIT E = vitamin E
VIT D = vitamin D
VIT C = vitamin C
FOL = folate
VIT B_6 = vitamin B_6
VIT B_{12} = vitamin B_{12}
PANT = pantothenic acid
CALC = calcium
IRON = iron
MAG = magnesium
PHOS = phosphorus
SOD = sodium
POTA = potassium
COP = copper
ZINC = zinc
SELE = selenium

BOX = box
CAK = cake
CI = cubic inch
CP = cup
EA = each
FO = fluid ounce
LG = large
LK = link
MD = medium
MDE = medium egg used
OZ = ounce
PC = piece
PKG = package
PKT = packet
POD = pod
PTY = patty
REB = regular bar
REG = regular
RG = ring

SET = set
SI = square inch
SL = slice
SM = small
STK = stick
STR = strip
SUG = sugar cone
SV = serving
SW = sandwich
TB = tablespoon
TS = teaspoon

mg = milligram
μg = microgram
IU = international unit
g = gram
NA = value not available

VITAMIN COUNTER	WEIGHT (g)	VIT A (IU)	BETA-C (μg)	VIT E (mg)	VIT D (μg)	VIT C (mg)	FOL (μg)	VIT B$_6$ (mg)	PANT (mg)	VIT B$_{12}$ (mg)
BEVERAGES										
Club soda (CP)	236.80	0	0	0	0	0	0	0	0	0
Coffee, brewed, hot or iced, without sugar (CP)	237	0	0	0	0	0	0.24	0	0	0
Coffee, decaffeinated, instant, dry powder (TS)	1	0	0	0	0	0	0	0	0	0
Coffee, instant, dry powder (TS)	0.9	0	0	0	0	0	0	0	0	0
Cola (CP)	246.40	0	0	0	0	0	0	0	0	0
Cola, diet, with aspartame (CP)	236.80	0	0	0	0	0	0	0	0	0
Cola, diet, with saccharin (CP)	240	0	0	0	0	0	0	0	0	0
Noncola (CP)	245.60	0	0	0	0	0	0	0	0	0
Noncola, diet, with aspartame (CP)	240	0	0	0	0	0	0	0	0	0
Noncola, diet, with saccharin (CP)	236.80	0	0	0	0	0	0	0	0	0
Noncola, diet, with saccharin, sodium free (CP)	236.80	0	0	0	0	0	0	0	0	0
Postum, dry powder (TS)	3.06	0	0	0.02	0	0	4.80	0.03	0.03	0
Root beer, cream soda, birch beer, near beer (CP)	246.40	0	0	0	0	0	0	0	0	0

VITAMIN COUNTER	WEIGHT (g)	VIT A (IU)	BETA-C (µg)	VIT E (mg)	VIT D (µg)	VIT C (mg)	FOL (µg)	VIT B$_6$ (mg)	PANT (mg)	VIT B$_{12}$ (mg)
Root beer, diet, with aspartame (CP)	240	0	0	0	0	0	0	0	0	0
Root beer, diet, with saccharin (CP)	240	0	0	0	0	0	0	0	0	0
Tea, herbal (CP)	237	0	0	0	0	0	1.42	0	0.02	0
Tea, hot or iced, with aspartame, reconstituted (CP)	238	0	0	0	0	0	4.50	0	0.02	0
Tea, hot or iced, with saccharin, reconstituted (CP)	238	0	0	0	0	0	6.90	0	0.02	0
Tea, hot or iced, without sugar, brewed (CP)	237	0	0	0	0	0	12.32	0	0.02	0
Tea, hot or iced, with sugar, reconstituted, presweetened, instant (CP)	240	0	0	0	0	0	8.88	0	0.02	0
Tea, instant, decaffeinated, dry powder (TS)	0.70	0	0	0	0	0	0.72	0.01	0.03	0
Tea, instant, decaffeinated, dry powder, with aspartame (TS)	0.80	0	0	0	0	4.68	0	0	0	0
Tea, instant, decaffeinated, dry powder, with sugar (TS)	3.80	0	0	0	0	0	0.47	0	0.02	0
Tea, instant, decaffeinated, with saccharin, dry powder (TS)	1.20	0	0	0	0	0	0.38	0	0.01	0
Tea, instant, dry powder (TS)	0.70	0	0	0	0	0	0.72	0.01	0.03	0

Food												
Tea, instant, dry powder, with aspartame (TS)	0.78	0	0	0	0	0	0	0	2.25	0	0.01	0
Tea, instant, dry powder, with saccharin (TS)	1.20	0	0	0	0	0	0	0	3.46	0	0.01	0
EGGS AND EGG PRODUCTS												
Egg, scrambled with whole milk (LG)	122.20	983.9	170.8	1.27	2.34	0.30			48.61	0.15	1.35	1.12
Egg, whole (LG)	50	317.5	57.03	0.37	0.63	0			23.50	0.07	0.63	0.50
Egg, yolk (LG)	16.60	322.8	57.93	0.36	0.67	0			24.24	0.06	0.63	0.52
Egg Beaters egg substitute, prepared as directed (CP)	210.14	2295.36	1004.27	1.39	4.28	0.03			147.6	0.27	3.70	3.32
Eggnog, commercial (CP)	254	894.0	223.5	0.38	3.07	3.81			2.29	0.13	1.07	1.14
Egg white (LG)	33.40	0	0	0	0	0			1	0	0.04	0.07
Scramblers egg substitute, prepared as directed (CP)	217.18	4827.95	2519.46	3.39	5.96	0.03			7.69	0.76	4.58	4.84
Second Nature egg substitute, prepared as directed (CP)	217.20	2428.53	986.1	3.05	4.47	0.41			127.9	0.33	3.19	1.91
FATS AND OILS												
Butter, salted (TS)	4.73	144.6	38.03	0.08	0.02	0			0.13	0	0.01	0.01

VITAMIN COUNTER	WEIGHT (g)	VIT A (IU)	BETA-C (µg)	VIT E (mg)	VIT D (µg)	VIT C (mg)	FOL (µg)	VIT B6 (mg)	PANT (mg)	VIT B12 (mg)
Butter, unsalted (TS)	4.73	144.6	38.03	0.08	0.02	0	0.14	0	0.01	0.01
Butter, whipped (TS)	3.15	96.33	25.51	0.05	0.02	0	0.09	0	0	0
Butter, whipped, unsalted (TS)	3.15	96.33	25.55	0.05	0.02	0	0.09	0	0	0
Lard, rendered (TS)	4.27	0	0	0.05	0	0	0	0	0	0
Margarine, corn, diet (40% fat) (TS)	4.80	246.6	52.85	0.44	0.53	0	0.03	0	0	0
Margarine, corn, liquid (80% fat) (TS)	4.70	207.3	31.07	0.81	0.52	0.01	0.06	0	0	0
Margarine, corn, spread (52% fat) (TS)	4.80	235.3	46.03	0.59	0.53	0	0.05	0	0	0
Margarine, corn, stick/tub (80% fat) (TS)	4.70	206.9	31.07	0.89	0.52	0.01	0.05	0	0	0
Margarine, corn, stick/tub (80% fat), unsalted (TS)	4.70	206.9	31.07	0.89	0.52	0.01	0.05	0	0	0
Margarine, corn, whipped (80% fat) (TS)	3.16	162.3	34.79	0.56	0.35		0.03	0	0	0
Margarine, safflower, stick/tub (80% fat) (TS)	4.70	206.9	31.07	0.43	0.52	0.01	0.05	0	0	0
Margarine, safflower, stick/tub (80% fat), unsalted (TS)	4.70	207.2	31.07	1.01	0.52	0.01	0.06	0	0	0
Margarine, soybean, diet (40% fat) (TS)	4.80	246.6	52.85	0.17	0.53	0	0.03	0	0	0
Margarine, soybean, spread (52% fat) (TS)	4.80	171.4	46.03	0.37	0.53	0	0.05	0	0	0

Margarine, soybean, stick/tub (80% fat) (TS)	4.70	206.9	31.07	0.40	0.52	0.01	0.05	0	0	0
Margarine, sunflower, diet (40% fat) (TS)	4.80	246.9	52.85	0.60	0.53	0.01	0.03	0	0	0
Margarine, sunflower, spread (52% fat) (TS)	4.80	179.9	12.86	0.82	0.53	0.01	0.04	0	0	0
Margarine, sunflower, stick/tub (80% fat) (TS)	4.70	207.3	31.07	1.21	0.78	0.01	0.05	0	0	0
Oil, canola (rapeseed) (TS)	4.54	0	0	0.92	0	0	0	0	0	0
Oil, coconut (TS)	4.54	0	0	0.02	0	0	0	0	0	0
Oil, cod liver (TS)	4.54	4540	271.8	1	11.35	0	0	0	0	0
Oil, corn (TS)	4.54	0	0	0.95	0	0	0	0	0	0
Oil, cottonseed (TS)	4.54	0	0	1.74	0	0	0	0	0	0
Oil, olive (TS)	4.50	0	0	0.54	0	0	0	0	0	0
Oil, palm (TS)	4.54	0	0	0.67	0	0	0	0	0	0
Oil, palm kernel (TS)	4.54	0	0	0.17	0	0	0	0	0	0
Oil, peanut (TS)	4.50	0	0	0.58	0	0	0	0	0	0
Oil, safflower (TS)	4.54	0	0	1.56	0	0	0	0	0	0
Oil, sesame (TS)	4.54	0	0	0.18	0	0	0	0	0	0
Oil, soybean, partially hydrogenated (TS)	4.54	0	0	0.68	0	0	0	0	0	0
Oil, sunflower seed (TS)	4.54	0	0	2.72	0	0	0	0	0	0

VITAMIN COUNTER	WEIGHT (g)	VIT A (IU)	BETA-C (µg)	VIT E (mg)	VIT D (µg)	VIT C (mg)	FOL (µg)	VIT B6 (mg)	PANT (mg)	VIT B12 (mg)
Olives, black (ripe) (MD)	4	16.12	9.65	0.05	0	0.04	0	0	0	0
Olives, green, plain or stuffed (MD)	4	12	7.20	0.06	0	0	0.04	0	0	0
Salad dressing, blue cheese, commercial (TB)	15.30	32.13	7.65	1.08	0.06	0.31	1.24	0.01	0.06	0.04
Salad dressing, blue cheese, low calorie, commercial (TB)	15.30	12.24	2.91	0	0.02	0.31	0.02	0	0.02	0
Salad dressing, French, commercial (TB)	15.60	10.45	6.24	0.97	0	0	0.65	0	0.02	0.02
Salad dressing, French, low calorie, commercial (TB)	16.30	264.3	158.2	0.02	0	0	0.25	0	0	0
Salad dressing, French, no salt added, commercial (TB)	16.30	0	0	0.15	0	0	0	0	0	0
Salad dressing, Italian, commercial (TB)	14.70	11.47	6.91	1.05	0.03	0	0.72	0	0.03	0.02
Salad dressing, Italian, low calorie, commercial (TB)	15	0	0	0.22	0	0	0	0	0	0
Salad dressing, mayonnaise type, commercial (33% fat) (TB)	14.70	32.34	5.88	0.72	0.04	0	0.92	0	0.04	0.03
Salad dressing, mayonnaise, commercial (79% fat) (TB)	13.80	38.64	6.90	1.62	0.04	0	1.06	0.08	0.03	0.03
Salad dressing, mayonnaise, imitation (19% fat) (TB)	15	18.15	3.30	0.43	0.04	0	0	0	0.03	0

Food									
Salad dressing, Thousand Island, commercial (TB)	15.60	49.92	22.93	0.82	0.04	0	0.98	0	0.04	0.03
Salad dressing, Thousand Island, low calorie, commercial (TB)	15.30	48.96	22.49	0.23	0.04	0	0.85	0	0.03	0.03
Salad dressing, yogurt based, commercial (TB)	15	18.67	11.13	0.31	0	0.34	0.44	0	0.02	0.01
Sandwich spread (TB)	15.30	15.30	2.75	0.91	0.05	0.11	0.15	0	0.02	0.01
Shortening, household (TS)	4.27	0	0	1.14	0	0	0	0	0	0
Tartar sauce (TB)	14.38	31.64	5.61	1.36	0.02	0.14	1.11	0.04	0.03	0.03

FRUITS AND FRUIT PRODUCTS

Food									
Apple, fresh, with skin (MD)	138	73.14	44.16	0.54	0	7.87	3.86	0.07	0.08	0
Apple juice, sweetened (CP)	248	0	0	0.02	0	2.18	0	0.07	0.07	0
Apple juice, unsweetened, bottled or canned (CP)	248	2.48	1.49	0.02	0	2.23	0.25	0.07	0.15	0
Apples, dried, uncooked (CP)	86	0	0	0.38	0	3.35	0	0.11	0.21	0
Applesauce, sweetened, canned (CP)	255	28.05	17.85	0.48	0	4.33	1.53	0.08	0.13	0
Applesauce, unsweetened (CP)	244	70.76	41.48	0.46	0	2.93	1.46	0.07	0.22	0
Apricots, dried, uncooked (CP)	130	9412	5647.20	1.20	0	3.12	13.39	0.21	0.97	0
Apricots, dried, unsweetened, cooked (CP)	250	5907.50	3545	0.82	0	4	0	0.27	0.52	0

VITAMIN COUNTER	WEIGHT (g)	VIT A (IU)	BETA-C (µg)	VIT E (mg)	VIT D (µg)	VIT C (mg)	FOL (µg)	VIT B$_6$ (mg)	PANT (mg)	VIT B$_{12}$ (mg)
Apricots, fresh (MD)	35.33	369.55	221.17	0.33	0	3.53	3.04	0.02	0.08	0
Apricots, sweetened, canned (CP)	258	3173.40	1904.04	2.37	0	8	4.39	0.13	0.23	0
Avocado (SM)	173	1058.76	634.91	2.16	NA	13.67	107.09	0.48	1.68	0
Banana, fresh (MD)	114	92.34	55.86	0.31	0	10.37	21.77	0.66	0.30	0
Blackberries, fresh (CP)	144	237.60	142.56	1.04	0	30.24	48.96	0.09	0.35	0
Blueberries, fresh (CP)	145	145	87	1.04	0	18.85	9.28	0.06	0.13	0
Cantaloupe, fresh (MD)	922.75	25375.62	15197.69	1.29	0	389.40	156.87	1.02	1.20	0
Cherries, fresh, sweet (CP)	145	310.30	185.60	0.19	0	10.15	6.09	0.06	0.19	0
Cherries, sweetened, canned (CP)	200	308	184	0.26	0	7.20	8.40	0.06	0.26	0
Cranberries, fresh (CP)	95	43.70	26.60	0	0	12.82	1.61	0.06	0.21	0
Cranberry-apple juice, sweetened (CP)	245	7.35	4.90	0.02	0	78.40	0.49	0.05	0.15	0
Cranberry juice, sweetened (CP)	253	10.12	6.07	0	0	89.56	0.51	0.05	0.15	0
Dates, dried (CP)	178	89	53.40	0	0	0	22.43	0.34	1.39	0
Figs, canned in heavy syrup (CP)	259	95.83	56.98	0	0	2.59	5.18	0.18	0.18	0
Figs, dried (CP)	199	264.67	159.20	0	0	1.59	14.92	0.44	0.86	0
Figs, fresh (MD)	50	71	42.50	0	0	1	3.50	0.05	0.15	0
Fruit-flavored drink or juice, low calorie (CP)	237	9.48	5.69	0	NA	76.31	0.47	0.05	0.14	0

Food										
Grapefruit juice, sweetened, frozen or canned (CP)	250	0	0	0.52	0	67.25	26	0.05	0.32	0
Grapefruit juice, unsweetened, fresh, frozen, or canned (CP)	247	17.29	9.88	0.52	0	72.12	25.69	0.05	0.32	0
Grapefruit sections, sweetened, canned (CP)	254	0	0	1.02	0	54.10	21.59	0.05	0.30	0
Grapefruit, fresh (MD)	291.20	361.09	215.49	0.70	0	100.17	29.70	0.12	0.82	0
Grape juice, sweetened, frozen (CP)	250	20	12.50	0	0	59.75	3.25	0.10	0.05	0
Grape juice, unsweetened (CP)	253	20.24	12.65	0	0	0.25	6.58	0.15	0.10	0
Grapes, fresh (CP)	160	116.80	70.40	0.54	0	17.28	6.24	0.18	0.03	0
Guava, fresh (MD)	90	712.80	426.82	1.01	0	165.15	12.60	0.13	0.13	0
Honeydew melon, fresh (MD)	1290	516	309.60	0	0	319.92	387	0.77	2.71	0
Kiwifruit, fresh (MD)	76	133	79.80	1.15	0	74.48	28.88	0.07	0.13	0
Kumquats, fresh (MD)	19	57.38	34.39	0	0	7.11	3.04	0.01	NA	0
Lemon, fresh (MD)	58	16.82	9.86	0	0	30.74	6.15	0.05	0.11	0
Lemonade or limeade, sweetened, other than fruit-flavored beverage mix (CP)	248	52.08	31.17	0	0	9.67	5.46	0.02	0.02	0
Lemon juice, unsweetened; fresh, frozen, bottled, or canned (1 whole or 4 wedges = 1.50 oz) (CP)	244	36.60	21.96	0.54	0	60.51	24.64	0.10	0.22	0

VITAMIN COUNTER	WEIGHT (g)	VIT A (IU)	BETA-C (µg)	VIT E (mg)	VIT D (µg)	VIT C (mg)	FOL (µg)	VIT B$_6$ (mg)	PANT (mg)	VIT B$_{12}$ (mg)
Mandarin orange, fresh (MD)	84	772.80	463.68	0	0	25.87	17.14	0.06	0.17	0
Mango, fresh (MD)	207	8060.58	4835.52	2.32	0	57.34	74.52	0.27	0.33	0
Nectarine, fresh (MD)	136	150.96	89.76	1.21	0	7.34	5.03	0.03	0.22	0
Nectars, apricot, sweetened (CP)	251	3303.16	1982.90	2.33	0	1.51	3.26	0.05	0.25	0
Nectars, peach, sweetened, canned (CP)	249	642.42	385.95	0.25	0	13.20	3.49	0.02	0.17	0
Orange, fresh (MD)	131	268.55	161.13	0.24	0	69.69	39.69	0.08	0.33	0
Orange juice, sweetened, canned or frozen (CP)	250	424.38	254.12	0.22	0	83.42	43.90	0.20	0.40	0
Orange juice, unsweetened, fortified with calcium (CP)	249	194.22	117.03	0.47	0	96.86	109.06	0.10	0.40	0
Orange juice, unsweetened; fresh, frozen, or canned (CP)	249	194.22	117.03	0.47	0	96.86	109.06	0.10	0.40	0
Papaya, fresh (CP)	140	397.60	238	0	0	86.52	53.20	0.03	0.31	0
Papaya juice, canned (CP)	250	277.50	167.50	0	0	7.50	5.25	0.02	0.12	0
Peach, fresh (MD)	87	465.45	279.27	1.17	0	5.74	2.96	0.02	0.15	0
Peaches, dried, unsweetened, cooked (CP)	258	508.26	304.44	0	0	9.55	0.26	0.10	0.46	0
Peaches, sweetened, canned or frozen (CP)	256	849.92	509.44	3.43	0	7.17	8.19	0.05	0.13	0

Food										
Pear, fresh (MD)	166	33.20	19.92	0.86	0	6.64	12.12	0.03	0.12	0
Pears, dried, unsweetened, cooked (CP)	255	107.10	63.75	0	0	10.20	3.06	0.08	0.18	0
Pears, sweetened, canned (CP)	255	0	0	1.43	0	2.80	3.06	0.03	0.05	0
Persimmons, Japanese, raw (MD)	168	3640.56	2184	0	0	12.60	12.60	0.17	NA	0
Pineapple, canned, unsweetened or juice pack (CP)	250	95	57.50	0.25	0	23.75	12	0.17	0.25	0
Pineapple, fresh (SL)	84	19.32	11.76	0.08	0	12.94	8.90	0.08	0.13	0
Pineapple, sweetened, canned (SL)	58	8.70	5.22	0.06	0	4.35	2.73	0.04	0.06	0
Pineapple juice, frozen or canned (CP)	250	12.50	7.50	0.05	0	26.75	57.75	0.25	0.25	0
Plum, fresh (MD)	66	213.18	128.04	0.47	0	6.27	1.45	0.05	0.12	0
Plums, sweetened, canned (CP)	258	668.22	399.90	1.81	0	1.03	6.45	0.08	0.18	0
Pomegranate, fresh (MD)	154	0	0	0	0	9.39	9.24	0.15	0.92	0
Prunes, dried, cooked (CP)	212	648.72	390.08	0.83	0	6.15	0.21	0.47	0.23	0
Prunes, dried, uncooked (CP)	161	3199.07	1919.12	2.33	0	5.31	5.96	0.42	0.74	0
Prune juice, bottled (CP)	256	7.68	5.12	0.84	0	10.50	1.02	0.56	0.28	0
Raisins (TB)	9.69	0.78	0.46	0.03	0	0.32	0.32	0.02	0	0
Raspberries, fresh (CP)	123	159.90	95.94	0.59	0	30.75	31.98	0.07	0.30	0
Raspberries, sweetened, canned or frozen (CP)	250	150	90	1.20	0	41.25	65	0.07	0.37	0
Rhubarb, stewed, unsweetened (CP)	240	256.80	153.77	0.43	0	12	19.68	0.05	0.19	0

VITAMIN COUNTER	WEIGHT (g)	VIT A (IU)	BETA-C (µg)	VIT E (mg)	VIT D (µg)	VIT C (mg)	FOL (µg)	VIT B₆ (mg)	PANT (mg)	VIT B₁₂ (mg)
Rhubarb, sweetened, cooked (CP)	240	165.60	98.40	0.48	0	7.92	12.72	0.05	0.12	0
Strawberries, fresh or frozen, unsweetened (CP)	149	40.23	23.84	0.36	0	84.48	26.37	0.09	0.51	0
Strawberries, sweetened, canned or frozen (CP)	255	61.20	35.70	0.59	0	105.57	37.99	0.08	0.28	0
Watermelon, fresh (SL)	482	1764.12	1060.40	0	0	46.27	10.60	0.67	1.01	0
GRAIN PRODUCTS										
Bagel, egg (MD)	55	17.60	3.30	0.33	0.05	0	13.20	0.02	0.20	0.05
Bagel, plain (MD)	55	0	0	0.19	0	0	13.20	0.02	0.20	0
Bagel, rye (MD)	55	0	0	0.13	0	0	31.27	0.05	0.24	0
Bagel, whole wheat (MD)	55	0	0	0.16	0	0	35.13	0.07	0.32	0
Barley, pearled, cooked with salt (CP)	157	12.03	7.21	0.02	0	0	12.58	0.14	0.16	0
Barley, pearled, dry (CP)	200	44	26.34	0.04	0	0	46	0.52	0.56	0
Biscuit, baking powder (MD)	45	33.51	3.10	1.56	0.17	0.15	7.33	0.02	0.16	0.06
Bran, unprocessed (TB)	3.75	0	0	0.07	NA	0	2.96	0.05	0.08	0
Bread, Boston brown (SL)	48	33.60	20.16	0.29	0	0	14.40	0.07	0.20	0
Bread, diet, with fiber added (SL)	23	0	0	0.50	0	0	9.66	0.01	0.04	0

Food										
Bread, egg (SL)	32.70	98.82	14.22	0.13	0.29	0.10	15.83	0.02	0.18	0.07
Bread, Italian (SL)	30	0	0	0.07	0	0	9.90	0.02	0.15	0
Bread, nut (SL)	48.90	57.47	9.15	0.51	0.22	0.31	9.14	0.04	0.19	0.09
Bread, oatmeal (SL)	35.50	5.11	3.06	0.41	0	0	14.96	0.02	0.17	0
Bread, pumpkin, without nuts (SL)	56.20	3268.81	1940.17	1.12	0.08	0.69	8.32	0.02	0.20	0.06
Bread, raisin (SL)	22.50	0.41	0.25	0.04	NA	0.17	7.87	0.01	0.10	0
Bread, rye (SL)	28.69	0	0	0.06	0	0	11.19	0.03	0.13	0
Bread, white (SL)	25	0	0	0.04	0	0	8.75	0.01	0.07	0
Bread, white, low sodium (SL)	25	0	0	0.04	0	0	8.75	0.08	0.11	0
Bread, whole wheat, low sodium (SL)	25	0	0	0.04	0	0	13.75	0.03	0.15	0
Bread, zucchini, without nuts (SL)	37.10	47.22	16.18	0.57	0.06	0.40	5.85	0.01	0.11	0.04
Buckwheat groats, cooked with salt (CP)	198	0	0	0.53	0	0	21.60	0.18	0.63	0
Buckwheat groats, dry (CP)	164	0	0	1.69	NA	0	68.88	0.57	2.02	0
Bulgur, cooked with salt (CP)	182	0	0	0.05	0	0	11.68	0.15	0.45	0
Bulgur, dry (CP)	140	0	0	0.15	0	0	37.80	0.48	1.46	0
Cereal, cream of rice, cooked with salt (CP)	244	0	0	0.02	0	0	10.96	0.07	0.22	0
Cereal, cream of wheat, instant, cooked with salt (CP)	241	0	0	0.34	0	0	14.22	0.02	0.19	0

VITAMIN COUNTER	WEIGHT (g)	VIT A (IU)	BETA-C (µg)	VIT E (mg)	VIT D (µg)	VIT C (mg)	FOL (µg)	VIT B$_6$ (mg)	PANT (mg)	VIT B$_{12}$ (mg)
Cereal, cream of wheat, regular, cooked with salt (CP)	251	0	0	0.33	0	0	12.35	0.05	0.20	0
Cereal, dry, All-Bran (CP)	85	2242.77	0	1.31	3.73	44.84	297.63	1.49	1.47	0
Cereal, dry, Apple Jacks (CP)	28.35	749.57	29.42	0.02	1.25	14.99	99.92	0.50	0.04	0
Cereal, dry, Cap'n Crunch (CP)	37	0	0	0.73	0	0	227.18	0.73	3.58	1.99
Cereal, dry, Cheerios (CP)	22.68	995.51	13.03	0.33	0.82	12.02	79.45	0.41	0.27	0
Cereal, dry, Cinnamon Toast Crunch (CP)	42.50	1873.82	0	0.86	1.50	22.49	150.02	0.75	0.16	0
Cereal, dry, Common Sense Oat Bran (CP)	37.80	1015.33	9.97	0.23	1.60	0	202.06	1	0.74	0
Cereal, dry, Cracklin' Oat Bran (CP)	56.70	1448.14	29.94	0.88	2.40	30	132.75	0.67	0.41	2.64
Cereal, dry, Frosted Flakes (CP)	37.80	1000.19	39.26	0.03	1.67	20	133.33	0.67	0.05	0
Cereal, dry, Frosted Mini-Wheats (CP)	56.70	0	0	0.28	0	0	201.56	1	0.47	3.99
Cereal, dry, Fruitful Bran (CP)	59.10	1131.56	0	1.02	2.09	0	149.71	0.75	0.44	2.25
Cereal, dry, Grape-Nuts (CP)	113.40	4999.81	0	1.47	5	0	400.30	2	1.08	6
Cereal, dry, Honeycomb (CP)	21.26	938.08	0	0.01	0.94	0	75.11	0.37	0.06	1.12
Cereal, dry, Just Right, with raisins, dates, and nuts (CP)	50.30	6631.27	24	26.84	1.60	0.16	534.52	2.67	13.33	8
Cereal, dry, Kellogg's Corn Flakes (CP)	28.35	749.57	0	0.04	1.25	14.99	100	0.50	0.16	0

Food										
Cereal, dry, Kix (CP)	18.90	830.56	0	0.02	0.83	10	66.73	0.33	0.11	0
Cereal, dry, Life (CP)	44	0	0	0.15	0	0	32.56	0.07	0.37	0
Cereal, dry, Oatmeal Raisin Crisp (CP)	68	2525.90	17.50	0.08	2.02	2.04	189.80	1.06	0.36	0
Cereal, dry, Product 19 (CP)	28.35	750.14	0	20.13	1.25	60.10	400.02	2.01	10	6.01
Cereal, dry, Raisin Bran (Ralston) (CP)	50.40	1664.65	0.12	5.09	1.32	0.08	130.10	0.86	0.49	2
Cereal, dry, Rice Chex (CP)	25.20	0	0	0.02	0	13.33	88.60	0.44	0.19	1.33
Cereal, dry, Rice Krispies (CP)	28.35	749.57	0	0.04	1.25	14.99	100	0.50	0.16	0
Cereal, dry, Special K (CP)	28.35	750.14	0	0.15	1.25	15.03	100.08	0.70	0.15	0.01
Cereal, dry, Total (CP)	33	5820.21	0	23.43	1.16	69.96	465.63	2.34	11.55	7
Cereal, dry, Wheat Chex (CP)	42.50	0	0	0.41	0	22.52	149.62	0.75	0.39	2.25
Cereal, dry, puffed rice (CP)	14	0	0	0.01	NA	0	2.66	0.01	0.04	0
Cereal, dry, puffed wheat (CP)	12	0	0	0.08	0	0	3.84	0.02	0.06	0
Coffeecake, yeast, without nuts, without topping (PC)	39.60	28.19	5.66	0.27	0.04	0.11	24.72	0.03	0.26	0.11
Cornbread (PC)	67.40	189.46	55.75	1.30	0.42	0.26	17.58	0.07	0.34	0.21
Corn grits, cooked with salt, regular or instant (CP)	242	0	0	0.05	0	0	1.91	0.05	0.17	0
Corn grits, dry (CP)	156	0	0	0.25	0	0	7.80	0.23	0.75	0
Cornmeal, cooked with salt (CP)	240	135.70	81.26	0.07	0	0	15.77	0.10	0.10	0
Cornmeal, dry (CP)	138	569.94	341.29	0.28	NA	0	66.24	0.36	0.43	0

VITAMIN COUNTER	WEIGHT (g)	VIT A (IU)	BETA-C (µg)	VIT E (mg)	VIT D (µg)	VIT C (mg)	FOL (µg)	VIT B$_6$ (mg)	PANT (mg)	VIT B$_{12}$ (mg)
Cornstarch (TB)	8	0	0	0	NA	0	0.16	0	0	0
Couscous, cooked with salt (CP)	179	0	0	0.09	0	0	10.72	0.05	0.66	0
Couscous, dry (CP)	184	0	0	0.33	0	0	36.80	0.20	2.28	0
Cracker, graham (PC)	3.50	0.07	0.04	0.03	0	0	0.74	0	0.02	0
Cracker, saltine (PC)	3.50	0	0	0.04	0	0	0.63	0	0.01	0
Cracker, saltine, unsalted top (PC)	3.50	0	0	0.05	0	0	0.77	0	0.01	0
Cracker, zwieback (PC)	3.50	2.03	0.36	0.03	0	0	0.70	0	0.02	0
Donut, cake (MD)	42	144.03	21.66	0.45	0.38	0.08	6.73	0.02	0.15	0.07
Donut, yeast (MD)	60	59.42	8.75	1.08	0.19	0.10	42.47	0.04	0.31	0.10
Flour, all-purpose (CP)	125	0	0	0.06	0	0	32.50	0.05	0.55	0
Flour, amaranth (whole grain) (CP)	195	0	0	NA	0	8.19	95.55	0.43	2.05	0
Flour, buckwheat (whole groat) (CP)	120	0	0	1.42	0	0	64.80	0.70	0.53	0
Flour, cake or pastry (CP)	109	0	0	0.05	0	0	20.71	0.03	0.50	0
Flour, corn, masa, enriched (CP)	114	0	0	0.17	0	0	27.36	0.42	0.75	0
Flour, rice (CP)	158	0	0	0.11	0	0	6.32	0.70	1.30	0
Flour, rice, brown (CP)	158	0	0	2.01	0	0	25.28	1.17	2.51	0
Flour, rye, medium (CP)	102	0	0	1.03	0	0	19.38	0.28	0.50	0

474

Food										
Flour, triticale (whole grain) (CP)	130	0	0	0.26	0	0	96.20	0.52	2.82	0
Flour, whole wheat (CP)	120	0	0	1.30	0	0	52.80	0.41	1.21	0
Hominy, canned (CP)	160	0	0	0.06	NA	0	1.60	0	0.24	0
Macaroni, whole wheat, cooked without salt (CP)	140	0	0	0.15	0	0	7	0.11	0.59	0
Matzo (PC)	3.50	0	0	0	0	0	0.50	0	0.02	0
Melba toast, unsalted (PC)	3.50	0	0	0	0	0	0.91	0	0.02	0
Millet, cooked with salt (CP)	240	0	0	0.14	0	0	64.75	0.29	0.65	0
Millet, dry (CP)	200	0	0	0.36	0	0	170	0.76	1.70	0
Muffin, bran, homemade (MD)	50	250.87	5.29	0.86	0.41	4.64	34.85	0.16	0.28	0.07
Muffin, corn, commercial mix or homemade (MD)	52	112.01	34.78	1.12	0.25	0.17	11.50	0.05	0.21	0.11
Muffin, English, whole wheat (MD)	58	55.58	5.15	0.59	0.28	0.26	45.25	0.08	0.41	0.10
Noodles, chow mein (CP)	45	38.25	6.87	2.07	0	0	9.90	0.05	0.24	0
Noodles, egg, cooked without salt (CP)	160	32	5.74	0.13	0.05	0	11.20	0.06	0.22	0.14
Noodles, macaroni, white, cooked without salt (CP)	140	0	0	0.04	0	0	9.80	0.04	0.15	0
Noodles, macaroni, whole wheat, cooked with salt (CP)	140	0	0	0.15	0	0	7	0.11	0.59	0
Noodles, manicotti, cooked without salt (CP)	140	0	0	0.04	0	0	9.80	0.06	0.15	0

VITAMIN COUNTER	WEIGHT (g)	VIT A (IU)	BETA-C (µg)	VIT E (mg)	VIT D (µg)	VIT C (mg)	FOL (µg)	VIT B$_6$ (mg)	PANT (mg)	VIT B$_{12}$ (mg)
Noodles, ramen, cooked, all varieties (CP)	227	17.02	10.21	1.66	0	0	7.99	0.07	0.16	0.13
Noodles, rice, cooked without salt (CP)	160	0	0	0.03	0	0	3.46	0.10	0.45	0.13
Noodles, rice, fried (CP)	9.45	0	0	0.62	0	0	0.11	0	0.02	0
Oat bran, cooked with salt (CP)	219	36.79	22.03	0.15	0	0	19.14	0.07	0.55	0
Oat bran, dry (CP)	94	94	56.29	0.40	0	0	48.88	0.15	1.40	0
Oatmeal, cooked with salt (CP)	234	38.05	22.79	0.58	0	0	12.05	0.05	0.47	0
Oatmeal, dry (CP)	81	81.81	48.99	1.25	0	0	25.92	0.10	1	0
Pancake, homemade, all varieties except whole wheat and buckwheat (MD)	40	76.96	10.20	0.48	0.28	0.19	7.26	0.02	0.20	0.13
Pancake, homemade, whole wheat (MD)	40	76.96	10.20	0.62	0.28	0.19	9.53	0.06	0.27	0.13
Quinoa (CP)	170	0	0	8.28	0	0	83.30	0.37	1.78	0
Rice, brown, cooked without salt (CP)	195	0	0	0.80	0	0	7.80	0.27	0.55	0
Rice, white, cooked without salt (CP)	158	0	0	0.05	0	0	4.74	0.14	0.62	0
Rice, wild, cooked without salt (CP)	164	0	0	0	0	0	42.64	0.21	0.25	0
Rice bran, dry (CP)	83	0	0	5.69	0	0	52.29	3.38	6.13	0
Rice cakes, plain, no salt added (PC)	9	0	0	0.13	0	0	1.89	0.01	0.09	0
Rice cakes, plain, salted (PC)	9	0	0	0.13	0	0	1.91	0.01	0.09	0
Roll, croissant (MD)	69.70	731.46	182.03	0.43	0.39	0.19	32	0.04	0.38	0.16

Food									
Roll, hamburger (MD)	43	0	0	0.03	0	0	16.77	0.03	0.13	0
Roll, hamburger, whole wheat (MD)	43	0	0	0.07	0	0	23.65	0.06	0.26	0
Roll, hard (MD)	37	0	0	0.15	0	0	9.25	0.02	0.11	0
Roll, hot dog (MD)	43	0	0	0.03	0	0	16.77	0.03	0.13	0
Roll, hot dog, whole wheat (MD)	43	0	0	0.07	0	0	23.65	0.06	0.26	0
Roll, kaiser (MD)	50	0	0	0.08	0	0	29.89	0.02	0.15	0
Roll, rye (MD)	36	0	0	0.07	0	0	14.04	0.03	0.16	0
Roll, sourdough (MD)	45	0	0	0.10	0	0	14.85	0.03	0.22	0
Roll, submarine (MD)	94	0	0	0.14	0.46	0	34.78	0.04	0.50	0
Roll, white, dinner (MD)	36	0	0	0.03	0.14	0.11	13.68	0.02	0.11	0.04
Roll, whole wheat (MD)	36	0	0	0.06	0	0	19.25	0.05	0.21	0
Rye (whole grain) (CP)	169	0	0	2.60	0	0	101.40	0.49	2.47	0
Stuffing, bread, all types except cornbread (CP)	114.20	50.54	30.27	4.84	0	3.11	29.27	0.08	0.25	0
Stuffing, cornbread (CP)	213.60	551.86	177.78	7.34	1.09	3.78	56.86	0.26	0.96	0.56
Tortilla, corn, fried (MD)	25.57	36.21	21.73	0.22	0	0	4.05	0.06	0.04	0
Tortilla, corn, plain (MD)	21.30	36.21	21.73	0.17	NA	0	4.05	0.06	0.04	0
Tortilla, flour, plain, commercial (PC)	42.50	0	0	0.05	NA	0	5.95	0.02	0.09	0
Tortilla, flour, whole wheat, commercial (PC)	36.90	0	0	0.44	0	0	8.61	0.07	0.20	0

VITAMIN COUNTER	WEIGHT (g)	VIT A (IU)	BETA-C (µg)	VIT E (mg)	VIT D (µg)	VIT C (mg)	FOL (µg)	VIT B₆ (mg)	PANT (mg)	VIT B₁₂ (mg)
Tortilla, taco shell (MD)	13	55.12	32.76	0.25	NA	0	3.77	0.04	0.04	0
Waffle, frozen, all varieties including bran (LG)	34	38.39	2.92	0.20	0.14	0.05	5.03	0.01	0.12	0.06
Waffle, homemade with whole milk, bran (PC)	75	135.85	30.11	1.14	0.67	0.49	20.80	0.17	0.60	0.30
Wheat, rolled, dry (CP)	94	0	0	1.20	0	0	73.32	0.37	0.86	0
Wheat germ (CP)	113	0	0	19.58	0.79	6.78	397.76	1.11	1.57	0
MEAT AND MEAT PRODUCTS (BEEF, FISH, AND POULTRY)										
Abalone, cooked, canned (OZ)	28.35	1.42	0.09	0.01	0.03	0.57	1.42	0.03	0.09	27.57
Anchovies, smoked, canned in oil (PC)	4	2.80	0.17	0.29	NA	0	0.50	0.01	0.04	0.04
Bacon, beef, kosher, cooked (SL)	6.50	0	0	0.03	0.08	2.01	0.52	0.02	0.03	0.25
Bacon, Canadian, cooked, drained (SL)	21	0	0	0.02	0	4.54	0.84	0.09	0.11	0.16
Bacon, low salt, cooked, drained (SL)	6.33	0	0	0.03	NA	2.12	0.32	0.02	0.07	0.11
Bacon, regular, cooked, drained (SL)	6.33	0	0	0.04	0	2.12	0.32	0.02	0.07	0.11
Bacon, turkey, cooked, drained (SL)	8	2.11	0.12	0.09	0	0	0.56	0.04	0.09	0.03
Beef, arm roast (9% fat), no visible fat, cooked (OZ)	28.35	0	0	0.07	0	0	2.27	0.12	0.10	0.57

Food									
Beef, chipped (OZ)	28.35	0	0	0.31	0	4.20	3.12	0.10	0.17	0.75
Beef, ground, regular (22.56% fat), cooked (OZ)	28.35	0	0	0.17	0.09	0	2.55	0.07	0.10	0.77
Beef, hamburger, ground chuck (20% fat), cooked (OZ)	28.35	0	0	0.11	0	0	3.12	0.10	0.09	0.73
Beef, pot roast (26% fat), cooked (moist heat) (OZ)	28.35	0	0	0.20	0	0	1.98	0.09	0.08	0.82
Beef, prime rib (30% fat), cooked (OZ)	28.35	0	0	0.22	0	0	1.98	0.07	0.10	0.66
Beef, rib eye steak (20% fat), cooked (OZ)	28.35	0	0	0.15	0	0	1.98	0.10	0.09	0.55
Beef, short ribs (42% fat), cooked (OZ)	28.35	0	0	0.31	0	0	1.42	0.06	0.07	0.74
Beef, top round roast/steak (5% fat), no visible fat, cooked (OZ)	28.35	0	0	0.04	0	0	3.40	0.16	0.14	0.70
Breakfast strips, beef, cooked (SL)	11.33	0	0	0.10	0.07	4.08	0.91	0.04	0.04	0.39
Breakfast strips, pork, cooked (SL)	11.33	0	0	0.05	0	4.92	0.45	0.04	0.10	0.20
Chicken, canned (OZ)	28.35	33.17	1.98	0.08	0	0.57	1.13	0.10	0.24	0.08
Chicken, dark meat, without skin, cooked (OZ)	28.35	10.21	0.57	0.18	0	0	2.41	0.10	0.35	0.10
Chicken, dark meat, with skin, cooked (OZ)	28.35	28.49	1.71	0.18	0	0	2.27	0.09	0.32	0.09
Chicken, light meat, without skin, cooked (OZ)	28.35	4.11	0.25	0.10	0	0	1.42	0.16	0.23	0.10

VITAMIN COUNTER	WEIGHT (g)	VIT A (IU)	BETA-C (µg)	VIT E (mg)	VIT D (µg)	VIT C (mg)	FOL (µg)	VIT B6 (mg)	PANT (mg)	VIT B12 (mg)
Chicken, light meat, without skin, without visible fat, cooked (OZ)	28.35	3.83	0.23	0.05	0	0	1.42	0.16	0.23	0.10
Chicken, light meat, with skin, cooked (OZ)	28.35	15.59	0.85	0.10	0	0	1.28	0.14	0.22	0.10
Chicken-fried steak (untrimmed beef round) (PC)	102.50	58.29	10.09	1.71	0.13	0.02	12.28	0.31	0.42	1.50
Chitterlings, cooked (CP)	161	0	0	0.61	NA	0	4.83	0.02	0.35	1.66
Clams, cooked or canned (MD)	12.50	71.25	4.27	0.20	0.01	2.76	3.60	0.01	0.08	12.36
Corned beef, canned (OZ)	28.35	0	0	0.10	0	0.43	2.55	0.04	0.18	0.46
Crab, all types, cooked, fresh or frozen (OZ)	28.35	1.70	0.10	0.35	NA	0.94	14.40	0.05	0.12	2.07
Crabmeat, canned (OZ)	28.35	1.42	0.09	0.35	NA	0.77	12.05	0.04	0.10	0.13
Duck, domestic, with skin, cooked (OZ)	28.35	59.53	3.69	0.23	0	0	1.70	0.05	0.31	0.09
Duck, domestic, without skin, cooked (OZ)	28.35	21.83	0	0.07	0	0	1.70	0.10	0.43	0.11
Fish, carp, cooked (OZ)	28.35	17.86	1.07	0.43	2.30	0.14	4.25	0.11	0.64	2.12
Fish, chinook salmon, smoked (OZ)	28.35	24.95	1.49	0.24	0.85	0	0.54	0.08	0.25	0.92
Fish, cisco, smoked (OZ)	28.35	267.34	16.01	0.43	0.85	0	0.60	0.08	0.09	1.21

Food										
Fish, cod, dried, salted, soaked in water, cooked (OZ)	28.35	15.03	0.90	0.08	0.41	0	0.58	0.04	0.16	0.08
Fish, flounder, cooked (OZ)	28.35	10.77	0.65	0.10	0.43	0	2.61	0.07	0.16	0.71
Fish, gefilte (PC)	102.70	78.32	8.69	0.46	1.85	0.66	8.97	0.21	0.45	0.77
Fish, haddock, smoked (OZ)	28.35	20.70	1.24	0.11	0.85	0	4.34	0.11	0.05	0.45
Fish, mackerel, Atlantic, cooked (OZ)	28.35	51.03	0	0.43	2.55	0.11	0.43	0.13	0.28	5.39
Fish, salmon, chinook (king) and sockeye (red), cooked (OZ)	28.35	34.02	2.04	0.38	3.54	0	4.90	0.07	0.25	0.34
Fish, salmon, pink, canned (CP)	177	97.35	5.82	2.05	22.12	0	27.26	0.53	0.97	7.79
Fish, salmon, pink, canned without salt (CP)	177	97.35	5.82	2.05	22.12	0	27.26	0.53	0.97	7.79
Fish, sardines, canned, drained (MD)	12	26.88	1.61	0.13	0.90	0	1.42	0.02	0.08	1.07
Fish, whitefish, cooked (OZ)	28.35	39.97	2.39	0.36	1.59	0.34	2.78	0.14	0.25	0.07
Fish fillet, breaded, commercial (approx. 18% fat) (OZ)	28.35	4.49	0.27	0.76	0.18	0	2.70	0.03	0.10	0.30
Fish stick, breaded, commercial (approx. 10% fat) (OZ)	28.35	3.75	0.22	0.43	0.15	0	3.13	0.03	0.09	0.25
Fowl, wild, cooked, with or without skin (OZ)	28.35	53.54	3.21	0.10	0	0.65	1.70	0.21	0.34	0.20
Frankfurter, beef, low salt (REG)	45	0	0	0.31	0	0	1.54	0.08	0.07	0.52
Frankfurter, beef, regular (REG)	45	0	0	0.34	0.27	10.84	1.80	0.05	0.13	0.69

VITAMIN COUNTER	WEIGHT (g)	VIT A (IU)	BETA-C (µg)	VIT E (mg)	VIT D (µg)	VIT C (mg)	FOL (µg)	VIT B6 (mg)	PANT (mg)	VIT B12 (mg)
Frankfurter, beef and pork, low salt, regular (REG)	45	2.05	0.12	0.19	0	0	1.04	0.06	0.12	0.30
Frankfurter, beef and pork, reduced fat (LK)	57	1.92	0.11	0.20	0	0	2.10	0.13	0.20	0.76
Frankfurter, beef and pork, regular (REG)	45	0	0	0.22	0.40	11.70	1.80	0.06	0.16	0.58
Frankfurter, chicken, regular (REG)	45	0	0	0.24	0	0	3.60	0.10	0.32	0.13
Game, wild, cooked (OZ)	28.35	0	0	0.15	0	0	1.13	0.14	0.23	3.40
Goose, domestic, with skin, cooked (OZ)	28.35	19.84	1.13	0.31	0	0	0.57	0.10	0.43	0.12
Herring, canned or smoked (MD)	40	51.20	3.06	0.92	10	0.40	5.48	0.16	0.35	7.48
Herring, pickled (PC)	15	129.15	7.73	0.34	3.75	0	0.36	0.03	0.01	0.64
Lamb, chop, arm (9% fat), no visible fat, cooked (OZ)	28.35	0	0	0.05	0	0	5.95	0.05	0.20	0.73
Lamb, chop, breast (36% fat), cooked (OZ)	28.35	0	0	0.04	0	0	0.85	0.04	0.11	0.28
Lamb, chop, loin (24% fat), cooked (OZ)	28.35	0	0	0.03	0	0	5.39	0.03	0.18	0.63
Lamb, crown roast (30% fat), cooked (OZ)	28.35	0	0	0.03	0	0	4.25	0.03	0.18	0.63
Lamb, leg (20% fat), cooked (OZ)	28.35	0	0	0.04	0	0	5.95	0.04	0.20	0.75

Lamb, shank roast (13% fat), cooked (OZ)	28.35	0	0	0.04	0	0	6.24	0.04	0.19	0.61
Liver, beef, cooked (OZ)	28.35	10115	605.69	0.18	0.32	6.52	61.52	0.26	1.30	20.13
Liver, calves or veal, cooked (OZ)	28.35	7621.33	456.37	0.10	0.07	8.79	215.18	0.14	0.65	10.35
Liver, chicken, cooked (OZ)	28.35	4642.31	281.23	0.41	0.06	4.48	218.29	0.16	1.53	5.50
Liver, lamb, cooked (OZ)	28.35	7071.91	423.47	0.22	0.14	1.13	20.70	0.14	1.12	21.69
Liver, pork, cooked (OZ)	28.35	5102.15	305.52	0.13	0.32	6.69	46.21	0.16	1.35	5.29
Liverwurst (SL)	18	4980.06	298.21	0.08	0.11	0	5.40	0.03	0.53	2.42
Lobster, cooked (MD)	104	90.48	5.42	1.53	NA	0	11.54	0.08	0.29	3.23
Luncheon meat, bologna, beef (SL)	28.35	0	0	0.22	0.28	6.04	1.42	0.04	0.08	0.40
Luncheon meat, bologna, beef and pork (SL)	28.35	0	0	0.02	0.28	5.95	1.42	0.05	0.08	0.38
Luncheon meat, bologna, pork (SL)	23	0	0	0.05	0.05	8.12	1.15	0.06	0.17	0.21
Luncheon meat, bologna, turkey or chicken (SL)	28.35	0	0	0.14	0	0	1.56	0.07	0.17	0.07
Luncheon meat, chicken breast (SL)	28.35	3.67	0.21	0.06	0	0	0.97	0.08	0.12	0.06
Luncheon meat, corned beef (SL)	17	0	0	0.01	0	0	1.22	0.06	0.05	0.25
Luncheon meat, pastrami, beef (OZ)	28.35	0	0	0.22	0	0.85	1.98	0.05	0.09	0.50
Luncheon meat, pastrami, turkey (SL)	28.35	0	0	0.10	NA	0	1.42	0.08	0.16	0.07
Luncheon meat, salami, beef (SL)	23	0	0	0.01	0.26	3.98	0.46	0.04	0.22	0.70

VITAMIN COUNTER

	WEIGHT (g)	VIT A (IU)	BETA-C (μg)	VIT E (mg)	VIT D (μg)	VIT C (mg)	FOL (μg)	VIT B$_6$ (mg)	PANT (mg)	VIT B$_{12}$ (mg)
Luncheon meat, salami, beef and pork (SL)	23	0	0	0.09	0.21	2.76	0.46	0.05	0.20	0.84
Luncheon meat, salami, beef and pork, low salt (SL)	28.35	76.74	0.29	0.14	0.35	0.21	1.98	0.03	0.17	0.31
Luncheon meat, salami, dry or hard, pork (SL)	10	0	0	0.01	0.15	0	0.20	0.05	0.11	0.28
Luncheon meat, salami, dry or hard, pork and beef (SL)	10	0	0	0.06	0.19	2.60	0.20	0.05	0.11	0.19
Luncheon meat, turkey breast (SL)	21	1.95	0.12	0.05	0	0	0.67	0.08	0.11	0.05
Oyster, raw (MD)	14	14	0.84	0.12	1.12	0.52	1.40	0.01	0.03	2.72
Oyster, cooked (MD)	7	12.60	0.75	0.06	0.56	0.42	0.98	0.01	0.02	2.45
Pepperoni, pork and beef (SL)	5.50	0	0	0.04	0	0	0.22	0.01	0.10	0.14
Pork, picnic shoulder (14% fat), fresh, no visible fat, cooked (OZ)	28.35	2.55	0.15	0.05	0	0.11	2.27	0.10	0.15	0.16
Pork, chop, center loin (21% fat), fresh, cooked (OZ)	28.35	2.55	0.15	0.07	0	0.09	1.42	0.11	0.18	0.19
Pork, chop, loin (23% fat), smoked, cooked (OZ)	28.35	0	0	0.07	0	6.24	0.85	0.06	0.22	0.30
Pork, chop, rib (25% fat), fresh, cooked (OZ)	28.35	2.55	0.15	0.09	0	0.06	1.13	0.11	0.14	0.21

Pork, ham, Polish (15% fat), smoked, cooked (OZ)	28.35	0	0	0.08	0	3.97	1.42	0.09	0.21	0.30
Pork, ham, extra lean (6% fat), smoked, cooked (OZ)	28.35	0	0	0.02	0	5.95	0.85	0.11	0.11	0.18
Pork, ham, rump (11% fat), fresh, no visible fat, cooked (OZ)	28.35	2.27	0.14	0.03	0	0.11	2.55	0.11	0.16	0.16
Pork, ham, shank (21% fat), smoked, cooked (OZ)	28.35	0	0	0.08	0	6.24	0.85	0.08	0.16	0.26
Pork, loin ribs (30% fat), fresh, cooked (OZ)	28.35	2.83	0.17	0.10	0	0	1.13	0.10	0.21	0.31
Pork, salt, cooked (SL)	17	0	0	0.11	0	0	0.14	0.01	0.02	0.04
Pork, smoked (5% fat), low salt (OZ)	28.35	0	0	0.01	0	5.95	0.85	0.11	0.11	0.18
Pork, tenderloin roast (5% fat), fresh, cooked (OZ)	28.35	1.98	0.12	0.02	0	0.11	1.70	0.12	0.20	0.16
Sausage, braunschweiger (SL)	18	2529.18	151.74	0.06	0.11	1.80	7.92	0.06	0.61	3.62
Sausage, chorizo (LK)	60	0	0	0.27	0	0	1.20	0.32	0.67	1.20
Sausage, Italian (LK)	68	0	0	0.21	0	1.36	3.40	0.22	0.31	0.88
Sausage, knackwurst or bratwurst (LK)	68	0	0	0.38	0	18.36	1.36	0.12	0.22	0.80
Sausage, Polish (LK)	75.60	0	0	0.29	0	0.76	1.51	0.14	0.34	0.74
Sausage, pork, fresh, cooked (LK)	13	0	0	0.02	0.26	0.26	0.26	0.04	0.09	0.22
Sausage, pork and beef, fresh, cooked (LK)	13	0	0	0.06	0.26	0	0.26	0.01	0.06	0.06

VITAMIN COUNTER	WEIGHT (g)	VIT A (IU)	BETA-C (µg)	VIT E (mg)	VIT D (µg)	VIT C (mg)	FOL. (µg)	VIT B₆ (mg)	PANT (mg)	VIT B₁₂ (mg)
Sausage, turkey, fresh, cooked (LK)	24	19.52	1.17	0.12	0	0	1.55	0.06	0.22	0.06
Sausage, turkey, smoked (OZ)	28.35	18.22	1.09	0.12	0	0	1.45	0.06	0.21	0.06
Sausage, Vienna, cooked (LK)	16	0	0	0.09	NA	0	0.64	0.02	0.06	0.16
Scallops, cooked (LG)	15	25.50	1.53	0.09	NA	0	2.55	0.02	0.02	0.20
Shrimp, cooked, canned without salt (OZ)	28.35	62.09	3.72	0.81	0.74	0.62	0.99	0.04	0.10	0.42
Shrimp, cooked, canned with salt (OZ)	28.35	17.01	0	0.71	0.74	0.65	0.51	0.03	0.06	0.32
Squid, cooked (OZ)	28.35	34.30	1.98	0.34	NA	1.75	1.20	0.02	0.15	0.48
Surimi (OZ)	28.35	18.71	1.32	0.10	NA	0	0.45	0.01	0.02	0.45
Sushi or sashimi (raw tuna) (OZ)	28.35	619.16	37.08	0.42	1.53	0	0.54	0.13	0.30	2.67
Tuna, canned, oil pack, drained (CP)	160	124.80	7.47	1.84	9.28	0	8.48	0.18	0.59	3.52
Tuna, canned, oil pack, drained, no salt added (CP)	160	124.80	7.47	1.84	9.28	0	8.48	0.18	0.59	3.52
Tuna, canned, water pack, drained (CP)	160	124.80	7.47	0.85	9.28	0	7.52	0.61	0.59	3.52
Tuna, canned, water pack, drained, low sodium (CP)	160	124.80	7.47	0.85	9.28	0	7.52	0.61	0.59	3.52
Tuna, canned, water pack, drained, no salt (CP)	160	124.80	7.47	0.85	9.28	0	7.52	0.61	0.59	3.52
Turkey breast, processed (OZ)	28.35	0	0	0.03	0.14	0	1.42	0.09	0.14	0.09

Food										
Turkey ham (OZ)	28.35	0	0	0.12	0	0	1.70	0.07	0.24	0.07
Veal, breast (25% fat), cooked (OZ)	28.35	0	0	0.01	0	0	3.69	0.09	0.36	0.41
Veal, cutlet (10% fat), cooked (OZ)	28.35	0	0	0.12	0	0	4.25	0.09	0.36	0.40
Veal, rib roast (14% fat), cooked (OZ)	28.35	0	0	0.10	0	0	3.69	0.07	0.36	0.41
Veal, rump roast (6% fat), cooked (OZ)	28.35	0	0	0.14	0	0	4.82	0.09	0.34	0.45

MILK, DAIRY, AND RELATED PRODUCTS

Food										
Buttermilk, 1% fat (CP)	245	80.85	22.05	0.05	0.07	2.40	12.25	0.07	0.66	0.54
Buttermilk, whole (CP)	240	336	84	0.17	0.05	2.35	12	0.12	0.67	1.32
Cheese foods and spreads, pasteurized processed, 20–26% fat (TB)	16	136	36.64	0.07	0.05	0	1.12	0.02	0.09	0.18
Cheese, 17–26% fat (feta) (OZ)	28.35	126.72	5.10	0.01	NA	0	9.07	0.12	0.27	0.48
Cheese, 22–28% fat (Camembert, Brie, Jarlsberg) (OZ)	28.35	261.67	20.41	0.14	NA	0	17.63	0.07	0.39	0.37
Cheese, 25–30% fat (Edam, Gouda, Romano, provolone, Tilsit) (OZ)	28.35	259.69	18.14	0.16	NA	0	4.59	0.02	0.08	0.43
Cheese, 26–31% fat (blue, Roquefort, Limburger, Liederkranz) (OZ)	28.35	204.40	13.61	0.17	NA	0	10.32	0.05	0.49	0.35
Cheese, 28–32% fat (Muenster, brick, Monterey Jack, fontina, Cheshire) (OZ)	28.35	317.52	22.11	0.18	NA	0	3.43	0.02	0.05	0.42

VITAMIN COUNTER

VITAMIN COUNTER	WEIGHT (g)	VIT A (IU)	BETA-C (µg)	VIT E (mg)	VIT D (µg)	VIT C (mg)	FOL (µg)	VIT B$_6$ (mg)	PANT (mg)	VIT B$_{12}$ (mg)
Cheese, 29–33% fat (process American) (OZ)	28.35	342.92	88.74	0.19	0.05	0	2.21	0.02	0.14	0.20
Cheese, 31–37% fat (cheddar, colby, Havarti) (OZ)	28.35	300.23	93.84	0.20	0.05	0	5.16	0.02	0.12	0.24
Cheese, Parmesan, fresh or dry (TB)	5	35.05	15	0.03	0.01	0	0.40	0	0.03	0.07
Cheese, imitation, low cholesterol, 19–26% fat (OZ)	28.35	257.98	68.04	2.57	0	0	5.10	0.02	0.11	0.24
Cheese, mozzarella, part skim milk, low moisture (OZ)	28.35	178.04	48.48	0.10	0.03	0	2.81	0.02	0.03	0.26
Cheese, ricotta, part skim milk (CP)	246	1062.72	194.34	0.42	0.10	0	32.23	0.05	0.59	0.71
Cheese, ricotta, whole milk (CP)	246	1205.40	317.34	0.66	0.20	0	30.01	0.10	0.52	0.84
Cottage cheese, 1% fat (CP)	226	83.62	22.60	0.05	0.05	0	28.02	0.16	0.47	1.42
Cottage cheese, 2% fat (CP)	226	158.20	42.94	0.09	NA	0	29.61	0.18	0.54	1.60
Cottage cheese, 2% fat, no salt added (CP)	226.80	158.76	43.09	0.09	0.05	0	29.71	0.18	0.54	1.61
Cottage cheese, 4% fat (CP)	210	342.30	94.50	0.19	0.04	0	25.62	0.15	0.44	1.30
Cottage cheese, 4% fat, no salt added (CP)	210	342.30	94.50	0.19	0.04	0	25.62	0.15	0.44	1.30
Cottage cheese, low fat (CP)	226	158.20	42.94	0.09	0.05	0	29.61	0.18	0.54	1.60

Food										
Cottage cheese, uncreamed (CP)	145	43.50	5.80	0.01	0	0	21.46	0.12	0.23	1.19
Cream, half and half (CP)	242	1050.28	278.30	0.27	0.19	2.08	6.05	0.10	0.70	0.80
Cream, heavy whipping (CP)	238	3498.60	880.60	1.50	3.09	1.38	8.81	0.07	0.59	0.43
Cream, light (CP)	240	1728	463.20	0.36	0.26	1.82	5.52	0.07	0.67	0.53
Cream, whipping (CP)	239	2693.53	738.51	1.58	2.99	1.46	8.84	0.07	0.62	0.45
Cream, whipping, unsweetened (TB)	7.50	84.52	23.17	0.05	0.09	0.05	0.28	0	0.02	0.01
Cream cheese, 35% fat (TB)	14	199.78	48.86	0.10	0.03	0	1.85	0.01	0.04	0.06
Cream cheese, Neufchâtel (TB)	14	158.76	32.80	0.07	0	0	1.58	0.01	0.08	0.04
Cream cheese, light, 18% fat (TB)	14.69	109.99	27.04	0.06	0.02	0	1.93	0.01	0.04	0.08
Ice cream, 7% fat (light), all flavors except chocolate or coffee (CP)	121.50	350.01	93.29	0.16	0.05	0.85	6.71	0.06	0.66	0.63
Ice cream, 7% fat (light), chocolate or coffee (CP)	121.50	354.27	93.29	0.16	0.05	0.91	13.41	0.07	0.63	0.57
Ice cream, 11% fat (average), all flavors except chocolate and coffee (CP)	132	539.88	145.20	0.26	0.08	0.79	6.60	0.07	0.77	0.51
Ice cream, 11% fat (average), chocolate or coffee (CP)	132	549.12	145.20	0.26	0.08	0.92	21.12	0.08	0.73	0.38
Ice cream, 16% fat (rich), all flavors except chocolate or coffee (CP)	148	951.64	239.76	0.41	0.13	1.04	7.40	0.06	0.53	0.53
Ice cream, 16% fat (rich), chocolate or coffee (CP)	148	951.64	239.76	0.41	0.13	1.04	7.40	0.06	0.53	0.53

VITAMIN COUNTER	WEIGHT (g)	VIT A (IU)	BETA-C (µg)	VIT E (mg)	VIT D (µg)	VIT C (mg)	FOL (µg)	VIT B$_6$ (mg)	PANT (mg)	VIT B$_{12}$ (mg)
Ice milk, hardened, 4% fat, all flavors except chocolate (CP)	132	217.80	56.76	0.09	0.04	1.06	7.92	0.08	0.66	0.88
Milk, 1% fat (CP)	244	500.20	26.84	0.05	2.49	2.37	12.44	0.10	0.78	0.90
Milk, 2% fat (CP)	244	500.20	46.36	0.07	2.49	2.32	12.44	0.10	0.78	0.88
Milk, canned, condensed, sweetened (CP)	306	1003.68	266.22	0.55	0.15	7.96	34.27	0.15	2.29	1.35
Milk, canned, evaporated skim, undiluted (CP)	256	1003.52	5.12	0	5.32	3.17	22.02	0.13	1.89	0.61
Milk, canned, evaporated whole, undiluted (CP)	252	612.36	191.52	0.40	5.24	4.74	19.91	0.13	1.61	0.40
Milk, low fat (CP)	244	500.20	46.36	0.07	2.49	2.32	12.44	0.10	0.78	0.88
Milk, powdered, nonfat, instant (TS)	1.42	33.65	0.10	0	0.16	0.08	0.71	0	0.05	0.06
Milk, powdered, nonfat, regular (TS)	2.50	59.22	0.17	0	0.27	0.14	1.24	0.01	0.08	0.10
Milk, skim (CP)	245	499.80	4.90	0	2.50	2.40	12.74	0.10	0.81	0.93
Milk, whole (CP)	244	307.44	81.50	0.10	2.49	2.29	12.20	0.10	0.76	0.88
Sherbet (CP)	192	145.92	38.40	0.08	0.02	8.26	7.68	0.06	0.29	0.25
Sour cream, low fat (CP)	248	1599.60	159.96	0.35	0.47	1.54	15.77	0.27	2.43	1.12
Whipped topping, aerosol, saturated vegetable fat (TB)	4.38	20.72	12.48	0	NA	0	0	0	0	0

Whipped topping, frozen, saturated vegetable fat (TB)	4.69	40.38	24.18	0	0	0	0	0	0	0
Whipped topping, powdered, reduced calorie, with aspartame (TB)	4.94	8.45	4.94	0.04	0	0.04	0	0	0.02	0.01
Yogurt, 1% fat, all flavors (CP)	245	862.40	154.35	0.10	0	1.71	22.05	0.05	0.64	0.98
Yogurt, 1% fat, sweetened with aspartame, all flavors (CP)	245	409.25	10.53	0.10	2.01	1.84	0.10	0.78	0.73	248.48
Yogurt, 2–4% fat, all flavors (CP)	245	311.15	78.40	0.17	0.05	1.57	0.22	22.29	0.10	0.96
Yogurt, 2–4% fat, unflavored or plain (CP)	245	301.35	79.62	0.17	0.05	1.30	18.13	0.07	0.96	0.91
Yogurt, frozen, 1–2% fat, all flavors except chocolate (CP)	193	88.78	21.23	0.04	0.04	1.27	17.95	0.08	0.95	0.91
Yogurt, frozen, 1–2% fat, chocolate (CP)	193	86.27	21	0.02	0.02	1.22	18.91	0.08	0.89	0.87
Yogurt, low fat, all flavors except coffee (CP)	245	112.70	26.95	0.05	0.05	1.62	22.78	0.10	1.20	1.15
Yogurt, low fat, coffee flavor (CP)	245	111.99	26.78	0.05	0.05	1.59	22.64	0.10	1.20	1.15
Yogurt, low fat, unflavored or plain (CP)	245	161.70	39.20	0.07	0	1.96	27.44	0.12	1.45	1.37
NUTS AND SEEDS										
Almonds, unsalted (CP)	142	0	0	22.83	0	0.85	83.35	0.16	0.67	0
Brazil nuts, unsalted (CP)	140	0	0	10.64	0	0.98	5.60	0.35	0.34	0
Cashews, salted (CP)	130	0	0	1.96	0	0	88.01	0.32	1.55	0

VITAMIN COUNTER	WEIGHT (g)	VIT A (IU)	BETA-C (µg)	VIT E (mg)	VIT D (µg)	VIT C (mg)	FOL (µg)	VIT B₆ (mg)	PANT (mg)	VIT B₁₂ (mg)
Cashews, unsalted (CP)	130	0	0	1.96	0	0	88.01	0.32	1.55	0
Chestnuts, unsalted (CP)	143	0	0	1.72	0	21.45	156.30	0.94	1.29	0
Coconut, fresh (PC)	45	0	0	0.04	0	1.48	11.88	0.02	0.13	0
Coconut, shredded, sweetened (TS)	1.94	0	0	0	0	0.01	0.16	0.01	0.01	0
Coconut, shredded, unsweetened (TS)	1.67	0	0	0	0	0.03	0.15	0.01	0.01	0
Filberts, hazelnuts, unsalted (CP)	135	90.45	54.16	32.29	0	1.35	96.93	0.82	1.55	0
Hickory nuts, unsalted (CP)	100	131	78.44	3.84	0	2	40	0.19	1.75	0
Macadamia nuts, salted (CP)	134	12.06	7.22	0	0	0	21.04	0.27	0.59	0
Peanut butter, no salt added, creamy or chunky (TS)	5.33	0	0	0.44	0	0	4.17	0.02	0.05	0
Peanut butter, with salt, creamy or chunky (TS)	5.33	0	0	0.44	0	0	4.17	0.02	0.05	0
Peanuts, salted (CP)	144	0	0	13.15	0	0	181.01	0.36	2	0
Peanuts, unsalted (CP)	144	0	0	13.15	0	0	181.01	0.36	2	0
Pecans, salted (CP)	110	141.90	84.97	2.91	0	2.20	43.34	0.21	1.89	0
Pecans, unsalted (CP)	108	138.24	82.78	2.86	0	2.16	42.34	0.21	1.85	0
Pine nuts, unsalted (CP)	120	34.80	20.84	4.25	0	2.40	69.36	0.13	0.25	0
Pistachio nuts, salted (CP)	128	304.64	182.41	6.67	0	9.34	75.65	0.32	1.55	0

Pumpkin seeds, salted (CP)	138	524.40	314.01	2.26	0	2.48	79.21	0.12	0.47	0
Pumpkin seeds, unsalted (CP)	138	524.40	314.01	2.26	0	2.48	79.21	0.12	0.47	0
Sesame seeds (TB)	8	5.28	3.16	0.18	0	0	7.68	0.01	0.05	0
Sunflower seeds, hulled, salted (CP)	144	72	43.11	72.19	0	2.02	327.46	1.11	9.71	0
Sunflower seeds, hulled, unsalted (CP)	144	72	43.11	72.19	0	2.02	327.46	1.11	9.71	0
Tahini (sesame butter) (TS)	5	3.35	2.01	0.90	0	0	4.88	0.01	0.03	0
Walnuts, unsalted (CP)	100	124	74.25	2.63	0	3.20	66	0.56	0.63	0

VEGETABLES AND LEGUMES

Artichokes, cooked, without salt (CP)	168	297.36	178.06	0.32	0	16.80	85.68	0.18	0.57	0
Arugula, raw (CP)	20	474.60	284.19	0.50	0	18.20	19.40	0.01	0.09	0
Asparagus, canned, drained solids, with salt (CP)	242	1285.02	769.46	2.20	0	44.53	231.35	0.27	0.34	0
Asparagus, fresh or frozen, cooked without salt (CP)	180	1472.40	881.68	2.59	0	43.92	242.46	0.04	0.29	0
Baked beans with franks, canned (CP)	257	248.47	148.78	1.16	0.33	16.55	83.06	0.23	0.33	0.49
Bamboo shoots, canned, cooked, with salt (CP)	131	10.48	6.27	0	0	1.44	4.19	0.18	0.12	0
Beans, kidney, dry, cooked or canned, without fat, without salt (CP)	177	0	0	0.14	0	2.12	229.39	0.21	0.39	0

VITAMIN COUNTER	WEIGHT (g)	VIT A (IU)	BETA-C (µg)	VIT E (mg)	VIT D (µg)	VIT C (mg)	FOL. (µg)	VIT B$_6$ (mg)	PANT (mg)	VIT B$_{12}$ (mg)
Beans, kidney, dry, cooked or canned, without fat, with salt (CP)	177	0	0	0.14	0	2.14	231.43	0.21	0.39	0
Beans, lima, cooked, fresh or frozen, without salt (CP)	170	323	193.41	0.49	0	21.76	36.04	0.20	0.27	0
Beans, lima, dry, cooked or canned, without fat, without salt (CP)	188	0	0	0.45	0	0	156.23	0.30	0.79	0
Beans, lima, dry, cooked or canned, without fat, with salt (CP)	188	0	0	0.45	0	0	156.79	0.30	0.79	0
Beans, navy, dry, cooked or canned, without fat, without salt (CP)	182	3.64	2.18	0.33	0	1.64	254.62	0.29	0.45	0
Beans, navy, dry, cooked or canned, without fat, with salt (CP)	182	3.64	2.18	0.33	0	1.64	254.36	0.29	0.45	0
Beans, northern, dry, cooked or canned, without fat, without salt (CP)	179	0	0	0.23	0	0	144.45	0.16	0.41	0
Beans, northern, dry, cooked or canned, without fat, with salt (CP)	179	0	0	0.23	0	0	144.45	0.16	0.41	0
Beans, pinto, dry, cooked or canned, without fat, without salt (CP)	171	3.42	2.05	0.02	0	3.59	294.12	0.26	0.48	0
Beans, pinto, dry, cooked or canned, without fat, with salt (CP)	171	3.45	2.07	0.02	0	3.63	296.55	0.26	0.48	0

Food	g								
Beans, yellow, canned, drained solids, with salt (CP)	136	142.80	85.50	0.39	0	6.53	43.25	0.05	0.18	0
Beans, yellow, cooked, fresh or frozen, without salt (CP)	135	151.20	90.54	0.39	0	11.07	11.07	0.08	0.07	0
Beets, Harvard (CP)	246	374.07	64.72	0.87	0.89	7.12	52.60	0.10	0.28	0.01
Beets, pickled (CP)	169	62.38	37.37	0.30	0	6.49	135.99	0.12	0.24	0
Beets, red, canned, drained solids, with salt (CP)	170	18.70	11.20	0.27	0	6.97	51.34	0.10	0.27	0
Beets, red, cooked, fresh or frozen, without salt (CP)	170	59.50	35.63	0.29	0	6.12	136	0.12	0.24	0
Broccoli, cooked, fresh or frozen, without salt (CP)	184	3481.28	2084.72	1.90	0	73.78	103.78	0.24	0.50	0
Broccoli, raw (CP)	88	1121.12	671.44	0.42	0	82.02	62.48	0.14	0.47	0
Brussels sprouts, cooked, fresh or frozen, without salt (CP)	155	912.95	546.67	1.32	0	70.83	156.86	0.45	0.53	0
Cabbage, Chinese (pak-choi), cooked, drained (CP)	170	4365.60	2614.60	0.20	0	44.20	69.02	0.29	0.14	0
Cabbage, Chinese (pak-choi), raw, shredded (CP)	70	2100	1257.20	0.09	0	31.50	45.99	0.13	0.06	0
Cabbage, Chinese (pe-tsai), cooked, drained (CP)	119	1150.73	689.01	0.14	0	18.80	63.55	0.21	0.10	0

VITAMIN COUNTER	WEIGHT (g)	VIT A (IU)	BETA-C (µg)	VIT E (mg)	VIT D (µg)	VIT C (mg)	FOL (µg)	VIT B₆ (mg)	PANT (mg)	VIT B₁₂ (mg)
Cabbage, Chinese (pe-tsai), raw, shredded (CP)	76	912	546.44	0.09	0	20.52	59.81	0.17	0.08	0
Cabbage, cooked, without salt (CP)	150	198	118.56	2.50	0	30.15	30	0.16	0.21	0
Cabbage, raw (CP)	70	93.10	55.75	1.17	0	22.54	30.10	0.07	0.10	0
Carrot, raw (CP)	110	17022.50	10192.60	0.49	0	10.23	15.40	0.16	0.22	0
Carrot juice (CP)	246	63347.46	37933.20	0.84	0	20.91	9.35	0.54	0.57	0
Carrots, canned, drained solids, with salt (CP)	146	20010.04	12041.93	0.61	0	3.94	13.43	0.16	0.19	0
Carrots, fresh or frozen, cooked, without salt (CP)	156	38304.24	22936.66	1.34	0	3.59	21.68	0.39	0.47	0
Cauliflower, fresh or frozen, cooked, without salt (CP)	180	39.60	23.71	0.07	0	56.34	73.80	0.16	0.18	0
Cauliflower, raw (CP)	100	19	11.38	0.04	0	46.40	57	0.22	0.65	0
Celery, raw (CP)	120	160.80	96.29	0.43	0	8.40	33.60	0.11	0.23	0
Chard, Swiss, fresh or frozen, cooked, without salt (CP)	175	5493.25	3289.37	0	0	31.50	15.05	0.14	0.28	0
Chickpeas, dry, cooked or canned, without fat, with salt (CP)	164	44.28	26.52	0.51	0	2.13	282.08	0.23	0.48	0

Food									
Chickpeas, dry, cooked or canned, without fat, without salt (CP)	164	44.28	26.52	0.51	0	2.13	282.08	0.23	0.48	0
Corn, ear, cooked (MD)	77	167.09	100.05	0.08	0	4.77	35.73	0.05	0.68	0
Corn, whole kernel, drained solids, canned, with salt (CP)	164	255.84	153.19	0.10	0	13.94	79.70	0.08	1.10	0
Corn, whole kernel, fresh or frozen, without salt (CP)	164	406.72	243.54	0.23	0	4.26	37.39	0.16	0.36	0
Cucumber, raw (CP)	104	223.60	133.89	0.14	0	5.51	13.52	0.04	0.19	0
Eggplant, cooked, boiled, without salt, diced (CP)	96	61.44	36.79	0.03	0	1.25	13.82	0.09	0.07	0
Endive, raw (CP)	29	594.50	355.99	0.13	0	1.88	41.18	0.01	0.26	0
Fennel, bulb, raw (CP)	87	203.41	121.80	NA	0	10.44	23.49	0.04	0.20	0
Garlic, fresh (TS)	3.12	0	0	0	0	0.97	0.10	0.04	0.02	0
Ginger root, raw (CP)	96	0	0	NA	0	4.80	10.75	0.15	0.19	0
Green beans, canned, drained solids, with salt (CP)	136	474.64	284.21	0.04	0	6.53	43.25	0.05	0.18	0
Green beans, fresh or frozen, cooked, without salt (CP)	135	712.80	426.83	0.11	0	11.07	11.07	0.08	0.07	0
Greens, collard, fresh or frozen, cooked, without salt (CP)	128	3490.56	2090.15	2.87	0	15.49	7.68	0.06	0.06	0
Greens, turnip, fresh or frozen, cooked, without salt (CP)	144	7917.12	4740.80	3.23	0	39.46	170.50	0.26	0.39	0

VITAMIN COUNTER	WEIGHT (g)	VIT A (IU)	BETA-C (µg)	VIT E (mg)	VIT D (µg)	VIT C (mg)	FOL (µg)	VIT B$_6$ (mg)	PANT (mg)	VIT B$_{12}$ (mg)
Jicama, cooked, without salt (CP)	135.20	25.69	15.39	0.07	0	19.06	10.82	0.05	0.16	0
Jicama, raw (CP)	130	0	0	0.16	0	26	71.50	0.03	0.06	0
Kohlrabi, fresh or frozen, cooked, without salt (CP)	165	57.75	34.58	0	0	89.10	19.96	0.25	0.26	0
Lentils, dry, cooked or canned, without fat, without salt (CP)	198	15.84	9.48	0.08	0	2.97	357.98	0.36	1.27	0
Lentils, dry, cooked or canned, without fat, with salt (CP)	198	15.68	9.39	0.08	0	2.95	354.52	0.36	1.25	0
Lettuce (CP)	55	181.50	108.68	0.24	0	2.14	30.80	0.02	0.03	0
Mushrooms, canned, drained solids, with salt (CP)	156	0	0	0.16	0	0	19.19	0.09	1.26	0
Mushrooms, fresh or frozen, cooked, without salt (CP)	156	0	0	0	0	6.24	28.39	0.14	3.37	0
Mushrooms, raw, whole or sliced (CP)	70	0	0	0.07	0	2.45	14.77	0.07	1.54	0
Okra, fresh or frozen, cooked, without salt (CP)	184	945.76	566.32	0	0	22.45	267.90	0.09	0.44	0
Onions, fresh or frozen, cooked, without salt (CP)	210	0	0	0.25	0	10.92	31.50	0.27	0.23	0
Onions, raw (CP)	160	0	0	0.19	0	10.24	30.40	0.19	0.18	0

Food									
Parsley, fresh (TB)	3.75	195	116.77	0.07	0	4.99	5.70	0	0.01	0
Parsnips, fresh or frozen, cooked, without salt (CP)	156	0	0	1.56	0	20.28	90.79	0.14	0.92	0
Peas and carrots, fresh or frozen, cooked, without salt (CP)	160	12417.60	7435.70	0.82	0	12.96	41.60	0.14	0.26	0
Peas, blackeye, dry, cooked or canned, without fat, without salt (CP)	171	25.65	15.36	0	0	0.68	355.51	0.17	0.70	0
Peas, blackeye, dry, cooked or canned, without fat, with salt (CP)	171	25.65	15.36	0	0	0.68	355.51	0.17	0.70	0
Peas, blackeye, fresh, cooked (CP)	165	1305.15	781.52	0	0	3.63	209.55	0.10	0.25	0
Peas, edible podded, fresh or frozen, cooked without salt (CP)	160	209.60	125.50	0.50	0	76.64	46.56	0.22	1.07	0
Peas, green, canned, drained solids, with salt (CP)	170	1305.60	781.80	0.03	0	16.32	75.31	0.10	0.22	0
Peas, green, fresh or frozen, cooked, without salt (CP)	160	1068.80	640	0.26	0	15.84	93.76	0.18	0.22	0
Peas, split, dry, cooked or canned, without fat, without salt (CP)	196	13.72	8.21	0.59	0	0.78	127.20	0.10	1.16	0
Peas, split, dry, cooked or canned, without fat, with salt (CP)	196	13.72	8.21	0.59	0	0.78	127.20	0.10	1.16	0
Pepper, chili, Mexican, canned (CP)	136	829.60	497.76	4.03	0	92.48	13.60	0.20	0.04	0

VITAMIN COUNTER	WEIGHT (g)	VIT A (IU)	BETA-C (µg)	VIT E (mg)	VIT D (µg)	VIT C (mg)	FOL (µg)	VIT B₆ (mg)	PANT (mg)	VIT B₁₂ (mg)
Pepper, chili, fresh, cooked, without salt (CP)	136	13158	7878.48	.94	0	263.84	22.28	0.34	0.07	0
Pepper, green, fresh or frozen, cooked, without salt (CP)	136	805.12	482.11	0.79	0	101.18	21.76	0.31	0.11	0
Pepper, green, raw (CP)	100	632	378.44	0.58	0	89.30	22	0.25	0.08	0
Pepper, red, fresh or frozen, cooked, without salt (CP)	136	5113.60	3061.36	0.79	0	232.56	21.76	0.31	0.11	0
Pepper, red, raw (CP)	100	5700	3420	0.58	0	190	22	0.25	0.08	0
Plantains, fresh, cooked, without salt (CP)	154	1399.86	838.24	7.70	0	16.79	40.04	0.37	0.35	0
Potatoes, French fried (REG)	4.20	0	0	0.12	0	0.49	0.59	0.02	0.03	0
Potatoes, French fried, without salt (REG)	4.20	0	0	0.12	0	0.49	0.59	0.02	0.03	0
Potatoes, baked, without skin, without salt (MD)	93	0	0	0.03	0	11.90	8.46	0.28	0.52	0
Potatoes, baked, with skin, without salt (CP)	122	0	0	0.05	0	15.74	13.42	0.43	0.67	0
Potatoes, boiled, without skin, without salt (CP)	156	0	0	0.06	0	11.54	13.88	0.42	0.80	0
Potatoes, boiled, with skin, without salt (MD)	142	0	0	0.04	0	14.74	12.57	0.40	0.62	0

Pumpkin, canned, cooked (CP)	245	54037.20	32357.15	2.60	0	10.29	30.13	0.15	0.98	0
Radicchio, raw (CP)	40	10.80	6.47	0.18	0	3.20	24	0.02	0.11	0
Radish, raw (CP)	116	9.28	5.56	0	0	26.45	31.32	0.08	0.10	0
Refried beans, canned (CP)	253	0	0	0.03	0	15.18	211.25	0.25	0.33	0
Romaine, raw (CP)	30	780	467.07	0.13	0	7.20	40.71	0.01	0.05	0
Rutabaga, fresh or frozen, cooked, without salt (CP)	170	953.70	571.08	0.25	0	31.96	25.50	0.17	0.27	0
Sauerkraut, cooked, canned, solids and liquid (CP)	236	42.48	25.44	3.94	0	34.69	55.93	0.31	0.21	0
Scallion, cooked (CP)	219	10312.71	6175.80	1.07	0	72.18	21.90	0.13	0.31	0
Scallion, raw (CP)	100	385	230.54	0.46	0	18.80	64	0.06	0.07	0
Seaweed, kelp, raw (CP)	80	92.80	55.57	0.72	0	9	144	0	0.51	0
Soybean curd (tofu) (OZ)	28.35	24.10	14.46	0.18	0	0.03	4.25	0.01	0.02	0
Soybeans, dry, cooked or canned, without salt (CP)	172	15.48	9.27	3.51	0	2.92	92.54	0.40	0.31	0
Soybeans, roasted (CP)	172	344	206.40	9.91	0	3.78	362.92	0.36	0.77	0
Soy flour (CP)	85	102	61.08	3.01	0	0	293.25	0.39	1.35	0
Spinach, canned, drained solids, with salt (CP)	214	18780.64	11245.89	0.04	0	30.60	209.29	0.21	0.11	0
Spinach, fresh or frozen, cooked, without salt (CP)	190	14789.60	8856.05	3.50	0	23.37	204.25	0.28	0.15	0

VITAMIN COUNTER	WEIGHT (g)	VIT A (IU)	BETA-C (µg)	VIT E (mg)	VIT D (µg)	VIT C (mg)	FOL (µg)	VIT B$_6$ (mg)	PANT (mg)	VIT B$_{12}$ (mg)
Spinach, raw (CP)	56	4705.12	2817.36	1.06	0	15.74	108.86	0.11	0.03	0
Sprouts, alfalfa, raw (CP)	33	51.15	30.63	0.18	0	2.71	11.88	0.01	0.18	0
Sprouts, soybean, raw (CP)	70	7.70	4.61	0.18	0	10.71	120.26	0.13	0.65	0
Squash, summer, all varieties, fresh or frozen, cooked, without salt (CP)	180	516.60	309.35	0.22	0	9.90	36.18	0.11	0.25	0
Squash, winter, all varieties, fresh or frozen, cooked, without salt (CP)	245	8714.65	5218.35	0.29	0	23.52	68.60	0.17	0.86	0
Sweet potato, canned, syrup pack, drained solids, with salt (CP)	196	14027.72	8400.56	0.86	0	21.17	15.48	0.12	0.78	0
Sweet potatoes, candied (MD)	132.50	25187.55	14942.98	1.02	0.78	28.05	26.02	0.28	0.77	0.01
Sweet potatoes, canned, vacuum pack, drained solids, with salt (CP)	200	15966	9560.48	0.88	0	52.80	33.20	0.38	1.04	0
Sweet potatoes, fresh or frozen, cooked, without salt (CP)	255	55646.10	33320.85	1.12	0	62.73	57.63	0.61	1.66	0
Tempeh, fresh or frozen (PTY)	226.80	1555.85	931.65	3.95	0	0	117.94	0.68	0.82	2.27
Tomatillos, raw (CP)	132	150.48	90.10	NA	0	15.44	9.24	0.08	0.20	0
Tomatoes, canned, no salt added (CP)	240	1449.60	868.03	3.05	0	36.24	18.72	0.22	0.41	0
Tomatoes, canned, with salt (CP)	240	1449.60	868.03	3.05	0	36.24	18.72	0.22	0.41	0
Tomatoes, fresh, cooked, without salt (CP)	240	1783.20	1067.78	3.05	0	54.72	31.20	0.22	0.70	0

Food									
Tomatoes, raw (CP)	180	1121.40	671.49	0.85	0	34.38	27	0.14	0.45	0
Tomatoes, sun dried (CP)	54	471.96	282.61	2.28	0	21.17	36.72	0.18	1.13	0
Tomatoes, sun dried, oil pack, drained (CP)	110	1414.60	847.07	3.64	0	111.98	25.30	0.35	0.53	0
Tomato juice, no salt added (CP)	242.64	1349.08	807.82	0	0	44.40	48.29	0.27	0.61	0
Tomato juice, salt added (CP)	242.64	1349.08	807.82	0.53	0	44.40	48.29	0.27	0.61	0
Tomato paste, canned, no salt added (CP)	262	6466.16	3871.94	4.93	0	110.83	58.69	1	1.96	0
Tomato paste, canned, with salt (CP)	262	6466.16	3871.94	4.93	0	110.83	58.69	1	1.96	0
Tomato sauce, canned, without fat, no salt added (CP)	245	2398.55	1436.26	3.45	0	32.09	23.03	0.37	0.76	0
Tomato sauce, canned, without fat, with salt (CP)	245	2398.55	1436.26	3.45	0	32.09	23.03	0.37	0.76	0
Turnips, fresh or frozen, cooked, without salt (CP)	156	0	0	0.05	0	18.10	14.35	0.11	0.22	0
Vegetable juice, cocktail, no salt added (CP)	242	2831.40	1695.45	0	0	67.03	51.06	0.34	0.65	0
Vegetable juice, cocktail, salt added (CP)	242	2831.40	1695.45	0	0	67.03	51.06	0.34	0.65	0
Water chestnuts, cooked, canned (CP)	140	0	0	0	0	8.40	8.12	0.22	0.31	0
Watercress, raw (CP)	34	1598	956.89	0.34	0	14.62	3.13	0.04	0.11	0
Zucchini, fresh or frozen, cooked, without salt (CP)	180	432	258.68	0.70	0	8.28	30.24	0.14	0.20	0
Zucchini, raw (CP)	130	442	264.67	0.51	0	11.70	28.73	0.12	0.10	0

MINERAL COUNTER

	CALC (mg)	IRON (mg)	MAG (mg)	PHOS (mg)	SOD (mg)	POTA (mg)	COP (mg)	ZINC (mg)	SELE (µg)
BEVERAGES									
Club soda (CP)	11.84	0.02	2.37	0	49.73	4.74	0.02	0.24	0.24
Coffee, brewed, hot or iced, without sugar (CP)	4.74	0.12	11.85	2.37	4.74	127.98	0.02	0.05	0.12
Coffee, decaffeinated, instant, dry powder (TS)	1.40	0.04	3.11	2.86	0.23	35.01	0	0	0.05
Coffee, instant, dry powder (TS)	1.27	0.04	2.94	2.73	0.33	31.81	0	0	0.12
Cola (CP)	7.39	0.07	2.46	29.57	9.86	2.46	0.02	0.02	0.49
Cola, diet, with aspartame (CP)	9.47	0.07	2.37	21.31	14.21	0	0.02	0.19	0
Cola, diet, with aspartame and saccharin blend (CP)	0	0.31	2.40	39	24	1.99	0.05	0.53	0
Cola, diet, with saccharin (CP)	9.60	-0.10	2.40	26.40	38.40	4.80	0.05	0.12	0
Noncola (CP)	4.91	0.17	2.46	0	27.02	2.46	0.02	0.12	0.25
Noncola, diet, with aspartame (CP)	9.60	0.31	2.40	9.60	22.10	4.80	0.05	0.53	0.24
Noncola, diet, with aspartame and saccharin blend (CP)	9.60	0.31	2.40	9.60	52.80	4.80	0.05	0.53	0.24
Noncola, diet, with saccharin (CP)	9.47	0.09	2.37	26.05	37.89	4.74	0.05	0.12	0.24

Food									
Noncola, diet, with saccharin, sodium free (CP)	9.47	0.09	2.37	26.05	37.89	4.74	0.05	0.12	0.24
Postum, dry powder (TS)	8.26	0.21	10.23	21.11	3.03	97.61	0.06	0.25	1.7
Root beer, cream soda, birch beer, near beer (CP)	12.32	0.12	2.46	0	32.03	2.46	0.02	0.17	0.25
Root beer, diet, with aspartame (CP)	5.90	0.96	2.40	5.93	45.60	69.60	0.05	0.53	0.24
Root beer, diet, with aspartame and saccharin blend (CP)	5.90	0.96	2.40	5.93	14.40	69.60	0.05	0.53	0.24
Root beer, diet, with saccharin (CP)	9.60	0.10	2.40	26.40	38.40	4.80	0.05	0.12	0.24
Tea, herbal (CP)	4.74	0.19	2.37	0	2.37	21.33	0.02	0.09	0.05
Tea, hot or iced, with aspartame, reconstituted (CP)	0.33	0.14	1.95	2.19	0	25.01	0	0	0.07
Tea, hot or iced, without sugar, brewed (CP)	0	0.05	7.11	2.37	7.11	87.69	0.02	0.05	0.05
Tea, hot or iced, with saccharin, reconstituted (CP)	0.50	0.21	3	3.36	25.13	61.19	0	0.02	0.12
Tea, hot or iced, with sugar, reconstituted, presweetened, instant (CP)	4.80	0.05	4.80	2.40	7.20	45.60	0.02	0.07	0.05
Tea, instant, decaffeinated, dry powder (TS)	0.38	0.03	2.54	3.09	0.91	46.17	0.01	0.02	0.03
Tea, instant, decaffeinated, dry powder, with aspartame (TS)	0.03	0	6.22	0	0.31	11.77	0	0	0.01
Tea, instant, decaffeinated, dry powder, with saccharin (TS)	0.28	0.01	1.27	1.55	4.94	23.09	0	0.01	0.02

MINERAL COUNTER

	CALC (mg)	IRON (mg)	MAG (mg)	PHOS (mg)	SOD (mg)	POTA (mg)	COP (mg)	ZINC (mg)	SELE (µg)
Tea, instant, decaffeinated, dry powder, with sugar (TS)	0.28	0.02	1.65	2.08	0.63	30.14	0.01	0.02	0.06
Tea, instant, dry powder (TS)	0.38	0.03	2.54	3.09	0.91	46.17	0.01	0.02	0.03
Tea, instant, dry powder, with aspartame (TS)	0.16	0.07	0.97	1.09	0	12.50	0	0.01	0.04
Tea, instant, dry powder, with saccharin (TS)	0.25	0.11	1.50	1.68	12.56	30.60	0	0.01	0.06
Tea, instant, dry powder, with sugar (TS)	0.11	0.01	0.42	0.53	0.19	8.22	0	0	0.05
EGGS AND EGG PRODUCTS									
Egg, scrambled with whole milk (LG)	88.14	1.45	14.73	208.09	740.37	170.29	0.01	1.23	24.53
Egg, whole (LG)	24.50	0.72	5	89	63	60.50	0	0.55	12
Egg, yolk (LG)	22.74	0.59	1.49	81.01	7.14	15.60	0	0.52	6.81
Egg Beaters egg substitute, prepared as directed (CP)	153.01	3.96	20.29	162.71	650.36	293.97	0.12	2.25	29.57
Eggnog, commercial (CP)	330.20	0.51	46.99	277.88	138.18	419.61	0.03	1.17	5.13
Egg white (LG)	2	0.01	3.67	4.34	54.78	47.76	0	0	4.68
Scramblers egg substitute, prepared as directed (CP)	165.23	2.90	21.01	174.17	633.35	368.21	0.18	3.23	21.26

Second Nature egg substitute, prepared as directed (CP)	165.24	4.30	64.32	100.08	537.61	418.36	0.02	2.43	30.4
FATS AND OILS									
Butter, salted (TS)	1.11	0.01	0.10	1.08	25.49	1.23	0	0	0.08
Butter, unsalted (TS)	1.11	0.01	0.10	1.08	0.52	1.23	0	0	0.08
Butter, whipped (TS)	0.74	0.01	0.07	0.72	16.98	0.82	0	0	0.05
Butter, whipped, unsalted (TS)	0.74	0.01	0.07	0.72	0.35	0.82	0	0	0.05
Lard, rendered (TS)	0	0	0	0	0	0	0	0	NA
Margarine, corn, diet (40% fat) (TS)	0.85	0	0.07	0.66	46.06	1.21	0	0	0.04
Margarine, corn, liquid (80% fat) (TS)	1.41	0	0.12	1.08	31.91	1.99	0	0.01	0.08
Margarine, corn, spread (52% fat) (TS)	0.96	0	0.08	0.72	46.90	1.34	0	0.01	0.05
Margarine, corn, stick/tub (80% fat) (TS)	1.25	0	0.11	1.08	44.34	1.99	0	0.01	0.08
Margarine, corn, stick/tub (80% fat), unsalted (TS)	1.25	0	0.11	0.95	1.32	1.77	0	0.01	0.08
Margarine, corn, whipped (80% fat) (TS)	0.84	0	0.07	0.64	34.09	1.19	0	0.01	0.05
Margarine, safflower, stick/tub (80% fat) (TS)	1.25	0	0.11	0.95	50.70	1.77	0	0.01	0.08
Margarine, safflower, stick/tub (80% fat), unsalted (TS)	1.41	0	0.12	1.08	0.66	1.99	0	0.01	0.08

MINERAL COUNTER	CALC (mg)	IRON (mg)	MAG (mg)	PHOS (mg)	SOD (mg)	POTA (mg)	COP (mg)	ZINC (mg)	SELE (µg)
Margarine, soybean, diet (40% fat) (TS)	0.85	0	0.07	0.66	46.06	1.21	0	0	0.04
Margarine, soybean, spread (52% fat) (TS)	0.29	0	0.08	0.38	37.25	1.10	0	0.01	0.05
Margarine, soybean, stick/rub (80% fat) (TS)	1.25	0	0.11	0.95	50.71	1.77	0	0.01	0.08
Margarine, sunflower, diet (40% fat) (TS)	0.86	0	0.07	0.67	28.80	1.34	0	0	0.04
Margarine, sunflower, spread (52% fat) (TS)	0.95	0	0.08	0.48	24.29	1.44	0	0.01	0.05
Margarine, sunflower, stick/rub (80% fat) (TS)	1.25	0	0.11	0.95	33.37	0.47	0	0.01	0.08
Oil, canola (rapeseed) (TS)	0	0	0	0	0	0	0	0	0
Oil, coconut (TS)	0	0	0.01	0	0	0	0	0.01	0
Oil, cod liver (TS)	0	0	NA	0	0	0	NA	NA	0.23
Oil, corn (TS)	0	0	0.02	0	0	0	0	0.01	0
Oil, cottonseed (TS)	0	0	0	0	0	0	0	0	0
Oil, olive (TS)	0.01	0.02	0	0.05	0	0	0	0	0.95
Oil, palm (TS)	0	0	0	0.01	0	0	0	0	0
Oil, palm kernel (TS)	0	0	0	0	0	0	0	0	0
Oil, peanut (TS)	0	0	0	0	0	0	0	0	0.41
Oil, safflower (TS)	0	0	0	0	0	0	0.01	0.01	0
Oil, sesame (TS)	0	0	0	0	0	0	0	0.01	0

Food									
Oil, soybean, partially hydrogenated (TS)	0	0	0	0	0	0	0.02	0.01	0
Oil, sunflower seed (TS)	0	0	0.03	0	0	0	0	0	0.48
Olives, black (ripe) (MD)	3.52	0.13	0.16	0.12	34.88	0.32	0.01	0.01	0
Olives, green, plain or stuffed (MD)	2.44	0.06	0.88	0.68	96	2.20	0.02	0	0
Salad dressing, blue cheese, commercial (TB)	12.39	0.03	0	11.32	167.38	5.66	0	0	3.22
Salad dressing, blue cheese, low calorie, commercial (TB)	5.35	0.02	1.63	3.67	173.50	4.44	0	0	0.83
Salad dressing, French, commercial (TB)	1.72	0.06	1.06	2.18	213.72	12.32	0	0.01	0
Salad dressing, French, low calorie, commercial (TB)	1.79	0.07	0.16	2.28	128.28	12.88	0	0.03	0.82
Salad dressing, French, no salt added, commercial (TB)	1.79	0.07	0	2.28	4.89	12.88	0	0.03	2.68
Salad dressing, Italian, commercial (TB)	1.47	0.03	0.09	0.73	115.69	2.20	0.01	0.02	2.28
Salad dressing, Italian, low calorie, commercial (TB)	0.30	0.03	0.27	0.75	118.05	2.25	0	0.02	2.63
Salad dressing, mayonnaise, commercial (79% fat) (TB)	2.48	0.07	0.14	3.86	78.44	4.69	0.03	0.02	0.86
Salad dressing, mayonnaise, imitation (19% fat) (TB)	0	0.03	0	0.01	74.55	1.50	0	0.02	2.56
Salad dressing, mayonnaise type, commercial (33% fat) (TB)	2.06	0.03	0.29	3.82	104.48	1.32	0	0.03	1.59

	CALC (mg)	IRON (mg)	MAG (mg)	PHOS (mg)	SOD (mg)	POTA (mg)	COP (mg)	ZINC (mg)	SELE (µg)
Salad dressing, Thousand Island, commercial (TB)	1.72	0.09	0.31	2.65	109.20	17.63	0	0.02	2.38
Salad dressing, Thousand Island, low calorie, commercial (TB)	1.68	0.09	0.11	2.60	153	17.29	0	0.02	0.95
Salad dressing, yogurt based, commercial (TB)	5.17	0.04	1.50	4.42	135	15.18	0.01	0.04	2.09
Sandwich spread (TB)	1.38	0.04	0.31	2.29	153	5.35	0	0	0.53
Shortening, household (TS)	0	0	0	0	0	0	0	0	0
Tartar sauce (TB)	2.59	0.13	0.46	4.60	101.67	11.22	0	0.03	1.89
FRUITS AND FRUIT PRODUCTS									
Apple, fresh, with skin (MD)	9.66	0.25	6.90	9.66	0	158.70	0.06	0.06	0.83
Apple juice, sweetened (CP)	16.96	0.89	7.24	17.04	7.29	287.85	0.50	0.27	0.52
Apple juice, unsweetened, bottled or canned (CP)	17.36	0.92	7.44	17.36	7.44	295.12	0.05	0.07	0.5
Apples, dried, uncooked (CP)	12.04	1.20	13.76	32.68	74.82	387	0.16	0.17	1.03
Applesauce, sweetened, canned (CP)	10.20	0.89	7.65	17.85	7.65	155.55	0.10	0.10	0.51
Applesauce, unsweetened (CP)	7.32	0.29	7.32	17.08	4.88	183	0.07	0.07	0.49
Apricots, dried, uncooked (CP)	58.50	6.11	61.10	152.10	13	1791.40	0.56	0.96	1.56

Food									
Apricots, dried, unsweetened, cooked (CP)	40	4.17	42.50	102.50	7.50	1222.50	0.37	0.65	1.07
Apricots, fresh (MD)	4.95	0.19	2.83	6.71	0.35	104.58	0.03	0.09	0
Apricots, sweetened, canned (CP)	23.22	0.77	18.06	30.96	10.32	361.20	0.21	0.28	0.52
Avocado (SM)	19.03	1.76	67.47	70.93	17.30	1036.27	0.45	0.73	1.73
Banana, fresh (MD)	6.84	0.35	33.06	22.80	1.14	451.44	0.11	0.18	1.25
Blackberries, fresh (CP)	46.08	0.82	28.80	30.24	0	282.24	0.20	0.39	0
Blueberries, fresh (CP)	8.70	0.25	7.25	14.50	8.70	129.05	0.09	0.16	0
Cantaloupe, fresh (MD)	101.50	1.94	101.50	156.87	83.05	2851.30	0.37	1.48	3.69
Cherries, fresh, sweet (CP)	21.75	0.57	15.95	27.55	0	324.80	0.13	0.09	0.58
Cherries, sweetened, canned (CP)	18	0.70	18	36	6	290	0.28	0.20	0.8
Cranberries, fresh (CP)	6.65	0.19	4.75	8.55	0.95	67.45	0.06	0.12	0.19
Cranberry-apple juice, sweetened (CP)	17.15	0.15	4.90	7.35	4.90	66.15	0.02	0.10	0.49
Cranberry juice, sweetened (CP)	7.59	0.38	5.06	5.06	5.06	45.54	0.05	0.18	0.15
Dates, dried (CP)	56.96	2.05	62.30	71.20	5.34	1160.56	0.52	0.52	3.38
Figs, canned in heavy syrup (CP)	69.93	0.73	25.90	25.90	2.59	256.41	0.28	0.28	0.85
Figs, dried (CP)	286.56	4.44	117.41	135.32	21.89	1416.88	0.62	1.01	4.52
Figs, fresh (MD)	17.50	0.18	8.50	7	0.50	116	0.03	0.07	0.2
Fruit-flavored drink or juice, low calorie (CP)	21.33	0.09	4.74	2.37	7.11	52.14	0.02	0.05	0.14
Grapefruit juice, sweetened, frozen or canned (CP)	20	0.90	25	27.50	5	405	0.12	0.15	0.05

MINERAL COUNTER

	CALC (mg)	IRON (mg)	MAG (mg)	PHOS (mg)	SOD (mg)	POTA (mg)	COP (mg)	ZINC (mg)	SELE (µg)
Grapefruit juice, unsweetened; fresh, frozen, or canned (CP)	17.29	0.49	24.70	27.17	2.47	377.91	0.10	0.22	0
Grapefruit sections, sweetened, canned (CP)	35.56	1.02	25.40	25.40	5.08	327.66	0.18	0.20	2.24
Grapefruit, fresh (MD)	34.94	0.26	23.30	23.30	0	404.77	0.15	0.20	2.53
Grape juice, sweetened, frozen (CP)	10	0.25	10	10	5	52.50	0.02	0.10	0.25
Grape juice, unsweetened (CP)	22.77	0.61	25.30	27.83	7.59	333.96	0.08	0.13	0
Grapes, fresh (CP)	17.60	0.42	9.60	20.80	3.20	296	0.14	0.08	0.32
Guava, fresh (MD)	18	0.28	9	22.50	2.70	255.60	0.09	0.21	0.54
Honeydew melon, fresh (MD)	77.40	0.90	90.30	129	129	3495.90	0.52	1.29	0
Kiwifruit, fresh (MD)	19.76	0.31	22.80	30.40	3.80	252.32	0.12	0.15	0.3
Kumquats, fresh (MD)	8.36	0.07	2.47	3.61	1.14	37.05	0.02	0.02	0.08
Lemon, fresh (MD)	15.08	0.35	4.64	9.28	1.16	80.04	0.02	0.03	0.23
Lemonade or limeade, sweetened, other than fruit-flavored beverage mix (CP)	7.44	0.40	4.96	4.96	7.44	37.20	0.05	0.10	0.25
Lemon juice, unsweetened; fresh, frozen, bottled, or canned (1 whole or 4 wedges = 1.50 oz) (CP)	26.84	0.32	19.52	21.96	51.24	248.88	0.10	0.15	0
Mandarin orange, fresh (MD)	11.76	0.08	10.08	8.40	0.84	131.88	0.03	0.20	0.17
Mango, fresh (MD)	20.70	0.27	18.63	22.77	4.14	322.92	0.23	0.08	0

Nectarine, fresh (MD)	6.80	0.20	10.88	21.76	0	288.32	0.10	0.12	0.54
Nectars, apricot, sweetened (CP)	17.57	0.95	12.55	22.59	7.53	286.14	0.18	0.23	0.28
Nectars, peach, sweetened, canned (CP)	12.45	0.47	9.96	14.94	17.43	99.60	0.17	0.20	0.65
Orange, fresh (MD)	52.40	0.13	13.10	18.34	0	237.11	0.05	0.09	1.93
Orange juice, sweetened, canned or frozen (CP)	19.40	1.07	26.67	33.95	4.92	424.60	0.15	0.17	14
Orange juice, unsweetened, fortified with calcium (CP)	289.41	0.25	24.90	39.84	2.49	473.10	0.10	0.12	14.94
Orange juice, unsweetened; fresh, frozen, or canned (CP)	22.41	0.25	24.90	39.84	2.49	473.10	0.10	0.12	14.94
Papaya juice, canned (CP)	25	0.85	7.50	0	12.50	77.50	0.02	0.37	NA
Papaya, fresh (CP)	33.60	0.14	14	7	4.20	359.80	0.03	0.10	NA
Peach, fresh (MD)	4.35	0.10	6.09	10.44	0	171.39	0.06	0.12	0.35
Peaches, dried, unsweetened, cooked (CP)	23.22	3.38	33.54	98.04	5.16	825.60	0.31	0.46	1.01
Peaches, sweetened, canned or frozen (CP)	7.68	0.69	12.80	28.16	15.36	235.52	0.13	0.23	0.77
Pear, fresh (MD)	18.26	0.41	9.96	18.26	0	207.50	0.18	0.20	1
Pears, dried, unsweetened, cooked (CP)	40.80	2.60	40.80	71.40	7.65	657.90	0.46	0.48	1.48
Pears, sweetened, canned (CP)	12.75	0.56	10.20	17.85	12.75	165.75	0.13	0.20	0.51
Persimmons, Japanese, raw (MD)	13.44	0.25	15.12	28.56	1.68	270.48	0.18	0.18	0.67
Pineapple juice, frozen or canned (CP)	42.50	0.65	32.50	20	2.50	335	0.22	0.27	0

MINERAL COUNTER	CALC (mg)	IRON (mg)	MAG (mg)	PHOS (mg)	SOD (mg)	POTA (mg)	COP (mg)	ZINC (mg)	SELE (µg)
Pineapple, canned, unsweetened or juice pack (CP)	35	0.70	35	15	2.50	305	0.22	0.25	0.25
Pineapple, fresh (SL)	5.88	0.31	11.76	5.88	0.84	94.92	0.09	0.07	0.46
Pineapple, sweetened, canned (SL)	8.12	0.23	9.28	4.06	0.58	60.90	0.06	0.07	0.58
Plum, fresh (MD)	2.64	0.07	4.62	6.60	0	113.52	0.03	0.07	0.13
Plums, sweetened, canned (CP)	23.22	2.17	12.90	33.54	49.02	234.78	0.10	0.18	0.7
Pomegranate, fresh (MD)	4.62	0.46	4.62	12.32	4.62	398.86	0.11	0.62	0.62
Prune juice, bottled (CP)	30.72	3.02	35.84	64	10.24	706.56	0.18	0.54	0
Prunes, dried, cooked (CP)	48.76	2.35	42.40	74.20	4.24	708.08	0.40	0.51	0.49
Prunes, dried, uncooked (CP)	82.11	3.99	72.45	127.19	6.44	1199.45	0.69	0.85	0.8
Raisins (TB)	4.75	0.20	3.20	9.40	1.16	72.77	0.03	0.03	0.05
Raspberries, fresh (CP)	27.06	0.70	22.14	14.76	0	186.96	0.09	0.57	0
Raspberries, sweetened, canned or frozen (CP)	37.50	1.62	32.50	42.50	2.50	285	0.25	0.45	0.5
Rhubarb, stewed, unsweetened (CP)	465.60	0.70	43.20	45.60	2.40	552	0.05	0.26	0.96
Rhubarb, sweetened, cooked (CP)	348	0.50	28.80	19.20	2.40	230.40	0.07	0.19	1.37
Strawberries, fresh or frozen, unsweetened (CP)	20.86	0.57	14.90	28.31	1.49	247.34	0.07	0.19	0.3

514

Strawberries, sweetened, canned or frozen (CP)	28.05	1.50	17.85	33.15	7.65	249.90	0.05	0.15	0.82
Watermelon, fresh (SL)	38.56	0.82	53.02	43.38	9.64	559.12	0.14	0.34	1.93
GRAIN PRODUCTS									
Bagel, egg (MD)	8.80	1.21	11	36.85	226.02	105.10	0.04	0.29	17.6
Bagel, plain (MD)	23.10	2.14	11	36.85	227.49	149.07	0.04	0.29	17.6
Bagel, rye (MD)	8.15	1.68	16.68	62.55	165.39	81.75	0.10	0.48	15.56
Bagel, whole wheat (MD)	10.04	1.96	26.96	86.09	165.73	97.81	0.12	0.65	19.88
Barley, pearled, cooked with salt (CP)	17.93	1.37	43.74	120.86	72.14	153.14	0.24	1.18	17.51
Barley, pearled, dry (CP)	58	5	158	442	18	560	0.84	4.26	64
Biscuit, baking powder (MD)	95.72	1.17	7.91	60.34	186.14	59.05	0.04	0.24	10.25
Bran, unprocessed (TB)	2.74	0.40	22.91	37.99	0.07	44.32	0.04	0.27	3.27
Bread, Boston brown (SL)	43.20	1.01	36	76.80	120.48	140.16	0.13	0.19	8.3
Bread, diet, with fiber added (SL)	17.94	0.61	9.66	29.90	101.66	21.62	0.08	0.25	3.71
Bread, egg (SL)	17.33	0.99	6.56	39.45	55.29	45.30	0.04	0.23	8.73
Bread, Italian (SL)	25.20	0.87	6.90	23.10	175.50	22.20	0.03	0.18	16.7
Bread, nut (SL)	62.92	0.94	13.52	61.30	122.52	71.09	0.10	0.33	8.14
Bread, oatmeal (SL)	7.63	1.11	12.64	46.30	68.25	48.76	0.06	0.30	8.33

MINERAL COUNTER

	CALC (mg)	IRON (mg)	MAG (mg)	PHOS (mg)	SOD (mg)	POTA (mg)	COP (mg)	ZINC (mg)	SELE (μg)
Bread, pumpkin, without nuts (SL)	14.60	0.97	7.30	32.52	171.76	53.89	0.04	0.20	6.97
Bread, raisin (SL)	15.97	0.65	5.62	19.57	82.12	52.42	0.03	0.14	6.75
Bread, rye (SL)	22.95	0.78	6.89	41.60	199.97	58.53	0.03	0.36	9.47
Bread, white (SL)	21	0.70	6.50	24.25	126.75	26.25	0.04	0.20	7.5
Bread, white, low sodium (SL)	18.75	0.63	5.25	26	2.50	29	0.03	0.15	7.5
Bread, whole wheat, low sodium (SL)	24.75	0.75	23.25	57	2.50	68.25	0.07	0.50	10.48
Bread, zucchini, without nuts (SL)	8.57	0.56	4.42	22.30	120.72	35.84	0.04	0.13	4.99
Buckwheat groats, cooked with salt (CP)	12.93	1.27	115.37	164.14	1176.87	164.87	0.32	1.25	2.69
Buckwheat groats, dry (CP)	27.88	4.05	362.44	523.16	18.04	524.80	1.02	3.97	8.2
Bulgur, cooked with salt (CP)	19.11	1.07	72.53	129.82	1093.42	177.63	0.15	0.84	27.35
Bulgur, dry (CP)	49	3.44	229.60	420	23.80	574	0.46	2.70	88.2
Cereal, cream of rice, cooked with salt (CP)	14.27	0.49	10.20	46.87	486.88	54.14	0.10	0.41	7.2
Cereal, cream of wheat, instant, cooked with salt (CP)	63.24	11.95	15.42	43.04	368.75	48.13	0.10	0.41	8.39
Cereal, cream of wheat, regular, cooked with salt (CP)	55.80	10.39	11.07	41.79	331.77	43.67	0.08	0.33	7.3
Cereal, dry, All-Bran (CP)	50.61	13.44	414.95	687.11	776.45	801.91	0.69	11.22	59.45
Cereal, dry, Apple Jacks (CP)	0.91	4.50	1.93	9	125.19	24.97	0.02	3.61	1.15

Cereal, dry, Cap'n Crunch (CP)	7.40	6.28	12.95	38.48	262.33	46.99	0.05	3.09	2.96
Cereal, dry, Cheerios (CP)	31.88	6.69	32.08	102.12	232.01	75.46	0.07	0.73	6.06
Cereal, dry, Cinnamon Toast Crunch (CP)	59.92	6.74	16.57	90.10	329.80	59.92	0.05	0.38	7.66
Cereal, dry, Common Sense Oat Bran (CP)	35.32	2.84	119.78	368.58	277.54	307.34	0.22	3	14.14
Cereal, dry, Cracklin' Oat Bran (CP)	15.36	10.80	60.67	175.55	342.20	156.73	0.12	5	14.21
Cereal, dry, Frosted Flakes (CP)	1.33	2.40	2.66	12	266.67	33.33	0.03	0	1.54
Cereal, dry, Frosted Mini-Wheats (CP)	21.64	3.61	75.16	200.99	5.69	205.54	0.37	2.99	2.9
Cereal, dry, Fruitful Bran (CP)	27.81	6.76	100.59	247.93	385.80	364.50	0.33	1.80	6.51
Cereal, dry, Grape-Nuts (CP)	41.96	32.43	107.73	283.50	661.12	352.67	0.50	4.81	10.09
Cereal, dry, Honeycomb (CP)	4.36	2.04	5.87	15.96	120	32.83	0.04	1.12	2.22
Cereal, dry, Just Right, with raisins, dates, and nuts (CP)	18.91	24	37.72	95.19	270.03	168.52	0.14	20	10.61
Cereal, dry, Kellogg's Corn Flakes (CP)	3.20	1.80	7.14	26.06	291.20	30.04	0.05	0.19	4.01
Cereal, dry, Kix (CP)	2.11	5.39	4.75	17.39	173.07	20.04	0.03	0	2.67
Cereal, dry, Life (CP)	144.76	12.57	72.16	251.68	241.12	266.20	0.26	1.30	NA
Cereal, dry, Oatmeal Raisin Crisp (CP)	33.74	8.88	61.54	229.30	342.44	231.42	0.26	1.28	23.86
Cereal, dry, Product 19 (CP)	3.40	18	10.49	39.97	324.89	44.23	0.08	15	3.4
Cereal, dry, Raisin Bran (Ralston) (CP)	18.14	5.90	75.97	176.93	374.59	223.22	0.21	1.45	28.72
Cereal, dry, Rice Chex (CP)	2.61	7.19	8.38	22.99	213.82	17.88	0.03	0.19	5.13
Cereal, dry, Rice Krispies (CP)	3.20	1.80	7.14	26.06	291.20	30.04	0.05	0.38	4.01

MINERAL COUNTER

MINERAL COUNTER	CALC (mg)	IRON (mg)	MAG (mg)	PHOS (mg)	SOD (mg)	POTA (mg)	COP (mg)	ZINC (mg)	SELE (µg)
Cereal, dry, Special K (CP)	8.22	4.51	15.59	55	229.92	49.05	0.13	3.74	16.16
Cereal, dry, Total (CP)	281.82	20.95	36.96	136.95	163.02	123.09	0.14	17.49	3.85
Cereal, dry, Wheat Chex (CP)	13.46	12.16	53.15	132.60	345.01	155.27	0.14	1.12	23.63
Cereal, dry, puffed rice (CP)	0.84	0.15	3.50	13.72	0.42	15.82	0.02	0.14	1.68
Cereal, dry, puffed wheat (CP)	3.36	0.57	17.40	42.60	0.48	41.76	0.05	0.28	14.4
Coffeecake, yeast, without nuts, without topping (PC)	31.20	1.06	8.33	53.10	139.87	67.17	0.05	0.34	8.88
Cornbread (PC)	121.47	1.46	14.25	93.27	273.35	97.02	0.03	0.44	10.02
Corn grits, cooked with salt, regular or instant (CP)	5.35	1.48	11.64	27.78	521.53	52.22	0.02	0.15	2.71
Corn grits, dry (CP)	3.12	6.10	42.12	113.88	1.56	213.72	0.11	0.64	10.92
Cornmeal, cooked with salt (CP)	5.90	1.37	14.28	27.60	255.96	53.28	0.02	0.24	2.33
Cornmeal, dry (CP)	6.90	5.70	55.20	115.92	4.14	223.56	0.11	0.99	9.66
Cornstarch (TB)	0.16	0.04	0.24	1.04	0.72	0.24	0	0	0.25
Couscous, cooked with salt (CP)	15.77	0.57	24.49	91.08	407.53	89.02	0.13	0.45	5.92
Couscous, dry (CP)	44.16	1.99	80.96	312.80	18.40	305.44	0.46	1.53	20.24
Cracker, graham (PC)	1.27	0.10	1.26	4.14	22.22	6.50	0.01	0.03	1.04
Cracker, saltine (PC)	0.73	0.17	0.63	3.15	40.84	4.20	0	0.02	0.43

Cracker, saltine, unsalted top (PC)	5.93	0.21	0.99	3.79	26.33	4.46	0.01	0.03	1.16
Cracker, zwieback (PC)	0.70	0.02	0.49	1.92	8.12	10.67	0	0.02	1.23
Donut, cake (MD)	34.29	0.87	5.25	37.84	85.09	35.73	0.03	0.20	7.9
Donut, yeast (MD)	20.03	1.33	9.26	57.23	76.42	65.85	0.08	0.34	11.18
Flour, all-purpose (CP)	18.75	5.80	27.50	135	2.50	133.75	0.17	0.87	48.75
Flour, amaranth (whole grain) (CP)	298.35	14.80	518.70	887.25	40.95	713.70	1.52	6.20	21.45
Flour, buckwheat (whole groat) (CP)	49.20	4.87	301.20	404.40	13.20	692.40	0.62	3.74	6.84
Flour, cake or pastry (CP)	15.26	7.98	17.44	92.65	2.18	114.45	0.15	0.68	5.45
Flour, corn, masa, enriched (CP)	160.74	8.22	125.40	254.22	5.70	339.72	0.19	2.03	17.1
Flour, rice (CP)	15.80	0.55	55.30	154.84	0	120.08	0.21	1.26	34.33
Flour, rice, brown (CP)	17.38	3.13	176.96	532.46	12.64	456.62	0.36	3.87	12.8
Flour, rye, medium (CP)	24.48	2.16	76.50	211.14	3.06	346.80	0.30	2.03	36.41
Flour, triticale (whole grain) (CP)	45.50	3.37	198.90	417.30	2.60	605.80	0.73	3.46	76.6
Flour, whole wheat (CP)	40.80	4.66	165.60	415.20	6	486	0.46	3.52	73.8
Hominy, canned (CP)	16	0.99	25.60	56	336	14.40	0.05	1.68	NA
Macaroni, whole wheat, cooked without salt (CP)	21	1.48	42	124.60	4.20	61.60	0.24	1.13	32.02
Matzo (PC)	0.46	0.10	0.88	3.10	0.06	3.91	0	0.02	1.55
Melba toast, unsalted (PC)	0.53	0.16	0.77	3.78	4.95	3.75	0	0.02	1.37
Millet, cooked with salt (CP)	10.90	2.28	88.78	217.15	1416.70	148.85	0.58	1.30	1.66

MINERAL COUNTER	CALC (mg)	IRON (mg)	MAG (mg)	PHOS (mg)	SOD (mg)	POTA (mg)	COP (mg)	ZINC (mg)	SELE (μg)
Millet, dry (CP)	16	6.02	228	570	10	390	1.50	3.36	4
Muffin, bran, homemade (MD)	27.62	1.89	46.04	100.72	203.27	120.39	0.09	1.30	11.07
Muffin, corn, commercial mix or homemade (MD)	75.25	1.09	10.02	60.49	145.35	65.73	0.03	0.29	7.42
Muffin, English, whole wheat (MD)	41.55	1.75	27.93	106.60	133.41	134.11	0.13	0.70	18.18
Noodles, chow mein (CP)	9	2.13	23.40	72.45	197.55	54	0.08	0.63	19.35
Noodles, egg, cooked without salt (CP)	19.20	2.54	30.40	110.40	11.20	44.80	0.14	0.99	28.66
Noodles, macaroni, white, cooked without salt (CP)	9.80	1.96	25.20	75.60	1.40	43.40	0.14	0.74	26.6
Noodles, macaroni, whole wheat, cooked with salt (CP)	21	1.48	42	124.60	179.20	61.60	0.24	1.13	32.02
Noodles, manicotti, cooked without salt (CP)	9.80	1.96	25.20	75.60	1.40	43.40	0.14	0.74	26.6
Noodles, ramen, cooked, all varieties (CP)	8.06	1.07	51.76	70.05	978.37	40	0.11	1.25	15.14
Noodles, rice, cooked without salt (CP)	11.20	0.96	14.05	11.20	1.42	40.35	0.08	0.56	7.26
Noodles, rice, fried (CP)	0.37	0.03	0.46	0.37	5.68	1.33	0.02	0.02	0.24
Oat bran, cooked with salt (CP)	25.14	1.99	87.45	269.98	234.26	208.25	0.15	1.16	10.34
Oat bran, dry (CP)	54.52	5.09	220.90	689.96	3.76	532.04	0.38	2.92	26.32
Oatmeal, cooked with salt (CP)	23.77	1.59	56.96	178.59	349.69	131.93	0.14	1.17	10.6

Oatmeal, dry (CP)	42.12	3.40	119.88	383.94	3.24	283.50	0.28	2.49	22.68
Pancake, homemade, all varieties except whole wheat and buckwheat (MD)	109.74	0.74	6.64	64.01	262.53	54.93	0.02	0.24	7.38
Pancake, homemade, whole wheat (MD)	113.47	0.64	22.42	95.46	263.50	99.33	0.06	0.54	10.17
Quinoa (CP)	102	15.72	357	697	35.70	1258	1.39	5.61	18.7
Rice, brown, cooked without salt (CP)	19.50	0.82	83.85	161.85	9.75	83.85	0.19	1.23	25.56
Rice, white, cooked without salt (CP)	15.80	1.90	18.96	67.94	1.58	55.30	0.11	0.77	9.95
Rice, wild, cooked without salt (CP)	4.92	0.98	52.48	134.48	4.92	165.64	0.20	2.20	1.62
Rice bran, dry (CP)	47.31	15.39	648.23	1391.91	4.15	1232.55	0.61	5.01	9.13
Rice cakes, plain, no salt added (PC)	0.99	0.13	11.79	32.40	2.34	26.10	0.04	0.27	4.19
Rice cakes, plain, salted (PC)	1.03	0.14	11.94	32.76	29.87	26.39	0.04	0.27	4.24
Roll, croissant (MD)	38.41	1.97	13.26	81.85	87.84	93.57	0.08	0.46	17.37
Roll, hamburger (MD)	59.34	0.90	12.04	35.26	217.58	40.85	0.07	0.39	12.47
Roll, hamburger, whole wheat (MD)	42.57	1.29	39.99	98.04	226.61	117.39	0.12	0.86	18.02
Roll, hard (MD)	17.39	1.04	11.10	34.04	231.25	35.89	0.06	0.33	10.73
Roll, hot dog (MD)	59.34	0.90	12.04	35.26	217.58	40.85	0.07	0.39	12.47
Roll, hot dog, whole wheat (MD)	42.57	1.29	39.99	98.04	226.61	117.39	0.12	0.86	18.02
Roll, kaiser (MD)	23.50	1.40	17	46	312.50	48.50	0.09	0.45	15.43
Roll, rye (MD)	28.80	0.98	8.64	52.20	250.92	73.44	0.04	0.46	11.88
Roll, sourdough (MD)	37.80	1.30	10.35	34.65	263.25	33.30	0.04	0.27	25.05

MINERAL COUNTER	CALC (mg)	IRON (mg)	MAG (mg)	PHOS (mg)	SOD (mg)	POTA (mg)	COP (mg)	ZINC (mg)	SELE (µg)
Roll, submarine (MD)	84.60	2.63	17.86	79.90	545.20	84.60	0.16	0.58	26.55
Roll, white, dinner (MD)	26.64	1.01	10.08	30.60	182.16	34.20	0.06	0.32	10.44
Roll, whole wheat (MD)	34.65	1.05	32.55	79.80	184.45	95.55	0.09	0.70	14.67
Rye (whole grain) (CP)	55.77	4.51	204.49	632.06	10.14	446.16	0.76	6.30	1.69
Stuffing, bread, all types except cornbread (CP)	67.23	1.84	21.30	68.27	731.13	187.37	0.11	0.54	17.27
Stuffing, cornbread (CP)	343.21	4.17	44.94	262.64	1178.26	387.30	0.13	1.26	27.55
Tortilla, corn, fried (MD)	43.66	0.40	13.84	57.30	37.91	37.06	0.06	0.30	1.45
Tortilla, corn, plain (MD)	43.66	0.40	13.84	57.30	37.91	37.06	0.06	0.30	1.45
Tortilla, flour, plain, commercial (PC)	25.78	1.59	12.62	57.37	159.80	42.07	0.13	0.60	7.65
Tortilla, flour, whole wheat, commercial (PC)	7.14	0.76	27.19	67.67	151.25	79.24	0.07	0.57	12.04
Tortilla, taco shell (MD)	18.46	0.34	13.52	30.03	63.05	31.59	0.04	0.17	0.88
Waffle, frozen, all varieties including bran (LG)	31.16	0.64	4.46	31.75	218.02	33.55	0.02	0.16	5.85
Waffle, homemade with whole milk, bran (PC)	183.90	2.17	73.11	216.04	669	233.80	0.13	1.18	19.88
Wheat, rolled, dry (CP)	37.60	3.19	114.68	356.26	1.88	365.66	0.43	2.50	59.22
Wheat germ (CP)	50.85	10.27	361.60	1294.98	4.52	1070.11	0.70	18.84	89.5

Abalone, cooked, canned (OZ)	2.83	0.51	13.61	32.89	85.33	31.18	0.06	0.60	3.55
Anchovies, smoked, canned in oil (PC)	9.28	0.19	2.76	10.08	146.72	21.76	0.01	0.10	0.8
Bacon, beef, kosher, cooked (SL)	0.91	0.21	1.69	23.79	66.36	15.34	0.01	0.40	2.62
Bacon, Canadian, cooked, drained (SL)	2.10	0.17	4.41	62.16	324.66	81.90	0.01	0.36	5.25
Bacon, low salt, cooked, drained (SL)	0.76	0.10	1.52	21.27	65.20	30.76	0.01	0.21	1.08
Bacon, regular, cooked, drained (SL)	0.76	0.10	1.52	21.27	101.03	30.76	0.01	0.21	1.08
Bacon, turkey, cooked, drained (SL)	0.72	0.17	2.32	32.32	207.84	33.12	0.01	0.24	1.3
Beef, arm roast (9% fat), no visible fat, cooked (OZ)	2.27	0.70	7.65	61.80	19.28	112.27	0.03	1.48	7
Beef, chipped (OZ)	1.70	1.28	9.07	49.33	984.03	125.87	0.05	1.49	15.03
Beef, ground, regular (22.56% fat), cooked (OZ)	3.12	0.69	5.67	48.48	23.81	85.05	0.02	1.44	7.37
Beef, hamburger, ground chuck (20% fat), cooked (OZ)	1.70	0.82	7.09	62.37	17.86	101.49	0.03	1.20	7.64
Beef, pot roast (26% fat), cooked (moist heat) (OZ)	3.69	0.62	6.24	49.61	17.58	92.14	0.03	1.58	8.54
Beef, prime rib (30% fat), cooked (OZ)	2.83	0.65	5.39	48.19	18.14	81.65	0.03	1.62	9.46
Beef, rib eye steak (20% fat), cooked (OZ)	2.55	0.63	6.52	55	17.86	98.94	0.03	1.30	5.1
Beef, short ribs (42% fat), cooked (OZ)	3.40	0.65	4.25	45.93	14.17	63.50	0.03	1.38	7.37

MINERAL COUNTER	CALC (mg)	IRON (mg)	MAG (mg)	PHOS (mg)	SOD (mg)	POTA (mg)	COP (mg)	ZINC (mg)	SELE (µg)
Beef, top round roast/steak (5% fat), no visible fat, cooked (OZ)	1.70	0.82	8.79	69.74	17.29	125.31	0.03	1.58	6.55
Breakfast strips, beef, cooked (SL)	1.02	0.36	3.06	26.74	255.26	46.68	0.01	0.72	3.83
Breakfast strips, pork, cooked (SL)	1.59	0.22	2.95	30.02	237.82	52.80	0.02	0.42	3.97
Chicken, canned (OZ)	3.97	0.45	3.40	31.47	142.60	39.12	0.01	0.40	4.35
Chicken, dark meat, with skin, cooked (OZ)	6.80	0.52	6.38	51.60	23.11	70.02	0.03	0.94	3.86
Chicken, dark meat, without skin, cooked (OZ)	6.66	0.52	6.66	54.29	24.38	75.13	0.03	1.03	3.86
Chicken, light meat, with skin, cooked (OZ)	5.10	0.36	7.23	57.83	19.56	72.58	0.01	0.46	5.32
Chicken, light meat, without skin, cooked (OZ)	4.82	0.34	7.80	61.66	19.99	78.25	0.01	0.46	4.79
Chicken, light meat, without skin, without visible fat, cooked (OZ)	4.82	0.34	7.80	61.52	19.99	78.25	0.01	0.46	3.71
Chicken-fried steak (untrimmed beef round) (PC)	15.07	2.35	22.82	181.52	385.82	304.33	0.13	3.84	23.39
Chitterlings, cooked (CP)	43.47	5.96	16.10	75.67	62.79	12.88	0.37	8.15	3.22
Clams, cooked or canned (MD)	11.50	3.49	2.25	42.25	14	78.50	0.09	0.34	1.57
Corned beef, canned (OZ)	3.40	0.59	3.97	31.47	285.20	38.56	0.02	1.01	5.39
Crab, all types, cooked, fresh or frozen (OZ)	29.48	0.26	9.36	58.40	79.10	91.85	0.18	1.20	14.46

Crabmeat, canned (OZ)	28.63	0.24	11.06	73.71	94.41	106.03	0.22	1.14	6.24
Duck, domestic, with skin, cooked (OZ)	3.12	0.77	4.54	44.23	16.73	57.83	0.07	0.53	3.86
Duck, domestic, without skin, cooked (OZ)	3.69	0.79	6.38	72.58	20.13	90.72	0.07	0.74	3.86
Fish, carp, cooked (OZ)	15.59	0.54	7.94	89.02	18.99	131.26	0.07	0.24	16.73
Fish, chinook salmon, smoked (OZ)	3.12	0.24	5.10	46.49	222.26	49.61	0.07	0.09	6.8
Fish, cisco, smoked (OZ)	7.37	0.14	4.82	42.52	136.36	83.07	0.06	0.09	9.36
Fish, cod, dried, salted, soaked in water, cooked (OZ)	7.99	0.29	7.47	64.92	146	11.06	0.01	0.16	12.32
Fish, flounder, cooked (OZ)	5.10	0.10	16.44	81.93	29.77	97.52	0.01	0.18	12.76
Fish, gefilte (PC)	17.86	0.62	24.33	154.95	159.48	247.55	0.06	0.48	24.74
Fish, haddock, smoked (OZ)	13.89	0.40	15.31	71.16	216.31	117.65	0.01	0.14	13.61
Fish, mackerel, Atlantic, cooked (OZ)	4.25	0.45	27.50	78.81	23.53	113.68	0.03	0.27	7.37
Fish, salmon, chinook (king) and sockeye (red), cooked (OZ)	12.19	0.19	8.79	96.67	21.55	180.31	0.02	0.20	7.37
Fish, salmon, pink, canned (CP)	377.01	1.49	60.18	582.33	980.58	577.02	0.18	1.63	132.75
Fish, salmon, pink, canned without salt (CP)	377.01	1.49	60.18	582.33	132.75	577.02	0.18	1.63	132.75
Fish, sardines, canned, drained (MD)	45.84	0.35	4.68	58.80	60.60	47.64	0.02	0.16	4.2
Fish, whitefish, cooked (OZ)	8.79	0.40	9.36	69.17	20.13	129.84	0.04	0.25	13.32
Fish fillet, breaded, commercial (approx. 18% fat) (OZ)	3.26	0.33	8.32	40.86	94.90	47.31	0.03	0.12	7.75

MINERAL COUNTER	CALC (mg)	IRON (mg)	MAG (mg)	PHOS (mg)	SOD (mg)	POTA (mg)	COP (mg)	ZINC (mg)	SELE (µg)
Fish stick, breaded, commercial (approx. 10% fat) (OZ)	3.36	0.43	7.75	37.71	158.79	43.08	0.03	0.13	7.78
Fowl, wild, cooked, with or without skin (OZ)	13.89	2.38	9.92	87.88	28.35	116.23	0.02	0.39	14.46
Frankfurter, beef, low salt (REG)	3.87	0.49	4.95	41.28	307.80	315.90	0.02	0.93	3.43
Frankfurter, beef, regular (REG)	9	0.64	1.35	39.15	461.70	74.70	0.03	0.98	4.05
Frankfurter, beef and pork, low salt, regular (REG)	10.61	0.36	4.68	51.55	300.15	307.80	0.02	0.84	5.87
Frankfurter, beef and pork, reduced fat (LK)	12.51	0.77	9.40	83.47	628.21	123.61	0.05	1.95	8.12
Frankfurter, beef and pork, regular (REG)	4.95	0.52	4.50	38.70	504	75.15	0.04	0.83	4.05
Frankfurter, chicken, regular (REG)	47.70	0.83	6.30	85.05	505.35	80.55	0.04	1.40	4.05
Game, wild, cooked (OZ)	1.98	1.27	6.80	64.07	15.31	94.97	0.09	0.78	13.89
Goose, domestic, with skin, cooked (OZ)	3.69	0.80	6.24	76.54	19.84	93.27	0.07	0.74	3.86
Herring, canned or smoked (MD)	33.60	0.60	18.40	130	367.20	178.80	0.05	0.54	10.8
Herring, pickled (PC)	11.55	0.18	1.20	13.35	130.50	10.35	0.01	0.08	4.05
Lamb, chop, arm (9% fat), no visible fat, cooked (OZ)	2.27	0.62	7.09	57.55	20.13	94.41	0.03	1.37	3.38
Lamb, chop, breast (36% fat), cooked (OZ)	2.55	0.31	5.10	44.23	13.95	63.82	0.05	1.02	5.42
Lamb, chop, loin (24% fat), cooked (OZ)	5.10	0.60	6.52	51.03	18.14	69.74	0.03	0.97	4.82

Food									
Lamb, crown roast (30% fat), cooked (OZ)	6.24	0.45	5.67	47.06	20.70	76.83	0.03	0.99	4.82
Lamb, leg (20% fat), cooked (OZ)	5.67	0.56	6.52	52.16	18.71	71.16	0.03	1.48	4.82
Lamb, shank roast (13% fat), cooked (OZ)	5.95	0.50	6.52	55.28	22.96	89.30	0.04	1.27	3.76
Liver, beef, cooked (OZ)	1.98	1.92	5.67	114.53	19.84	66.62	1.28	1.72	15.88
Liver, calves or veal, cooked (OZ)	1.98	0.74	5.39	90.44	15.03	58.12	2.25	2.70	17.86
Liver, chicken, cooked (OZ)	3.97	2.40	5.95	88.45	14.46	39.69	0.10	1.23	10.21
Liver, lamb, cooked (OZ)	2.27	2.35	6.24	119.07	15.88	62.65	2	2.24	25.51
Liver, pork, cooked (OZ)	2.83	5.08	3.97	68.32	13.89	42.52	0.18	1.91	18.14
Liverwurst (SL)	4.68	1.15	2.16	41.40	154.80	30.60	0.04	0.41	10.44
Lobster, cooked (MD)	63.44	0.41	36.40	192.40	395.20	366.01	2.02	3.04	82.16
Luncheon meat, bologna, beef (SL)	3.40	0.47	3.40	24.95	278.11	44.51	0.01	0.61	4.82
Luncheon meat, bologna, beef and pork (SL)	3.40	0.43	3.12	25.80	288.89	51.03	0.02	0.55	4.82
Luncheon meat, bologna, pork (SL)	2.53	0.18	3.22	31.97	272.32	64.63	0.02	0.47	6.9
Luncheon meat, bologna, turkey or chicken (SL)	14.74	0.45	4.11	33.59	266.77	62.80	0.01	0.50	9.36
Luncheon meat, chicken breast (SL)	3.40	0.21	4.42	35.74	334.02	51.04	0.01	0.26	2.69
Luncheon meat, corned beef (SL)	0.97	0.29	3.36	25.10	204.01	45.14	0.01	0.57	2.38
Luncheon meat, pastrami, beef (OZ)	2.55	0.54	5.10	42.52	347.85	64.64	0.02	1.21	5.39
Luncheon meat, pastrami, turkey (SL)	2.55	0.47	3.97	56.70	296.26	73.71	0.01	0.61	9.36
Luncheon meat, salami, beef (SL)	2.07	0.50	3.22	25.99	270.48	51.52	0.03	0.50	4.6

MINERAL COUNTER	CALC (mg)	IRON (mg)	MAG (mg)	PHOS (mg)	SOD (mg)	POTA (mg)	COP (mg)	ZINC (mg)	SELE (µg)
Luncheon meat, salami, beef and pork (SL)	2.99	0.61	3.45	26.45	244.95	45.54	0.05	0.49	4.6
Luncheon meat, salami, beef and pork, low salt (SL)	43.54	0.20	5.29	49.11	199.87	199.87	0.01	0.40	3.45
Luncheon meat, salami, dry or hard, pork (SL)	1.30	0.13	2.20	22.90	226	37.80	0.02	0.42	3.3
Luncheon meat, salami, dry or hard, pork and beef (SL)	0.80	0.15	1.70	14.20	186	37.80	0.01	0.32	3.3
Luncheon meat, turkey breast (SL)	2.74	0.16	3.97	29.24	290.43	37.17	0.01	0.22	2.3
Oyster, raw (MD)	6.30	0.93	6.58	18.90	29.54	21.84	0.62	12.71	7.98
Oysters, cooked (MD)	6.30	0.84	6.65	14.21	29.54	19.67	0.53	12.71	3.43
Pepperoni, pork and beef (SL)	0.55	0.08	0.88	6.54	112.20	19.08	0	0.14	1.81
Pork, picnic shoulder (14% fat), fresh, no visible fat, cooked (OZ)	1.70	0.26	6.24	60.67	13.61	98.09	0.01	0.75	2.42
Pork, chop, center loin (21% fat), fresh, cooked (OZ)	4.25	0.28	6.24	72.86	16.73	95.82	0.03	0.87	2.62
Pork, chop, loin (23% fat), smoked, cooked (OZ)	1.98	0.25	3.69	44.23	275.85	55	0.02	0.69	13.16
Pork, chop, rib (25% fat), fresh, cooked (OZ)	9.64	0.31	5.67	59.53	8.50	92.42	0.02	0.94	2.77

Food									
Pork, ham, Polish (15% fat), smoked, cooked (OZ)	2.27	0.39	4.82	68.89	266.77	101.21	0.04	0.71	11.73
Pork, ham, extra lean (6% fat), smoked, cooked (OZ)	2.27	0.42	3.97	55.57	341.05	81.36	0.02	0.82	9.7
Pork, ham, rump (11% fat), fresh, no visible fat, cooked (OZ)	1.70	0.28	6.80	62.94	14.17	102.91	0	0.80	2.23
Pork, ham, shank (21% fat), smoked, cooked (OZ)	2.83	0.27	3.97	62.65	303.91	73.14	0.03	0.71	6.8
Pork, loin ribs (30% fat), fresh, cooked (OZ)	13.32	0.52	6.80	73.99	26.37	90.72	0.04	1.30	3.38
Pork, salt, cooked (SL)	1.36	0.27	1.70	20.40	206.04	7.14	0.01	0.14	7.14
Pork, smoked (5% fat), low salt (OZ)	1.13	0.31	5.10	73.14	234.74	248.35	0.02	0.53	9.7
Pork, tenderloin roast (5% fat), fresh, cooked (OZ)	1.70	0.42	7.94	73.43	15.88	123.89	0.01	0.75	1.91
Sausage, braunschweiger (SL)	1.62	1.68	1.98	30.24	205.74	35.82	0.04	0.51	3.96
Sausage, chorizo (LK)	4.80	0.95	10.80	90	741	238.80	0.05	2.05	15
Sausage, Italian (LK)	16.32	1.02	12.24	115.60	626.96	206.72	0.05	1.63	17
Sausage, knackwurst or bratwurst (LK)	7.48	0.62	7.48	66.64	686.80	135.32	0.04	1.13	17
Sausage, Polish (LK)	9.07	1.09	10.58	102.82	662.26	179.17	0.07	1.46	18.9
Sausage, pork and beef, fresh, cooked (LK)	1.30	0.15	1.56	13.91	104.65	24.57	0.01	0.24	1.95
Sausage, pork, fresh, cooked (LK)	4.16	0.16	2.21	23.92	168.22	46.93	0.02	0.32	1.95

MINERAL COUNTER	CALC (mg)	IRON (mg)	MAG (mg)	PHOS (mg)	SOD (mg)	POTA (mg)	COP (mg)	ZINC (mg)	SELE (µg)
Sausage, turkey, fresh, cooked (LK)	4.99	0.35	4.57	35.35	234.27	48.02	0.02	0.65	2.66
Sausage, turkey, smoked (OZ)	4.80	0.33	4.32	33	253.09	44.83	0.02	0.60	2.49
Scallops, cooked (LG)	17.25	0.45	10.35	50.70	39.75	71.40	0.01	0.23	13.6
Sausage, Vienna, cooked (LK)	1.60	0.14	1.12	7.84	152.48	16.16	0	0.26	5.28
Shrimp, cooked, canned without salt (OZ)	11.06	0.88	9.64	38.84	63.50	51.60	0.05	0.44	18.14
Shrimp, cooked, canned with salt (OZ)	16.73	0.78	11.62	66.06	651.77	59.53	0.09	0.36	18.14
Squid, cooked (OZ)	11.91	0.25	12.19	61.80	16.44	91.85	0.60	0.57	22.71
Surimi (OZ)	2.55	0.07	12.19	79.95	244.94	31.75	0.01	0.09	12.76
Sushi or sashimi (raw tuna) (OZ)	2.27	0.29	14.17	72.01	11.06	71.44	0.03	0.17	29.37
Tuna, canned, oil pack, drained (CP)	20.80	2.22	49.60	497.60	566.40	331.20	0.11	1.44	124.8
Tuna, canned, oil pack, drained, no salt added (CP)	20.80	2.22	49.60	497.60	80	331.20	0.11	1.44	124.8
Tuna, canned, water pack, drained (CP)	19.20	5.12	46.40	297.60	569.60	502.40	0.02	0.70	165.76
Tuna, canned, water pack, drained, low sodium (CP)	19.20	5.12	46.40	297.60	324.80	502.40	0.02	0.70	165.76
Tuna, canned, water pack, drained, no salt (CP)	19.20	5.12	46.40	297.60	80	502.40	0.02	0.70	165.76
Turkey breast, processed (OZ)	2.55	0.19	5.95	60.67	112.55	70.31	0.01	0.43	4.04

Turkey ham (OZ)	2.83	0.78	4.54	54.15	282.37	92.14	0.03	0.83	14.46
Veal, breast (25% fat), cooked (OZ)	3.12	1.11	7.94	66.06	24.66	138.91	0.07	0.93	3.4
Veal, cutlet (10% fat), cooked (OZ)	3.69	0.26	7.37	63.22	23.53	99.51	0.04	0.95	3.4
Veal, rib roast (14% fat), cooked (OZ)	3.12	0.27	6.24	55.85	26.08	83.63	0.03	1.16	3.4
Veal, rump roast (6% fat), cooked (OZ)	7.65	0.33	7.65	64.07	25.80	100.93	0.04	1.22	3.4

MILK, DAIRY, AND RELATED PRODUCTS

Buttermilk, 1% fat (CP)	285.18	0.12	26.83	218.54	257	370.68	0.02	1.03	2.52
Buttermilk, whole (CP)	273.60	0.24	31.20	211.20	230.40	369.60	0.07	0.98	2.47
Cheese, 17–26% fat (feta) (OZ)	139.62	0.18	5.45	95.60	316.41	17.52	0.01	0.82	3.12
Cheese, 22–28% fat (Camembert, Brie, Jarlsberg) (OZ)	109.88	0.09	5.66	98.26	238.62	52.90	0.01	0.67	3.12
Cheese, 25–30% fat (Edam, Gouda, Romano, provolone, Tilsit) (OZ)	207.24	0.12	8.44	151.84	273.58	53.21	0.01	1.06	3.12
Cheese, 26–31% fat (blue, Roquefort, Limburger, Liederkranz) (OZ)	149.57	0.09	6.50	109.83	395.57	72.66	0.01	0.75	3.12
Cheese, 28–32% fat (Muenster, brick, Monterey Jack, fontina, Cheshire) (OZ)	203.35	0.12	7.75	132.59	177.95	38.10	0.01	0.80	3.97
Cheese, 29–33% fat (process American) (OZ)	142.03	0.11	6.31	178.04	405.52	45.93	0.01	0.85	3.69

MINERAL COUNTER	CALC (mg)	IRON (mg)	MAG (mg)	PHOS (mg)	SOD (mg)	POTA (mg)	COP (mg)	ZINC (mg)	SELE (µg)
Cheese, 31–37% fat (cheddar, colby, Havarti) (OZ)	147.99	0.19	7.88	122.47	175.91	27.90	0.01	0.88	5.1
Cheese, imitation, low cholesterol, 19–26% fat (OZ)	136.36	0.14	6.01	106.03	395.48	41.67	0.01	0.57	3.52
Cheese, mozzarella, part skim milk, low moisture (OZ)	207.32	0.07	7.45	148.58	149.60	26.89	0.01	0.89	4.15
Cheese, Parmesan, fresh or dry (TB)	68.78	0.05	2.54	40.35	93.07	5.35	0	0.16	1
Cheese, ricotta, part skim milk (CP)	669.12	1.08	36.33	449.20	306.76	307.50	0.07	3.30	15.6
Cheese, ricotta, whole milk (CP)	509.22	0.93	27.80	388.93	206.89	257.32	0.05	2.85	17.24
Cheese foods and spreads, pasteurized processed, 20–26% fat (TB)	90.88	0.10	4.89	130.24	257.60	41.60	0.01	0.45	2.69
Cottage cheese, 1% fat (CP)	137.63	0.32	12.07	302.39	917.56	193.23	0.07	0.86	11.75
Cottage cheese, 2% fat (CP)	154.81	0.36	13.56	340.13	917.56	217.41	0.07	0.95	11.75
Cottage cheese, 2% fat, no salt added (CP)	155.36	0.36	13.61	341.33	45.36	218.18	0.07	0.95	11.79
Cottage cheese, 4% fat (CP)	126	0.29	11.05	276.78	850.08	177.03	0.06	0.78	10.92
Cottage cheese, 4% fat, no salt added (CP)	126	0.29	11.05	276.78	42	177.03	0.06	0.78	10.92
Cottage cheese, low fat (CP)	154.81	0.36	13.56	340.13	917.56	217.41	0.07	0.95	11.75
Cottage cheese, uncreamed (CP)	45.96	0.33	5.71	150.80	18.56	46.98	0.04	0.68	7.54
Cream, half and half (CP)	253.86	0.17	24.61	230.38	98.49	313.63	0.02	1.23	1.33

Cream, heavy whipping (CP)	153.75	0.07	16.73	148.51	89.49	179.45	0.02	0.55	0.48
Cream, light (CP)	230.88	0.10	20.76	191.76	95.04	292.08	0.02	0.65	0.48
Cream, whipping (CP)	165.87	0.07	17.28	146.03	81.98	231.35	0.02	0.60	0.48
Cream, whipping, unsweetened (TB)	5.20	0	0.54	4.58	2.57	7.26	0	0.02	0.01
Cream cheese, 35% fat (TB)	11.19	0.17	0.90	14.62	41.37	16.72	0	0.08	0.7
Cream cheese, light, 18% fat (TB)	19.83	0.10	0.94	18.73	81.66	15.84	0	0.07	0.76
Cream cheese, Neufchâtel (TB)	10.54	0.04	1.06	19.08	55.92	15.97	0	0.07	0.57
Ice cream, 7% fat (light), all flavors except chocolate or coffee (CP)	162.81	0.11	17.68	130.49	100.61	250	0.01	0.68	8.54
Ice cream, 7% fat (light), chocolate or coffee (CP)	151.22	0.62	26.83	131.71	98.17	280.48	0.09	0.62	8.54
Ice cream, 11% fat (average), all flavors except chocolate and coffee (CP)	168.96	0.12	18.48	138.60	105.60	262.68	0.03	0.91	9.24
Ice cream, 11% fat (average), chocolate or coffee (CP)	143.88	1.23	38.28	141.24	100.32	328.68	0.18	0.77	9.24
Ice cream, 16% fat (rich), all flavors except chocolate or coffee (CP)	173.16	0.07	16.28	140.60	82.88	235.32	0.03	0.59	10.36
Ice cream, 16% fat (rich), chocolate or coffee (CP)	173.16	0.07	16.28	140.60	82.88	235.32	0.03	0.59	10.36
Ice milk, hardened, 4% fat, all flavors except chocolate (CP)	183.48	0.13	19.80	143.88	112.20	278.52	0.01	0.58	9.24

MINERAL COUNTER	CALC (mg)	IRON (mg)	MAG (mg)	PHOS (mg)	SOD (mg)	POTA (mg)	COP (mg)	ZINC (mg)	SELE (µg)
Milk, 1% fat (CP)	300.12	0.12	33.72	234.73	123.22	380.88	0.02	0.95	9.44
Milk, 2% fat (CP)	296.70	0.12	33.35	232.04	121.76	376.74	0.02	0.95	7.27
Milk, canned, condensed, sweetened (CP)	867.51	0.58	78.49	775.10	388.62	1136.48	0.03	2.88	5.72
Milk, canned, evaporated skim, undiluted (CP)	741.12	0.74	69.12	498.94	294.40	848.64	0.05	2.30	3.2
Milk, canned, evaporated whole, undiluted (CP)	657.22	0.48	60.96	510.30	266.62	763.81	0.05	1.94	3.15
Milk, low fat (CP)	296.70	0.12	33.35	232.04	121.76	376.74	0.02	0.95	7.27
Milk, powdered, nonfat, instant (TS)	17.48	0	1.66	13.98	7.79	24.22	0	0.06	0.24
Milk, powdered, nonfat, regular (TS)	30.75	0.01	2.93	24.60	13.71	42.61	0	0.11	0.42
Milk, skim (CP)	302.33	0.10	27.83	247.20	126.17	405.72	0.02	0.98	11.64
Milk, whole (CP)	291.34	0.12	32.79	227.90	119.56	369.66	0.02	0.93	2.93
Sherbet (CP)	103.68	0.27	15.36	76.80	88.32	184.32	0.06	0.92	1.21
Sour cream, low fat (CP)	319.92	0.50	85.19	319.92	240.56	560.01	0	2.73	1.93
Whipped topping, aerosol, saturated vegetable fat (TB)	0.23	0	0.04	0.80	2.69	0.84	0	0	0
Whipped topping, frozen, saturated vegetable fat (TB)	0.30	0.01	0.08	0.36	1.19	0.85	0	0	0

Whipped topping, powdered, reduced calorie, with aspartame (TB)	3.26	0	0.70	4.64	6.58	8.08	0	0.01	0
Yogurt, 1% fat, all flavors (CP)	323.40	1.96	34.30	269.50	102.90	475.30	0.02	0.98	4.53
Yogurt, 1% fat, sweetened with aspartame, all flavors (CP)	248.48	0.27	27.07	206.09	108.22	392.51	0.12	0.83	10.71
Yogurt, 2–4% fat, all flavors (CP)	1.13	365.05	0.17	34.30	286.65	139.65	465.50	0.02	1.76
Yogurt, 2–4% fat, unflavored or plain (CP)	295.71	0.12	28.37	232.50	113.68	378.77	0.02	1.45	3.06
Yogurt, frozen, 1–2% fat, all flavors except chocolate (CP)	293.17	0.14	28.12	230.44	112.71	375.38	0.15	1.43	5.11
Yogurt, frozen, 1–2% fat, chocolate (CP)	288.11	0.87	53.27	259.82	109.30	440.50	0.37	1.74	6
Yogurt, low fat, all flavors except coffee (CP)	372.15	0.17	35.70	292.53	143.08	476.52	0.20	1.81	6.49
Yogurt, low fat, coffee flavor (CP)	370.39	0.20	36.87	291.97	142.34	488.70	0.20	1.81	6.52
Yogurt, low fat, unflavored or plain (CP)	447.37	0.20	42.75	351.57	171.99	572.81	0.02	2.18	3.80
NUTS AND SEEDS									
Almonds, unsalted (CP)	377.72	5.20	420.32	738.40	15.62	1039.44	1.33	4.15	6.67
Brazil nuts, unsalted (CP)	246.40	4.76	315	840	2.80	840	2.48	6.43	2261
Cashews, salted (CP)	53.30	5.33	331.50	553.80	813.80	689	2.82	6.17	26
Cashews, unsalted (CP)	53.30	5.33	331.50	553.80	22.10	689	2.82	6.17	26

MINERAL COUNTER	CALC (mg)	IRON (mg)	MAG (mg)	PHOS (mg)	SOD (mg)	POTA (mg)	COP (mg)	ZINC (mg)	SELE (µg)
Chestnuts, unsalted (CP)	95.81	3.40	105.82	250.25	52.91	1409.98	0.93	0.50	2.57
Coconut, fresh (PC)	6.30	1.09	14.40	50.85	9	160.20	0.19	0.49	6.3
Coconut, shredded, sweetened (TS)	0.29	0.04	0.97	2.08	5.08	6.54	0.01	0.04	0.28
Coconut, shredded, unsweetened (TS)	0.43	0.06	1.50	3.44	0.62	9.07	0.01	0.03	0.43
Filberts, hazelnuts, unsalted (CP)	253.80	4.41	384.75	421.20	4.05	600.75	2.04	3.24	4.32
Hickory nuts, unsalted (CP)	61	2.12	173	336	1	436	0.74	4.31	8.1
Macadamia nuts, salted (CP)	60.30	2.41	156.78	268	348.40	440.86	0.40	1.47	NA
Peanut butter, no salt added, creamy or chunky (TS)	1.81	0.09	8.37	17.22	0.91	38.43	0.03	0.13	0.53
Peanut butter, with salt, creamy or chunky (TS)	1.81	0.09	8.37	17.22	25.48	38.43	0.03	0.13	0.53
Peanuts, salted (CP)	126.72	2.64	266.40	744.48	623.52	982.08	1.87	9.55	10.08
Peanuts, unsalted (CP)	126.72	2.64	266.40	744.48	8.64	982.08	1.87	9.55	10.08
Pecans, salted (CP)	37.40	2.32	141.90	323.40	831.60	394.90	1.32	6.05	12.87
Pecans, unsalted (CP)	38.88	2.30	138.24	314.28	1.08	423.36	1.27	5.91	12.64
Pine nuts, unsalted (CP)	9.60	3.67	280.80	42	86.40	753.60	1.24	5.14	NA
Pistachio nuts, salted (CP)	89.60	4.06	166.40	609.28	998.40	1241.60	1.55	1.74	576
Pumpkin seeds, salted (CP)	59.34	20.62	736.92	1617.36	793.50	1112.28	1.90	10.27	7.73

Pumpkin seeds, unsalted (CP)	59.34	20.62	736.92	1617.36	24.84	1112.28	1.90	10.27	7.73
Sesame seeds (TB)	10.48	0.62	27.76	62.08	3.20	32.56	0.12	0.82	0.06
Sunflower seeds, hulled, salted (CP)	167.04	9.75	509.76	1015.20	1123.20	992.16	2.52	7.29	87.84
Sunflower seeds, hulled, unsalted (CP)	167.04	9.75	509.76	1015.20	4.32	992.16	2.52	7.29	87.84
Tahini (sesame butter) (TS)	21.30	0.45	4.75	36.60	5.75	20.70	0.08	0.23	2.5
Walnuts, unsalted (CP)	94	2.44	169	317	10	502	1.39	2.73	7.4

VEGETABLES AND LEGUMES

Artichokes, cooked, without salt (CP)	75.60	2.17	100.80	144.48	159.60	594.72	0.39	0.82	1.18
Arugula, raw (CP)	32	0.24	9.40	10.40	5.40	73.80	0.02	0.09	0.3
Asparagus, canned, drained solids, with salt (CP)	38.72	4.43	24.20	104.06	943.80	416.24	0.24	0.97	9.83
Asparagus, fresh or frozen, cooked without salt (CP)	41.40	1.15	23.40	99	7.20	392.40	0.31	1.01	10.75
Baked beans with franks, canned (CP)	137.19	4.06	77.95	261.93	1163.08	643.96	0.23	3.98	16.55
Bamboo shoots, canned, cooked, with salt (CP)	10.48	0.42	5.24	32.75	9.17	104.80	0.14	0.85	NA
Beans, kidney, dry, cooked or canned, without fat, without salt (CP)	49.56	5.20	79.65	251.34	3.54	713.31	0.42	1.89	3.65
Beans, kidney, dry, cooked or canned, without fat, with salt (CP)	50.48	5.26	80.71	253.57	425.76	719.74	0.42	1.91	3.72

MINERAL COUNTER

	CALC (mg)	IRON (mg)	MAG (mg)	PHOS (mg)	SOD (mg)	POTA (mg)	COP (mg)	ZINC (mg)	SELE (µg)
Beans, lima, cooked, fresh or frozen, without salt (CP)	37.40	2.31	57.80	107.10	90.10	693.60	0.08	0.75	0.24
Beans, lima, dry, cooked or canned, without fat, without salt (CP)	31.96	4.49	80.84	208.68	3.76	955.04	0.43	1.79	4.55
Beans, lima, dry, cooked or canned, without fat, with salt (CP)	32.58	4.51	81.52	209.43	449.85	958.59	0.43	1.79	4.61
Beans, navy, dry, cooked or canned, without fat, without salt (CP)	127.40	4.51	107.38	285.74	1.82	669.76	0.53	1.93	8.41
Beans, navy, dry, cooked or canned, without fat, with salt (CP)	127.76	4.51	107.63	285.45	431.67	669.18	0.53	1.93	8.44
Beans, northern, dry, cooked or canned, without fat, without salt (CP)	161.10	6.62	112.77	202.27	10.74	1004.19	0.52	2.47	7.8
Beans, northern, dry, cooked or canned, without fat, with salt (CP)	161.10	6.62	112.77	202.27	433.18	1004.19	0.52	2.47	7.8
Beans, pinto, dry, cooked or canned, without fat, without salt (CP)	82.08	4.46	94.05	273.60	3.42	800.28	0.44	1.85	12.59
Beans, pinto, dry, cooked or canned, without fat, with salt (CP)	83.23	4.50	95.18	275.86	411.07	806.98	0.44	1.86	12.72
Beans, yellow, canned, drained solids, with salt (CP)	35.36	1.22	17.68	25.84	341.36	148.24	0.05	0.39	0

Beans, yellow, cooked, fresh or frozen, without salt (CP)	60.75	1.11	28.35	32.40	17.55	151.20	0.09	0.84	0
Beets, Harvard (CP)	30.58	3.30	33.81	33.61	313.09	277.96	0.12	0.41	16.81
Beets, pickled (CP)	39.48	1.84	49.18	69.29	398.98	564.41	0.15	0.66	36.17
Beets, red, canned, drained solids, with salt (CP)	25.50	3.09	28.90	28.90	231.20	251.60	0.10	0.36	1.53
Beets, red, cooked, fresh or frozen, without salt (CP)	27.20	1.34	39.10	64.60	130.90	518.50	0.12	0.59	1.53
Broccoli, cooked, fresh or frozen, without salt (CP)	93.84	1.12	36.80	101.20	44.16	331.20	0.07	0.55	1.51
Broccoli, raw (CP)	42.24	0.77	22	58.08	23.76	286	0.04	0.35	1.5
Brussels sprouts, cooked, fresh or frozen, without salt (CP)	37.20	1.15	37.20	83.70	35.65	503.75	0.11	0.56	3.49
Cabbage, Chinese (pak-choi), cooked, drained (CP)	158.10	1.77	18.70	49.30	57.80	630.70	0.03	0.29	3.48
Cabbage, Chinese (pak-choi), raw, shredded (CP)	73.50	0.56	13.30	25.90	45.50	176.40	0.01	0.13	1.54
Cabbage, Chinese (pe-tsai), cooked, drained (CP)	38.08	0.36	11.90	46.41	10.71	267.75	0.04	0.21	2.62
Cabbage, Chinese (pe-tsai), raw, shredded (CP)	58.52	0.24	9.88	22.04	6.84	180.88	0.03	0.17	1.67
Cabbage, cooked, without salt (CP)	46.50	0.25	12	22.50	12	145.50	0.01	0.13	1.86

MINERAL COUNTER	CALC (mg)	IRON (mg)	MAG (mg)	PHOS (mg)	SOD (mg)	POTA (mg)	COP (mg)	ZINC (mg)	SELE (µg)
Cabbage, raw (CP)	32.90	0.41	10.50	16.10	12.60	172.20	0.01	0.13	1.57
Carrot, raw (CP)	29.70	0.55	16.50	48.40	38.50	355.30	0.05	0.22	3.19
Carrot juice (CP)	59.04	1.13	34.44	103.32	71.34	718.32	0.12	0.44	6.57
Carrots, canned, drained solids, with salt (CP)	36.50	0.93	11.68	35.04	351.86	261.34	0.15	0.38	1.9
Carrots, fresh or frozen, cooked, without salt (CP)	48.36	0.97	20.28	46.80	102.96	354.12	0.20	0.47	1.28
Cauliflower, fresh or frozen, cooked, without salt (CP)	30.60	0.74	16.20	43.20	32.40	250.20	0.04	0.23	5.76
Cauliflower, raw (CP)	22	0.44	15	44	30	303	0.04	0.28	3.2
Celery, raw (CP)	48	0.48	13.20	30	104.40	344.40	0.04	0.16	1.32
Chard, Swiss, fresh or frozen, cooked, without salt (CP)	101.50	3.95	150.50	57.75	313.25	960.75	0.28	0.58	45.5
Chickpeas, dry, cooked or canned, without fat, without salt (CP)	80.36	4.74	78.72	275.52	11.48	477.24	0.57	2.51	6.4
Chickpeas, dry, cooked or canned, without fat, with salt (CP)	80.36	4.74	78.72	275.52	398.52	477.24	0.57	2.51	6.4
Corn, ear, cooked (MD)	1.54	0.47	24.64	79.31	13.09	191.73	0.04	0.37	1.17

Food									
Corn, whole kernel, drained solids, canned, with salt (CP)	8.20	1.41	32.80	106.60	529.72	319.80	0.10	0.64	0.66
Corn, whole kernel, fresh or frozen, without salt (CP)	3.28	0.49	29.52	77.08	8.20	227.96	0.05	0.57	1.97
Cucumber, raw (CP)	14.56	0.27	11.44	20.80	2.08	149.76	0.03	0.21	6.55
Eggplant, cooked, boiled, without salt, diced (CP)	5.76	0.34	12.48	21.12	2.88	238.08	0.11	0.14	6.43
Endive, raw (CP)	15.08	0.24	4.35	8.12	6.38	91.06	0.03	0.23	3.77
Fennel, bulb, raw (CP)	42.63	0.26	14.79	43.50	45.24	360.18	0.06	0.17	NA
Garlic, fresh (TS)	5.65	0.05	0.78	4.77	0.53	12.51	0.01	0.04	0.81
Ginger root, raw (CP)	17.28	0.48	41.28	25.92	12.48	398.40	0.22	0.33	NA
Green beans, canned, drained solids, with salt (CP)	35.36	1.22	17.68	25.84	341.36	148.24	0.05	0.39	1.22
Green beans, fresh or frozen, cooked, without salt (CP)	60.75	1.11	28.35	32.40	17.55	151.20	0.09	0.84	2.02
Greens, collard, fresh or frozen, cooked, without salt (CP)	29.44	0.20	8.96	10.24	20.48	167.68	0.04	0.14	2.94
Greens, turnip, fresh or frozen, cooked, without salt (CP)	197.28	1.15	31.68	41.76	41.76	292.32	0.36	0.20	1.41
Jicama, cooked, without salt (CP)	14.87	0.77	14.87	21.63	5.41	182.52	0.07	0.20	NA
Jicama, raw (CP)	19.50	0.78	20.80	23.40	7.80	227.50	0.05	0.43	0

MINERAL COUNTER	CALC (mg)	IRON (mg)	MAG (mg)	PHOS (mg)	SOD (mg)	POTA (mg)	COP (mg)	ZINC (mg)	SELE (µg)
Kohlrabi, fresh or frozen, cooked, without salt (CP)	41.25	0.66	31.35	74.25	34.65	561	0.21	0.51	NA
Kohlrabi, raw (CP)	33.60	0.56	26.60	64.40	28	490	0.18	0.04	NA
Lentils, dry, cooked or canned, without fat, without salt (CP)	37.62	6.59	71.28	356.40	3.96	730.62	0.49	2.51	7.39
Lentils, dry, cooked or canned, without fat, with salt (CP)	37.78	6.53	70.98	352.93	467.50	723.63	0.49	2.49	7.35
Lettuce (CP)	10.45	0.27	4.95	11	4.95	86.90	0.02	0.12	0.44
Mushrooms, canned, drained solids, with salt (CP)	17.16	1.23	23.40	102.96	663	201.24	0.36	1.12	8.42
Mushrooms, fresh or frozen, cooked, without salt (CP)	9.36	2.71	18.72	135.72	3.12	555.36	0.78	1.36	10.78
Mushrooms, raw, whole or sliced (CP)	3.50	0.87	7	72.80	2.80	259	0.34	0.51	7.7
Okra, fresh or frozen, cooked, without salt (CP)	176.64	1.23	93.84	84.64	5.52	430.56	0.18	1.14	0.74
Onions, fresh or frozen, cooked, without salt (CP)	46.20	0.50	23.10	73.50	6.30	348.60	0.15	0.44	6.51
Onions, raw (CP)	32	0.35	16	52.80	4.80	251.20	0.10	0.30	4.96
Parsley, fresh (TB)	5.17	0.23	1.87	2.17	2.10	20.77	0.01	0.04	0.02

Food									
Parsnips, fresh or frozen, cooked, without salt (CP)	57.72	0.90	45.24	107.64	15.60	572.52	0.22	0.41	11.54
Peas, blackeye, dry, cooked or canned, without fat, without salt (CP)	41.04	4.29	90.63	266.76	6.84	475.38	0.46	2.21	28.18
Peas, blackeye, dry, cooked or canned, without fat, with salt (CP)	41.04	4.29	90.63	266.76	410.40	475.38	0.46	2.21	28.18
Peas, blackeye, fresh, cooked (CP)	211.20	1.85	85.80	84.15	6.60	689.70	0.21	1.70	31.18
Peas, edible podded, fresh or frozen, cooked without salt (CP)	67.20	3.15	41.60	88	6.40	384	0.13	0.59	8.98
Peas, green, canned, drained solids, with salt (CP)	34	1.61	28.90	113.90	372.30	294.10	0.14	1.21	0.97
Peas, green, fresh or frozen, cooked, without salt (CP)	38.40	2.51	46.40	144	139.20	268.80	0.22	1.50	0.91
Peas, split, dry, cooked or canned, without fat, without salt (CP)	27.44	2.53	70.56	194.04	3.92	709.52	0.35	1.96	0.98
Peas, split, dry, cooked or canned, without fat, with salt (CP)	27.44	2.53	70.56	194.04	466.48	709.52	0.35	1.96	0.98
Peas and carrots, fresh or frozen, cooked, without salt (CP)	36.80	1.50	25.60	78.40	108.80	252.80	0.13	0.72	1.1
Pepper, chili, Mexican, canned (CP)	9.52	0.68	19.04	23.12	1595.28	254.32	0.14	0.23	2.72
Pepper, chili, fresh, cooked, without salt (CP)	23.26	1.55	32.30	56.30	9.04	416.16	0.22	0.38	2.72

MINERAL COUNTER	CALC (mg)	IRON (mg)	MAG (mg)	PHOS (mg)	SOD (mg)	POTA (mg)	COP (mg)	ZINC (mg)	SELE (μg)
Pepper, green, fresh or frozen, cooked, without salt (CP)	12.24	0.63	13.60	24.48	2.72	225.76	0.08	0.16	2.99
Pepper, green, raw (CP)	9	0.46	10	19	2	177	0.06	0.12	2.2
Pepper, red, fresh or frozen, cooked, without salt (CP)	12.24	0.63	13.60	24.48	2.72	225.76	0.08	0.16	2.99
Pepper, red, raw (CP)	9	0.46	10	19	2	177	0.06	0.12	2.2
Plantains, fresh, cooked, without salt (CP)	3.08	0.89	49.28	43.12	7.70	716.10	0.11	0.20	3.08
Potatoes, French fried (REG)	0.48	0.02	1.32	2.66	6.77	21.82	0.01	0.02	0.07
Potatoes, French fried, without salt (REG)	0.53	0.02	1.33	2.66	0.33	21.82	0.01	0.02	0.07
Potatoes, baked, without skin, without salt (MD)	4.65	0.33	23.25	46.50	4.65	363.63	0.20	0.27	1.05
Potatoes, baked, with skin, without salt (CP)	12.20	1.66	32.94	69.54	9.76	509.96	0.37	0.39	1.61
Potatoes, boiled, without skin, without salt (CP)	12.48	0.48	31.20	62.40	7.80	511.68	0.27	0.42	1.62
Potatoes, boiled, with skin, without salt (MD)	11.98	1.56	30.98	65.15	9.32	477.72	0.34	0.37	1.52
Pumpkin, canned, cooked (CP)	63.70	3.41	56.35	85.75	12.25	504.70	0.27	0.42	NA
Radicchio, raw (CP)	7.60	0.12	5.20	16	8.80	120.80	0.14	0.25	0.6
Radish, raw (CP)	24.36	0.34	10.44	20.88	27.84	269.12	0.05	0.35	2.32
Refried beans, canned (CP)	116.38	4.48	98.67	212.52	1072.72	994.29	1.04	3.47	13.81

Romaine, raw (CP)	10.80	0.33	1.80	13.50	2.40	87	0.01	0.07	NA
Rutabaga, fresh or frozen, cooked, without salt (CP)	81.60	0.90	39.10	95.20	34	554.20	0.07	0.59	0.17
Sauerkraut, cooked, canned, solids and liquid (CP)	70.80	3.47	30.68	47.20	1559.96	401.20	0.24	0.45	0.24
Scallion, cooked (CP)	131.40	0.96	43.80	67.89	8.76	529.98	0.13	0.92	5.04
Scallion, raw (CP)	72	1.48	20	37	16	276	0.08	0.39	2.3
Seaweed, kelp, raw (CP)	134.40	2.28	96.80	33.60	186.40	71.20	0.10	0.98	NA
Soybean curd (tofu) (OZ)	29.77	1.52	29.20	27.50	1.98	34.30	0.05	0.23	0.09
Soybeans, dry, cooked or canned, without salt (CP)	175.44	8.84	147.92	421.40	1.72	885.80	0.71	1.98	10.32
Soybeans, roasted (CP)	237.36	6.71	249.40	624.36	280.36	2528.40	1.43	5.40	27.02
Soy flour (CP)	175.10	5.41	364.65	419.90	11.05	2137.75	2.48	3.33	7.65
Spinach, canned, drained solids, with salt (CP)	271.78	4.92	109.14	94.16	419.44	479.36	0.39	0.98	2.55
Spinach, fresh or frozen, cooked, without salt (CP)	277.40	2.89	131.10	91.20	163.40	566.20	0.27	1.33	2.75
Spinach, raw (CP)	55.44	1.52	44.24	27.44	44.24	312.48	0.07	0.30	0.67
Sprouts, alfalfa, raw (CP)	10.56	0.32	8.91	23.10	1.98	26.07	0.05	0.30	NA
Sprouts, mung bean, canned, cooked, without salt (CP)	17.36	0.53	11.16	39.68	173.60	33.48	0.20	0.35	NA

MINERAL COUNTER	CALC (mg)	IRON (mg)	MAG (mg)	PHOS (mg)	SOD (mg)	POTA (mg)	COP (mg)	ZINC (mg)	SELE (µg)
Sprouts, soybean, raw (CP)	46.90	1.47	50.40	114.80	9.80	338.80	0.30	0.82	NA
Squash, summer, all varieties, fresh or frozen, cooked, without salt (CP)	48.60	0.65	43.20	70.20	1.80	345.60	0.18	0.70	0
Squash, winter, all varieties, fresh or frozen, cooked, without salt (CP)	34.30	0.81	19.60	49	2.45	406.70	0.22	0.64	3.18
Sweet potato, canned, syrup pack, drained solids, with salt (CP)	33.32	1.86	23.52	49	76.44	378.28	0.33	0.31	1.23
Sweet potatoes, candied (MD)	49.97	0.86	28.48	68.34	262.74	605.69	0.29	0.37	1.13
Sweet potatoes, canned, vacuum pack, drained solids, with salt (CP)	44	1.78	44	98	106	624	0.28	0.36	1.4
Sweet potatoes, fresh or frozen, cooked, without salt (CP)	71.40	1.15	51	140.25	25.50	1206.15	0.54	0.74	1.78
Tempeh, fresh or frozen (PTY)	210.92	5.13	158.76	467.21	13.61	832.36	1.52	4.11	13.61
Tomatillos, raw (CP)	9.24	1.19	26.40	51.48	1.32	353.76	0.11	0.29	5.28
Tomatoes, canned, no salt added (CP)	62.40	1.46	28.80	45.60	31.20	530.40	0.26	0.38	2.28
Tomatoes, canned, with salt (CP)	62.40	1.46	28.80	45.60	391.20	530.40	0.26	0.38	2.28
Tomatoes, fresh, cooked, without salt (CP)	14.40	1.34	33.60	74.40	26.40	669.60	0.22	0.26	2.28
Tomatoes, raw (CP)	9	0.81	19.80	43.20	16.20	399.60	0.13	0.16	2.34
Tomatoes, sun dried (CP)	59.40	2.99	104.76	192.24	1131.30	1850.58	0.77	1.07	8.73

546

Food									
Tomatoes, sun dried, oil pack, drained (CP)	51.70	2.61	89.10	152.90	292.60	1721.50	0.52	0.86	10.43
Tomato juice, no salt added (CP)	21.84	1.41	26.69	46.10	24.26	533.81	0.24	0.34	0
Tomato juice, salt added (CP)	21.84	1.41	26.69	46.10	875.93	533.81	0.24	0.34	0
Tomato paste, canned, no salt added (CP)	91.70	7.83	133.62	206.98	170.30	2441.84	1.55	2.10	13.83
Tomato paste, canned, with salt (CP)	91.70	7.83	133.62	206.98	2069.80	2441.84	1.55	2.10	13.83
Tomato sauce, canned, without fat, no salt added (CP)	34.30	1.89	46.55	78.40	73.50	908.95	0.49	0.61	2.74
Tomato sauce, canned, without fat, with salt (CP)	34.30	1.89	46.55	78.40	1482.25	908.95	0.49	0.61	2.74
Turnips, fresh or frozen, cooked, without salt (CP)	34.32	0.34	12.48	29.64	78	210.60	0.09	0.31	1.4
Vegetable juice, cocktail, no salt added (CP)	26.62	1.02	26.62	41.14	55.66	467.06	0.48	0.48	0.48
Vegetable juice, cocktail, salt added (CP)	26.62	1.02	26.62	41.14	883.30	467.06	0.48	0.48	0.48
Water chestnuts, cooked, canned (CP)	25.20	0.70	4.21	100.80	19.60	215.60	0.04	0.24	NA
Watercress, raw (CP)	40.80	0.07	7.14	20.40	13.94	112.20	0.03	0.04	NA
Zucchini, fresh or frozen, cooked, without salt (CP)	23.40	0.63	39.60	72	5.40	455.40	0.16	0.32	1.8
Zucchini, raw (CP)	19.50	0.55	28.60	41.60	3.90	322.40	0.08	0.26	3.9

Index

Prologue

In twenty-four hours, the killing would be over.

Morrissey savored the words: *the killing, over*.

He tipped back his chair and let the slow, broad sweep of the ceiling fan cool him. Ah, Froggie's, ah, the first beer of the evening—the first beer of the *last* evening. He pressed the icy Kronenbourg to his face, groaning with pleasure. Picking his soaked shirt away from his chest, he concentrated on coolness, the caress of the fan. Another hour before Vandiver got off shift. In the meantime, what was he supposed to do with this fantastic feeling?

He grinned around the room, then sobered, shocked at his breach of manners. It was like giggling at a funeral. He might be going home, but these poor devils were still stuck here. For them, the killing was not over. The misery of it rose from their pores. They hunched motionless over the teakwood bar, slumped around the tables as though gassed by the blue haze of cigarette smoke. He knew most of them—medical corps officers from the Saigon base hospital. He'd seen their eyes too often in his own mirror—moist, peeled negatives of death.

Well, screw it.

He jumped onto the table, swinging his arms and kicking a salt shaker off before he caught his balance. Some men at the bar turned and gave a few derisive claps.

"Thank you, thank you . . ." He waited until everyone was looking at him, the men at the tables too. "As you know," he said, "after twelve months of debauchery here at Mr. Dang's Froggie Bistro, Vandiver and I have run out of steam. We're packing it in."

"Rear echelon mother fuckers!" someone yelled.

Morrissey grinned and waited for the ripple of laughter to die down. "You're half right. West Virginny is about as rear echelon as it gets. But that part about mothers—you'll have to ask Madame Tho." He nodded toward the curtained door at the back of the room.

Tho stepped from the curtains, swept her robes around her, and bowed to the hoots and applause like the noblest of courtesans. Her face beamed under the heavy makeup. "Not in mother business," she said, "but you pay extra, we pretend."

There was more laughter, hearty this time.

Morrissey shouted, "Hooch for everyone, Mr. Dang. Captain Vandiver will pay you when he gets here." The men laughed again and then began to cheer. He jumped down, waving clasped hands over his head until the cheers died down and they began pressing in on Dang.

He restored the shaker to its place and sat down again, listening to the clamor of drink orders. Ah, that was better—noise, life. He craned his neck as Mr. Dang slipped toward him through the crowd. Good—Dang was bringing the usual two bourbons. Morrissey swallowed in anticipation. He hadn't thought he'd *need* a drink tonight, not with his natural high over going home. But he did.

Dang looked nervous, nibbling his lower lip with stained teeth. "Captain . . . you say . . . Vandiver pay?"

Morrissey dug a wad of bills from his pocket and dropped it on the tray. Dang beamed and set the drinks in their customary places. "Sank you, Captain. Good luck in U.S.A."

The weary, wrinkled smile slipped past Morrissey's defenses, paining him. He squeezed Dang's arm. It felt fragile, just fatless skin over bone. The old man looked half eaten away, as if the miseries brought here by his patrons had turned on him. Will I really miss the old hooch-waterer? Morrissey wondered. Palest damn Jack Daniels in Saigon.

But he said, "Thanks for taking such good care of us— *Cám ơn ông Đang kinh Dang.*" He traded bows with Dang, extending the courtesy of lowered eyes and sober expression until he knew the old man was gone. Then he gazed into his shot glass, tapping the rim and admiring the ripple of brown and gold under the light. I've abused you, old friend, he thought. You've been my whore. But I'll treat you right tonight. We'll have one last dance together at Froggie's for old times' sake.

He offered the glass to the room before drinking: To 149 Cliff Street, Ridgetown, West Virginia. To the elm in the backyard, the streaks of cat piss on the basement windows, and the front step that always creaks. *To home.*

He held the first sip, letting it sting his tongue. What would it be like tomorrow? I will get on the plane, he thought. I will fly out of Bien Hoa. The sky will be blue, and there will be no shelling. I will come down in the U.S. of A., America the beautiful. Janet will be there, waiting for me . . .

Suddenly he was almost breathless. He swallowed more bourbon. Janet, Janet. What would she feel like? Soft against his chest, firm along his legs. Her hair would have a faint herbal smell from that shampoo she always used. When they kissed, he would lick her lip gloss and taste cinnamon. Later, she would wrap her legs around his waist and . . . Morrissey realized he was rising under the table and groaned. No, it was too soon, twenty-four hours, still too far away, he'd go ape-shit if he went on thinking about her now.

He sat, grinning. Okay, a month in the sack with my wife. Then Alan and I will set up the medical clinic in that old storefront on Jackson Street. A nice family practice, all clean and easy. No more bossing thirty men. I'll do all the lab work myself. I'll write reports that say women are pregnant or not pregnant. I'll tell Alan whether his fat old pa-

tients have too much cholesterol. When a kid drags his ass in
from Ridgetown High, I'll see whether its mono or just a
bad cold.

Morrissey envisioned the long brick L of Ridgetown
High—tan shades behind grimy windows, the flagpole in
front blackened by lightning. He and Alan would cruise
over there the first Sunday they were back. Sneak in through
the boiler room. Find out if the two of them could still pop
the lockbar on the football cabinet. Then hit the field, run
some patterns. Yeah, the ''Deadly Deuce'' strikes again,
still the best quarterback-end duo in Ridgetown High history. Maybe some kids from the current team would be
hanging out. Let them watch him and Alan read each others'
minds. Coach could never teach them that. You could practice pass routes all day, but when you and the other guy were
closer than brothers, that's when the magic happened.

Morrissey tried to picture the kids on the sideline. Thick
necks, coal dust under their nails, watching him and Alan
with awe under their adolescent deadpans. The picture
would not come clear. Instead he saw the kid at the hospital
yesterday, and his stomach plunged down inside him. *Oh,
shit*. He pressed his fingers against his eyelids until he saw
red splotches. In his fingertips he could feel the heat of the
kid's forehead: temp, 107°, high enough to boil the brain.
Had to move fast, get a make on the infection. The kid
hadn't even noticed when the scalpel cut into his foot. Then,
back at the lab, leaning over the microscope . . .

Morrissey twitched the shot glass to his mouth. The bourbon burned all the way down. It only sharpened the memory: the ugly swarm of *E. coli* bacteria straight from the
bowels of some Vietcong. Human shit. That's what the sons
of bitches had put on the spike before they'd hid it under the
leaves for the kid to step on.

Morrissey's throat tightened with pain. The poor, damned
kid. Too skinny to be a marine. Dark-frame glasses sliding
down his nose. Pimply face. So young. He hadn't lasted the
night. Dead like the others, an average of two lost kids every
week for twelve fucking months, and not a thing could be
done.

The great Dr. Morrissey, he thought bitterly. Number One in his class. Gregor Mendel Award for the best Ph.D. dissertation in genetics. Chief of labs for the biggest army hospital in all of 'Nam. Hot stuff. For a year, countless milliliters of blood and urine, sputum samples, and bone and tissue-mass biopsies from thousands of suffering ex–high school kids had passed under his supervision. He had been the base hospital's ultimate diagnostician.

And a hundred of his kids had died. Not such hot stuff.

Sweat began to pour down Morrissey's face. He spread his fingers; tried to relax his hands. It was pointless to feel so furious. The kids had died and there would be more of them. He had done his best, and there was no one else to blame, nothing *behind* it all to smash back at. Might as well scream at the sky for raining.

Disgusted, he thumped his empty shot glass onto its side, watched it circle to a stop. Damn it, this was Froggie's. No lab thoughts allowed here—his most sacred rule, and he couldn't seem to make it stick anymore.

Yes, it was time to get out.

Morrissey's throat began itching for another drink. He picked up Vandiver's glass and checked his watch as he sipped. 8:10. Come on, old buddy. Let's *party*!

And there Alan was, ducking to get in the door, golden hair sweat-plastered straight back. Morrissey felt his face split in a ridiculous grin. Vandiver grinned back and threw him a comic salute. Chairs scraped as men stood to shout out greetings. A few officers broke away from the bar to intercept Alan at the door. Morrissey shook his head, amused. All this fuss, and the big bastard hadn't even jumped up on a table.

He didn't have to. Look at him: Alan pushed up a bow wave of well-being wherever he went, bowling people over and sweeping them along in his wake—not just tonight, but every night. The truth was, Vietnam had not fazed Alan. He'd waded in a year ago, rolled up his sleeves, and started plunging his giant hands into the wreckage of kids' chests. Spitting in death's eye, and laughing every night afterward. Making the rest of them laugh too.

Morrissey watched with pity the other officers converging around Alan. *They* were losing him tonight. Instinctively they crowded around for a last clap on the back, a final joke. Over their heads, Vandiver gave him a helpless smile. He responded with the O.K. sign, conscious of a relief almost uncomfortable in its intensity: *he* was not losing Alan tonight.

He closed his eyes, walling out the noisy good cheer around Alan that was really grief. With his eyes shut, he immediately noticed a spicy aroma. Delicious, some kind of meat, probably charcoaled *thit heo* from one of the braziers on the street. The smell must have drifted in when the door opened. Morrissey realized his mouth was watering. Had he eaten tonight? No. The aroma grew stronger and he opened his eyes to find Vandiver waving the meat under his nose.

"Brought you some supper. Roast pork."

Morressey accepted the *thit heo* stick, surprised at how good it made him feel, like a kid at Christmas.

"Eat, man, eat. You're as skinny as a 'Cong."

Morrissey took a bite. It was tough and overdone, but Alan was watching him like a worried nanny. He chewed with what he hoped was the proper gusto. Vandiver beamed. "That's it, dig in. Janet's going to bust her easel over my head when she sees how thin I let you get. Better she should ease her bust over my head."

Morrissey laughed and almost choked on the meat.

Alan picked up his bourbon and gave the level a calculating squint. "Am I that late? Almost a centimeter."

"Evaporation," Morrissey said, dropping the remains of the *thit heo* under the table for Dang's dog.

"Evaporation my ass." Vandiver drained the glass and smacked his lips. "Let's dance."

"What would the men say?"

"No, jarhead. Those two over there."

Morrissey followed Vandiver's nod to where two of Madame Tho's joygirls sat at a table. One of them caught him looking and smiled. He felt heat rising up from his collar.

"No thanks. Not my type."

"You only have one type, Peter old boy."

Alan sounded almost wistful. Was he remembering what it had been like to dance with Janet, hold Janet? You could have married her, Morrissey thought. But you didn't—

He cut the thought off. "You go ahead." He watched Vandiver approach the women and bow gracefully. One of the joygirls smiled and stood. Alan pulled the other one up too. Beyond him, Morrissey noticed a young Vietnamese man sitting at the table across from the joygirls, staring at them. Odd, a Vietnamese man his age coming into Froggie's, a notorious hangout of American army officers. The guy looked mad, glaring like he was about to lunge across the table at Alan and the women. Morrissey tensed. Music started—the Rolling Stones. The man buried his head in a newspaper. Then other officers got up to look for dance partners, blocking him from view.

Morrissey relaxed. The guy probably objected to his countrywomen being in a place like this, letting a foreigner—a big yellow-haired *Ngư ờ i dāman*—touch them. A legitimate beef.

Morrissey ordered two more Jack Daniels. When his was gone, he started on Alan's. He noticed that things were beginning to soften around the edges and tilt slightly. He felt a rubbery smile on his lips. Trying to erase it only twisted it into an outright simper.

When he looked up, Vandiver was sitting across from him again, grinning.

"Wha's so funny, apeface?"

"Today they medevaced a guy in from up the pike," Vandiver said. "General's son, as a matter of fact. A Captain Stanhouse. The battalion aid surgeon missed some bleeders. Bastard was gray as wax, just about gone when I zipped him open again. I saved his ass. It made me feel good."

"You dreaming about how you can make his daddy pay off?" Morrissey said. But then he reached across and grabbed Vandiver's wrist, squeezing down hard. "Good going."

"Hey." Vandiver gave him a close look. "Take it easy."

"Right," Morrissey said. "We're almost there. Tomorrow, we're bailing out of this butcher shop."

"Yeah," Alan said without enthusiasm.

Morrissey saw that the two Vietnamese joygirls were back at their table, chattering and batting their eyelashes at Vandiver's back. The angry young Vietnamese man was gone, though. What was that under the table where he'd sat? A black briefcase. Morrissey labored to remember. Had the guy been carrying a briefcase? Better check the thing out. He started to get up, settling back when Vandiver caught his arm.

"Yeah," Alan repeated. "Tomorrow, the killing is over. We're going home, but that doesn't mean we'll forget. We were here. We saw what we saw. We can run, but we can't hide."

Morrissey glanced at the briefcase and back at Alan, torn between the two. "Speak for yourself. I aim to stick my head just as far down into the sand of Ridgetown, West Virginia, as it'll go."

Vandiver smiled. "You do and old Roger Blotz will come along and pick your pocket and then kick your ass."

Morrissey laughed and felt the tension blow out of him. He pictured Blotz, Ridgetown's most dedicated derelict, weaving down Main Street.

Tomorrow.

There was probably nothing in the briefcase but papers. He'd just take it out carefully and set it in the alley next to Froggie's, then call the MPs.

He stood. "I'm going to check something."

Vandiver gave a knowing grunt. "Take the girl on the left. She loves your black hair. Thinks you're an Indian. I told her your father was Geronimo."

Morrissey nodded absently and gave Vandiver's shoulder a squeeze on the way past.

There was a brilliant flash. Pain jammed through his eardrums. The room veered on its side and spun around him. He felt the floor striking him, front, back, front, back. Something crunched into his shin. He screamed at the pain, saw dark things blossoming.

He lay still and listened to the clanging inside his head, loud and meaningless. He watched the shelves behind the bar lean slowly forward. The bottles skittered silently over the bar and broke in noiseless cascades on the floor.

He turned his head the other way and saw a smoking crater in the floor where the briefcase had been sitting.

A bomb. The briefcase *was* a bomb.

Alan!

Morrissey tried to sit up. He gasped as pain exploded in his shin. Shit—broken! He screamed for Alan. His voice seemed to vanish, as though the room had sucked it away. His eardrums must have been ruptured.

He scrabbled across the floor, dragging his broken leg. A shattered half-moon of table blocked his way, and he flung it aside. Beyond it he saw a slim arm with gold and silver bracelets lying in his path. The arm was attached to nothing. The fingers twitched.

He put his head down and choked back the vomit. He crawled over the arm. There! Under the other half of the table, Alan's long legs sticking out. He hurled away the rest of the table and stared at Alan's face. So peaceful, as though he were sleeping. He groped Alan's wrist. No pulse. Alan's chest was still, no rise or fall.

Horror pumped through him. Alan was dead.

He tipped Vandiver's head back and cleared the tongue from blocking the windpipe. Pinching off the nostrils, he forced air into the slack mouth. "Breathe," he groaned.

He bent over Alan's chest and rhythmically pumped the sternum. He counted off fifteen beats, then stopped and fed Alan more air before going back to the heart massage.

Smoke rolled down around his face. Heat seared his back. The place was on fire! He had to get them both out of here, now. He set his heels to drag Alan away, and pain exploded up from his leg. Everything went gray. He clenched his teeth and the room knitted back into focus. His face was drenched with sweat. It was no use; he'd never be able to drag Alan's weight.

They'd *both* die.

Morrissey felt a kick of panic in his chest and legs and

knew he could make it alone, squirm and whip across the floor like a snake if he had to, *now*!

He grabbed Alan's shirt, holding himself in place. He started punching Vandiver's sternum again, then began to choke. He hunched down to get better air and lost leverage, his elbows giving way, the heel of his hand sliding to the side of Vandiver's chest. He forced himself to straighten again. Spasms of coughing tore at his throat. His arms were dead meat, barely jolting his shoulders with each thrust.

Alan drew a shuddering breath.

"Yes!" Morrissey yelled. He grabbed Alan's arms and tried to pull him along the floor. He was too weak. Please, he prayed, I can't lose him now. He doubled over, coughing his lungs out, and collapsed on top of Alan. Everything went gray again, and then he saw Janet's face inches away in the floorboards. He tried to reach for it, but his arm wouldn't move. Good-bye, he thought. I love you.

He felt hands encircling his chest, pulling at him. He fought them, trying to hang onto Alan. They pried his hands loose and dragged him over the buckling floorboards of the bistro into the street. He saw more men, Vietnamese police in white suits carrying Vandiver out behind him. He struggled up, standing on one leg, watching one of the policemen bend over Vandiver and press an ear to his chest. The man smiled and nodded up at him, giving the O.K. sign, and he knew in his mind that Alan was all right.

But he began to shake. The war was over, he thought. I was going. It isn't fair.

He hopped to a lightpole, clutching it hard against him to stop the quaking that seemed to come from his bones. He became aware of hands pulling at his arms again—policemen, gesturing and chattering at him in Vietnamese. Their voices were muffled, but he could make out the words: "Please, sir, we must get you to hospital, examine your leg."

No, he couldnot leave this place yet, leave Alan.

He waved them off, pushed their hands away, pretending not to understand. At last they left, shaking their heads.

He edged from the lightpole to a parked Citroën, leaning

against the hood. He watched them carry Vandiver to the ambulance. He tried not to blink. He would be all right as long as he could see Alan. One of Alan's arms dangled from the stretcher, his fingers dragging on the ground. Then he was out of sight inside. The siren began to blast and the wagon lunged away from the curb. It disappeared around a corner. Morrissey lurched over the hood of the Citroën, reaching after the ambulance, realizing he was losing control, seeing red, feeling pulses of pain from his fists, someone screaming through his throat.

Vision returned in a rush. He was leaning over the hood of the Citroën. The front windshield was punched out. He saw his fists still pounding the dash inside the window. He stopped and stared at the beads of glass all over the front seat and floor. His knuckles were numb and slippery with blood. He took long, deep breaths. After a minute he was able to look back at Froggie's. The bistro was only a burning shell now. He watched a roof timber fall, shooting sparks against the black sky. He strained to see into the glowing cavern, searching, feeling his teeth bare in a snarl. What was he looking for? A prancing goat-thing, with gloating, crimson eyes and the smell of rot in its lungs?

No. That was not death. He'd seen death already. A hundred kids. For a year he'd looked into their blood, their piss, and their tissues, torn, burned, poisoned. He'd watched their faces as the cells ran down and stopped inside them.

And he'd planned to walk away.

There could be no walking away now.

Just a few seconds, but looking down at Alan's dead face, he had learned how death was going to feel when it got really close.

It was no longer a pain he could stand.

He would have to fight. Fighting would be his life.

But how?

There must be ways. He was trained for it—perhaps better than any man alive. He would find the ways.

"I'm coming after you," he said. He spat toward the fire.

28
DAYS

Chapter 1

Washington, D.C.
2000 hours:

"Uno!" June squealed.

Tsong threw down her single card in disgust. Morrissey looked at his handful and groaned. "Dead last again."

He listened to June and Tsong giggle. The crawl of nerve in his stomach eased.

"Another game, Daddy," Tsong said.

"No, it's bedtime."

"We'll let you win." June tugged at his wrist pleadingly, leaning close to his face. He felt his eyes crossing, blurring her hair into a red torch.

"The sandman's coming," he said. "You have to be in bed so you won't fall down."

Tsong regarded him with sober, dark eyes. He held out his free hand to her. The warmth of her fingers filled him with love. So small and perfect. June let go and ran off to fetch her cushion. She brought it back and held it up to his face: plastic lips, a lush red, inflated to the bursting point.

"Kiss Marilyn," she instructed.

"I'd rather kiss you," he said, and did.

He squeezed both girls to him, nuzzling their soft faces, smelling soap and the fabric softener in their pajamas. He

15

wanted to hold them all night. He could be content just to sit here hugging their warm little bodies and gazing at the Poohbear in the rocker, getting slowly high on the sweet Play-doh vapors that leaked from the toybox. But that could not be.

The L-6 rats were ready.

Why wasn't *he* ready? This time was the hardest yet.

He felt June whopping Tsong with the lip cushion behind his back. "Come on. Off to bed with you. I'll tuck you in."

He followed them up the stairs. When he finished tucking June in, he went across the hall and settled on the edge of Tsong's bed. She still looked somber.

"Daddy, where are you going tonight?"

"Just the lab, honey."

"Are you going to do genetics?"

He smiled, pleased. "Yes."

"What are genetics?"

He folded his hands over one knee and drew a breath. "Let's see. Genetics is what makes you like you are. Everybody's got tiny things inside their body called genes. They decide whether you'll have red hair like June's or black hair like yours. They decide what color your eyes will be, and your skin, and what your face will look like."

"Do the genes vote?"

Morrissey laughed. "Sort of. Together, they make a code. What that code says, that's what you are: a little girl with black hair and pretty brown eyes, or a cat, or an elephant. Everything alive has its own genetic code . . ." He realized he was getting too technical. "Anyway, I work with genes. I study that code and try to change it a little bit so that people won't get cancer." *And other reasons*, he added silently.

"Could you make a sandman so he wouldn't get people?"

Morrissey hesitated, noticing that her lips were pressed tight to keep from trembling. She's scared of the sandman, he realized. And you've been hitting her with it every night. "The sandman won't get you, honey."

"June said he's big and cold and made of sand. She said he's like a zombie and he comes walking after you . . ."

"June was teasing you, honey. The sandman is just a nice man who comes around and sprinkles sand in your eyes to help you be sleepy. That way you can go to bed and have nice dreams and not be tired the next day. But it's only a story. The sandman isn't real."

"You'll keep him away?"

Morrissey sighed, then looked reassuring. "You bet."

She snuggled down and he kissed her and pulled the blanket up to her chin.

In the hall he thought: *Kids*, and smiled. When *you* were a kid, he reminded himself, you were scared of deer because of the big horns.

He checked to make sure June's light was still out, then went past their bedrooms to the attic steps. A bar of golden light fell through the trap and he thought, Beam me up, Scotty. The old fracture site in his leg pained him a little on the steep fold-down ladder. As his head and shoulders cleared the trap, he drew in the heady musk of old linseed oil and turpentine from the paintings stacked around the walls. The varnished oak floorboards stretched away from his eyes, a sheet of glare under the klieg lights.

He rested his arms on the floor at the top of the ladder. Janet was standing in front of a blank canvas, her back to him, head cocked. Her hair swung down to the side, a gorgeous blend of chestnut and deep brown under the blaze of lights. He saw that she was wearing one of his old sweatshirts, the hem falling halfway to her knees. It pleased him—a small, unconscious gesture of intimacy.

He watched her avidly. If only he could peek into her mind right now—see the colors swirl, the ideas take form. Later she'd pull some of them from the blankness of the canvas. But it would be fascinating to see them now, uncensored. How did she choose and shape? He couldn't even draw a decent stick-man.

Ah, well. There was always his woodworking. He thought longingly of the birdhouse that waited unfinished on his worktable.

He began to feel an unpleasant pull at the top of his vision. He looked beyond Janet to the ceiling. There, behind the coronas of the kliegs: the black slits of the skylights. They seemed to focus on Janet like the eyes of a beast.

His neck prickled. *A beast, hungry, waiting for Janet.* He stared at the eyes until they became skylights again.

Janet came over and bent to kiss him. "Time for the biopsy?"

"Yes."

"Good luck. Call me the minute you know."

He pulled her face to him again and closed his eyes, smelling her hair, feeling her eyelashes against his cheek, still conscious of the dark beyond the skylights. It can't have you, he thought. Never.

"I'll call you," he said. If it works, he added silently.

On his way in, Morrisey saw a light in Alan's office and cursed silently. Alan must still be at work in the radiation lab. A rotten stroke of luck. What if Alan dropped by to shoot the breeze when he was in the middle of the biopsy? It would start him wondering. Alan knew Morrissey's latest cancer study was just under way; there'd be no reason to biopsy rats yet.

Christ! He'd have to put the biopsy off a night. No. He couldn't stand that. He was ready now. He had to know.

Then Morrissey recalled the MP guards he'd seen outside the lab for the past few weeks. It would be all right. Alan wouldn't come by. Alan obviously had his own secret to worry about.

As Morrissey hurried through his shower-and-change routine, he dulled the clamor of his nerves by puzzling over Alan. What *was* Alan doing in that radiation lab with the marine guards? Why would Alan keep his research from his best friend?

Morrissey saw the irony of the question and grunted. Irony or not, hiding his research from Alan wasn't the same thing at all. For one thing, *his* secrecy was for Alan's own protection. As head of Army Labs, Colonel Vandiver would be put in a difficult position if he *knew* his star civilian employee was using the army's billion-dollar equipment for unauthorized work.

And if L-6 worked, it would be more dangerous than a thousand 50-megaton bombs. It had to be controlled. The only way to guarantee that was to tell no one—no one at all.

Alan, on the other hand, had no such excuses. He could not possibly be working on anything as earthshaking as L-6. And Alan always told him everything.

Morrissey had to laugh at himself. What conceit! He was like the man with five mistresses who kicked his wife out for a one-night stand. He toweled off and slipped into one of the white zip-suits, with its pajamalike booties. As he tugged the drawstring of the hood around his ears, he smelled the familiar, bleachy tang of disinfectant. Tonight it knifed straight to his gut, twanging his agonized stomach back to full pitch.

Outside his lab door he saw a smashed cricket on the cement floor. He looked away at once, irritated. That lout Harvey Goins again, and his murderous, hungry boots.

He locked the door behind him and pulled the L-6 notebook from the safe. How black it looked on the lab table, with the stainless steel gleaming all around it. Like a Bible on some futuristic altar.

Morrissey's mouth went dry and his heart began to pound. He wanted L-6 to be it; God, how he wanted it.

He tried to imagine it and could not, and realized he wasn't just nervous. He was afraid, damn it—scared stiff. He could see only failure tonight, and that he didn't have to imagine. He could remember it all too well. Five other nights like this one, five other L-genes. Five failures.

He rolled his head around, trying to ease the tension in his neck. He opened the notebook and thumbed quickly past the pages of notes and formulas to the back of the book. On the last page were the 104 names. The leftmost column started with Spec 4 John Ewald and the rightmost ended with Captain Alan Vandiver. He looked down the columns, noting the checkmarks. Only fourteen names remained unchecked. Twelve years since 'Nam and he'd found the families of all but fourteen. Still, it was disappointing. He'd planned to be

through long before now. But some of them were hard to
find, and, with the passing years, it didn't get any easier.

He remembered his last visit, the small, irrelevant details
standing out with unwanted clarity in his mind: walking
down the dim hall of the apartment in Denver; the dirty fin-
gerprints all around the doorknob; the black-haired woman
in the bathrobe, with the tell-tale spiderwebs of vein on her
cheeks and nose. She was rosy with false health—gin on her
breath and it wasn't noon yet. Even the black hair had come
from a bottle.

*Mrs. Specht? I'm Peter Morrissey. I knew your son
Jimmy. It was just for a short time. He was in the hospital in
Saigon while I was there. I was with him, off and on, those
last few days. I tried to help him all I could, but it wasn't
enough. He seemed like a very good kid.*

Morrissey turned away from the book. He waited until his
stomach stopped paining him.

He looked at Alan's name and felt better. The one name
he wouldn't have to check off. But it belonged there, at the
bottom of the list. Alan had been dead. No heartbeat, no
pulse.

Morrissey stared around the lab. "Are you here?" he said
softly. "You son of a bitch."

He heard nothing but the whisper of air through the filters.

He smiled grimly. *Poor Doc Morrissey. One of those
Vietnam vets, you know. They all came back a little crazy.
He likes to pretend death's an actual thing that crawls inside
and eats you. Poor bastard. He's all right most of the time.
Just humor him—and don't make any loud noises.*

Morrissey slammed the notebook shut and shoved it back
in the safe.

He went into the animal room, to the last rolling cart of rat
cages. He checked the tape label to make sure the animal-
care men hadn't switched the carts during cleanup. CANCER
STUDY, CONTROL RATS. Cancer study control rats—right.

Like hell!

Almost reverently, he slid the closest cage drawer out.
The rat was curled up, sleeping atop the mix in its feed jar.

He lifted it gently by the nape of the neck and watched it uncurl, smelling the pleasant, malty odor of the feed dust in its hair. He stroked its back, trying to absorb some of its sleepy calm. The rat peered nearsightedly at him. Its rear leg blurred as it tried to scratch its side. He laughed, and some of his tension evaporated.

What the hell. He would just do it now and see.

He shaved a patch of hair away from the rat's pink belly. Then he scraped the skin with the edge of the blade and drew it over the end of a slide, transferring the film of epidermal cells. He eased the rat back into its cage, and inspected the glass pipette to make sure its delicate tip was unbroken. Good thing he'd remembered to draw it last week, before his nerves had started to fray. Last time he'd been unable to stop his hands shaking. He'd ruined four glass rods and burned his fingers before getting the dropper narrow enough.

Morrissey picked up pinpoint droplets of dye with the pipette and tinted the rat cells on the slide. He put the slide under the scope and flipped on the stage light.

Here we go!

He eased the focus knobs around until he saw the cells from the rat jitter into view. If the gene was there, it would appear as a tiny dot of green stain.

He felt cold sweat rolling down his forehead. *Just do it!*

He looked. There was nothing.

He sat back, rubbed the sweat from his eyes, and looked again. He held himself still a moment. Then he let himself go, punching at the black tube of the microscope. He pulled up an inch away. His fist shook with frustration and he slammed it on the table.

He couldn't take it!

He rubbed the aching heel of his fist. For God's sake, what was he doing wrong? The cells in culture had performed perfectly. So why hadn't L-6 taken hold in the living animal? He would go back to the safe, get out the L-6 notes and go through them again.

But he made no move toward the safe. He sat, head down.

After a moment he began sluggishly to fight off the despair. *Misery is chemical.* He grimaced at how familiar the

phrase was becoming. He must go through the rest of it anyway. It was important to analyze now, to stop the internal
chain reaction of misery. You didn't see the stain, he told
himself. You realized that nothing had happened in the L-6
cells. Then you *said* something to yourself—*you failed, you
miserable S.O.B.*

Mistake: As soon as you make the harsh judgment against
yourself, your brain sent signals to the hypothalamus, the pi-
tuitary; other endocrine glands. Adrenaline and other hormones spurted into your bloodstream. The seratonin balance
shifted in your brain.

You felt like shit.

Once you'd set the chemicals loose, they were beyond
your control. You couldn't regulate your endocrine glands
with your conscious mind—not directly. But you *could* control your thoughts.

That was the trick—to catch yourself, keep from thinking
you dumb shit over and over. Then the balance would gradually shift back. Your cells would convert the corrosive
chemicals to harmless sludge that would drain out of the
bloodstream. You would feel better.

It took time and vigilance. The more vigilance, the less
time.

Okay, he thought, you feel terrible. It will pass. You will
try again and do better.

The old fatalistic calm began to settle over Morrissey. He
could take it.

L-6 was the past now. Time to go home.

Tomorrow he would start planning L-7.

He reached for the microscope switch, his arm as heavy
as lead. His finger stopped above the switch, unable to do
this final small thing and officially admit defeat.

All right, one last look. He bent over the scope and saw
the band.

He stared at it, uncomprehending at first, and then caught
up in growing excitement. There *was* something! Not a dot
of stain, but a faint pink circle around the cell border. So
faint that he had missed it the first time.

Morrissey switched to the intermediate power lens, bringing a group of cells into focus. The back of his eye began to itch and he sat back, closing both eyes. He waited, controlling his impatience. No good straining himself blind. He bent over the scope again.

It was there in every cell—a very faint pink band.

Sweat poured out, soaking his shirt. He rocked on the stool, driven by spurts of energy. He stood, knocking the stool over backward. He started to caper around the lab, and stopped short, wincing at the stab of pain from the old fracture site. He leaned against a table and massaged the leg, squeezing hard in his excitement. *Yeah! Crazy Viet Nam vet who thought he could beat death. Now we would all fucking see!*

Okay. Be calm. *Think*.

Point one: The L-6 gene was *not* a failure. It had already performed an operation in the rat cells. He'd hoped simply to see the gene in place. But this was better—it was already working!

Point two: This band wasn't one of the effects he'd expected. He hadn't seen it in the petri-dish cells. But these cells came directly from a living animal, not from the artificial environment of a petri dish. Some variation could be expected.

Point three—what was point three? Plans: Tomorrow evening, after everyone left, he could see if the pink band was also there in the L-6 dogs. Then, in the next week, he could set up a battery of tests to determine whether the band was actually shielding the cell. Radiation, toxins, the whole spectrum.

Then for the coup de grace: waiting for a cell division and looking for aging errors. If there were none, then he'd done it. L-6—*Life-Six!* A giddy smile transfixed his face.

Janet! She'd said to call her the minute he knew. He reached for the phone. No, he couldn't do this over the phone. What time was it? 10:40. If he hurried, he could get to a 7-Eleven before it closed and pick up some champagne. Probably nothing at a 7-Eleven but André. No matter—André would taste like Dom Perignon tonight!

By the door Morrissey saw a tiny dark movement at his

feet and jumped back. He smiled to himself—it was only a cricket. What a bundle of nerves.

Yeah, a cricket, and if it was still there in the morning, Harvey Goins would stomp it flat.

Morrissey got out his clear plastic cup and crawled after the cricket, cursing himself for a mush-hearted fool and thinking of cold champagne. It took him ten minutes to trap the cricket under the cup. Bye-bye, champagne.

Resisting the urge to give the cup a vindictive shake, he took the cricket down the hall and put it in Dr. Pancek's lab, out of range of Harvey Goins's boots.

27
DAYS

Chapter 2

0750 hours:

Vandiver waited while the master sergeant swung the safe
door shut on him. When he was alone and closed in, he sat.

He looked down the length of the table to the photo above
the Chairman's place: Warren Maddock posed at his desk in
the Oval Office. Vandiver remembered the day two years
ago: Secret Service men smuggling Maddock into the Pentagon basement before dawn. The President sitting there at the
other end of the table, under his own photo. Vandiver
straightened now, the muscles of his back and legs coming
alert with the memory of him standing to attention to accept
command of Project Parasol from the President of the
United States. He flexed his fingers, enjoying the tingle of
blood and nerve, the feeling of strength in his hands. Project
Parasol: so secret it was known to only a dozen men, so important that it could save 165 million lives; so dangerous
that a single premature leak of its success to Soviet intelli-
gence could lose those same 165 million lives.

And it was *his*.

Vandiver filled his lungs, relishing the damp, basement
scent that the air conditioners could not scrub out. The smell
of bunkers. It touched him with yearning. If only this could

be his day of victory. He imagined himself facing the generals and saying, *Gentlemen, we have the shielding material.* The most important words anyone could ever speak in this room. By the sacred Virgin, he *would* say them. But not today.

Damn it, how much longer?

Vandiver heard the massive door whispering open and stood to attention as General Stanhouse and the two major generals entered. Behind the generals was the Deputy Secretary of Defense and a stranger—a slender man in an elegant European-tailored suit. Vandiver tried not to gape at him in surprise. The only civilians cleared for Project Parasol were the Deputy Secretary and the Secretary of Defense.

Surprise turned to vague suspicion. Who was this guy?

Vandiver sized the man up in discreet glances. First impression—negative. He looked too cocky, wearing a fixed smile of superiority. This man thought he was better than other men—better and *smarter*. He showed it even now, in the select company of this room.

A prick, Vandiver thought.

He looked to Stanhouse for a clue. The old general looked tight-lipped and unhappy. He's been trying to catch my eye, Vandiver realized. He wants to get something across to me; he's almost in pain with it. What is it?

Stanhouse sighed and looked at the other men. "All right, gentlemen. Let's get started. Deputy Secretary Pennylegion, I don't believe Colonel Vandiver has met Dr. Fitch."

Pennylegion scrunched his fat body around in the chair. Disgusting, Vandiver thought, keeping his face carefully neutral. Soft. He can't even master his own body.

And he's the most powerful man in this room.

The Deputy Secretary gestured: "Dr. Vandivah, Dr. Fitch, head of Bah-log Lab'ratories. Dr. Fitch, Dr. Vandivah, head of the Army Radiobah-ology Labs."

Vandiver returned the civilian's nod, running the Deputy Secretary's introduction through again, with the heavy southern drawl filtered out: Bah-log—*Biolog Laboratories. Civilian experts in radiobiology. They'd landed a bunch of fat government contracts since Maddock came to office.*

There'd been something in the Post *about Fitch. Wasn't he an old classmate of Pennylegion's?*

All at once Vandiver realized what was in the Chairman's eyes: pity.

Stanhouse said, "Alan—Colonel, for the benefit of Dr. Fitch, could you please summarize Project Parasol before you proceed with your interim report."

Vandiver stood slowly. Damn it, the president of a competitor lab, here—with no advance word to him. A consultant? Or worse?

Vandiver swallowed, trying to wet his dry throat. "Okay, Dr. Fitch. We've been trying to formulate a new material to block radiation and fallout from a nuclear attack. Of course, lead and a few other heavy, bulky materials will do this already. But we want a material that is lightweight, flexible, and cheap. We need something we can mass-produce for homeowners, landlords, commercial building management, and so on. Something people can tack up in their basements in an hour . . ."

Worse—it was worse. Fitch was not here to consult. Fitch was here to replace him.

Vandiver glared at the Deputy Secretary, furious. You fat bureaucrat. You found another government contract for your old buddy, Dr. Fitch.

Vandiver went on, trying not to bite off the words. "We believe that the Soviets are considering a pre-emptive nuclear strike. Apparently, because of their clear superiority in civil defense, some of the top Soviet generals think they can win a nuclear war with us. It *is* true that more of their people would survive an exchange—especially one that they started with a sneak attack. That's why Project Parasol was initiated. We hope this civil-defense gap will be closed with the new shielding material. If the Russians do decide to hit us, many more people will be killed by radiation than by all the immediate firestorm, blast, and drag effects combined. But if we can shield these potential victims, we could cut the casualties from a possible high of one hundred and sixty-five million to perhaps thirty-five million."

"That's still a staggering figure, Colonel."

Vandiver stared at Fitch. The jerk-off! Fitch had to know what the figures meant. Lord help them all if he didn't understand even that much. "Of course it's staggering," he said. "But the point is, if the Soviets knew we could prevent a hundred and thirty million casualties, they'd know we'd come out of an exchange in much better shape than they. They'd have to throw out any idea of a pre-emptive strike. So we're really talking about going from one hundred and sixty-five million to zero casualties.

"Of course, absolute secrecy is necessary—especially at the moment we succeed in the lab. If the Russians learned we had such a material before we got it in place, they would hit us at once."

Fitch looked down, avoiding his eyes. Vandiver heard Pennylegion shift uncomfortably. Chew on that, Deputy Secretary. Then think about bringing another lab in on the secret.

"Thank you for the summary, Colonel," Stanhouse said. "Proceed with your report."

Yes, Vandiver thought bitterly. Proceed, and give Pennylegion his opening. "We still don't have the final breakthrough we're all looking for, but I'm sure we're getting close. Since the last report, we've tested eight more variants of the new alloy I briefed you on last time. We've reduced the porosity by half again. We've kept it lightweight and cheap to make—"

Pennylegion lifted his hand. "Yes, yes, Colonel. But can it withstand radiation at the four-hundred-and-fifty-roentgen level?"

Vandiver fought to hide his contempt. This lawyer, this born talker. How he could roll the scientific terms off his tongue. But he understood nothing about science, or he could not dream of shifting the contract. "No sir," Vandiver said. "Not yet."

"Then when?"

"I think very soon. Unfortunately, with scientific breakthroughs, there is no way to be sure of the timing."

"Ah seem to remember you sayin' you'd run *nine* variants during the extension period?"

"Yes, sir. The ninth is almost ready for testing, but we had a piece of bad luck. We're temporarily out of lab rats to test the shielding effectiveness. At the moment, our supplier of laboratory rats can't fill our orders for more animals."

"Even if you had the rats now," Pennylegion said, "is there any reason to think your ninth variant would be any less a failure than the other eight?"

Vandiver felt the blood rushing to his face. He saw Stanhouse glaring at Pennylegion. A deliberate insult. The fat bastard wanted him to lose his temper, make it easier. He would *not* lose his temper. "We don't think of the first eight materials as failures, sir. They have been stepping-stones to the present level of progress. The ninth variant may very well be—"

The Deputy Secretary waved again, and Vandiver imagined grabbing the fat wrist, twisting it until the fingers spread into claws.

"I may as well be frank with you right from the top, Colonel. Save us going round and round. Defense is opposed to any further extension of this contract to Army Labs."

Vandiver clenched his hands behind his back.

"We have another worry now," Pennylegion went on. "The coming election may affect the Russians' thinking. The White House is confident that Governor Howard isn't going to win, of course, but even the outside possibility of a hawk being elected is going to sensitize the Russians even more. Gentlemen, we think the pre-emptive strike option is tempting them. Army Labs has clearly failed to produce an adequate shielding material, and the White House thinks it's time for some new blood—a fresh approach, completely different from the one we've been taking. I've been talking to Larry—Dr. Fitch—for several weeks, and I'm convinced that Biolog has devised such an approach—"

"Excuse me, sir."

Pennylegion sighed. "Yes, Colonel?"

"If the committee believes Biolog has a promising approach, why not fund both them and Army Labs?"

Pennylegion rolled his eyes. "Now, the Colonel knows that's not possible. We have to live with the budgetary appropriation we've been given. There's not enough money for both labs to proceed.''

Vandiver felt the muscles of his back and neck turning rigid with frustration. How could he make this man understand what he was risking? ''Sir, it's unthinkable to stop Army Labs this close to the goal and start over cold. Army Labs brought in the finest minds in our country for this project. Dr. Hisle, Dr. Wintermeier, Dr. Pancek—all the others. America has not assembled so much talent in one place since the Manhattan Project. With all respect to Dr. Fitch and Biolog, no one can possibly be in a better position to succeed than Army Labs. We've got to stand behind my people, sir. I'd stake my professional reputation on them.''

''Perhaps you already have, Colonel,'' Pennylegion said.

Vandiver looked down, humiliated and sick. He heard Stanhouse grunt. One of the other generals started digging in his briefcase, making the papers snap. Vandiver realized that the other men—the military men—were embarrassed too. One of their own was taking a drubbing from a civilian. There was no way he could win. His shoulders turned heavy, trying to drag him down. He resisted the urge to lean forward on the table.

''I think we should hear from Dr. Fitch now,'' Pennylegion said.

Vandiver saw Stanhouse nod. The old man looked ill. He's taking this as hard as I am, Vandiver thought. Through his pain, he felt a pang of sympathy. Poor old George. He must have wanted desperately to head this off. But Pennylegion had the real power. There would have been nothing the Chairman could do.

Vandiver groped behind him for the back of his chair. His legs felt weak. He concentrated on keeping them from dumping him.

Fitch stood. ''I've prepared a slide presentation,'' he said, ''to introduce the new line of research we've been charting at Biolog.''

I won't ever sit here again, Vandiver thought numbly.

The lights went dim. He stared at the first slide. It showed a smashed cityscape. The devastation was total except for a building in the middle distance, miraculously still standing. In the foreground was the charred body of a child, legs and arms raised, as if in a doomed effort to hold off the sky.

"Hiroshima," Fitch intoned. "The building you see still standing in the middle caught our attention . . ."

Fitch's voice droned on and on. More slides, more Japanese corpses. Vandiver stared, filled with helpless anger. If the Kremlin listened to the wrong generals, these could become American corpses—American old men and women, American babies—burnt and twisted.

Vandiver watched each slide. When he could think of helpful comments, he made them. When it was over, he wished Fitch luck.

He had a dim impression of wandering the corridors of the Pentagon. Then he was sitting in his car. He looked around the gleaming acreage of the Pentagon's parking lot. How had he gotten here? Christ it was hot. He leaned forward, unsticking his back from the car seat. He realized his fingers were rubbing the white diamond of hair where the back of his head had hit the wall in the Froggie Bistro.

Hope stirred in him. Yes, Froggie's. Every day he lived was borrowed time. He'd known that from the moment he'd come out of the coma. This was his second life, a life that had to make a difference. Project Parasol was that difference.

Determination flowed back into him. Somehow he must find more test rats. The lab could finish the ninth material in the next two days. It would take at least that long for the contract to be officially transferred to Biolog. In those few days he could make one last try. If he succeeded, today's meeting would be undone. Project Parsol would remain on track.

But where could they get laboratory rats? He'd already contacted all the other labs that might have extras.

Vandiver punched the steering wheel with excitement. *Control rats!* Of course! He could take control rats already being used in some other Army Labs study. They would be practically as good as new rats.

It would be expensive. Losing animals in midstream

would mean starting the affected study over again. It would
cause a hell of a ruckus. It could stain the rest of his career.

But Pennylegion made it necessary. Switching the contract now was virtually as bad as starting over from
scratch—worse, with that smug bastard Fitch in charge.

When the bombs starting falling, 165 million people
would die.

So which study should he stop?

Hadn't Peter just started a new study a few weeks ago?
Yes. The cost of destroying the project at this early point
would be relatively small. The untreated control group of
Peter's study was large, forty rats if he remembered right.
He could put these together with his own few remaining ani-
mals and have enough for statistical significance.

But could he push aside Peter's work for a last chance to
save Project Parasol?

Yes, that was the beauty of it: Peter would accept his need
without tantrums or questions. What were friends for?

Vandiver squared his shoulders. He started the Porsche
and sped away from the Pentagon parking lot.

Acknowledgments

I take pleasure in acknowledging the important contributions of the following people to this work: Lt. Colonel John Gaither, U.S.A.; Mr. Harris Eisenhardt; Dr. Richard Setton; and special thanks to Dr. Faye Austin of the National Institutes of Health.

I am most grateful to my wife, Dr. Nancy L. Spruill, for her many hours of editing and her special insights.

I would also like to thank my literary agent, Dr. Al Zuckerman, for his instruction, his patience, and his faith.

Finally, heartfelt thanks to my good friend and fellow novelist, Dr. F. Paul Wilson, for giving my manuscript the parallax view.